2

Acupuncture in Practice

Neither the publishers nor the author will be liable for any loss of damage of any nature occasioned to or suffered by any person acting or refraining from acting as a result of reliance on the material contained in this publication.

For Churchill Livingstone:

Commissioning editor: Inta Ozols
Project manager: Valerie Burgess
Project development editor: Valerie Bain
Design direction: Judith Wright
Project controller: Pat Miller
Copy editor: Anita Hible
Indexer: Liza Weinkove
Sales promotion executive: Maria O'Connor

Acupuncture in Practice
Case History Insights from the West

Edited by

Hugh MacPherson PhD
Principal, Northern College of Acupuncture, York, UK

Ted J. Kaptchuk OMD
Associated Director, Center for Alternative Medicine Research,
Beth Israel Hospital, and Instructor in Medicine,
Harvard Medical School, Boston, USA

Foreword by

Giovanni Maciocia
Acupuncturist and Medical Herbalist
Amersham, Buckinghamshire, UK

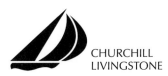

CHURCHILL
LIVINGSTONE

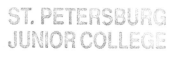
NEW YORK, EDINBURGH, LONDON, MADRID, MELBOURNE, SAN FRANCISCO AND TOKYO 1997

CHURCHILL LIVINGSTONE
Medical Division of Pearson Professional Limited

Distributed in the United States of America by Churchill
Livingstone Inc., 650 Avenue of the Americas, New York,
N.Y. 10011, and by associated companies, branches and
representatives throughout the world.

First published 1997

ISBN 0 443 05049 X

British Library Cataloguing in Publication Data
A catalogue record for this book is available from the British
Library.

Library of Congress Cataloging in Publication Data
A catalog record for this book is available from the Library
of Congress.

Note
Medical knowledge is constantly changing. As new
information becomes available, changes in treatment,
procedures, equipment and the use of drugs and herbs
become necessary. The editors/authors/contributors and the
publishers have, as far as it is possible, taken care to
ensure that the information given in this text is accurate and
up-to-date. However, readers are strongly advised to
confirm that the information, especially with regard to drug
and herb usage, complies with latest legislation and
standards of practice.

The
publisher's
policy is to use
**paper manufactured
from sustainable forests**

Produced by Longman Singapore Publishers (Pte) Ltd.
Printed in Singapore

Contents

Foreword

The 'Chinese Medicine' section of every bookshop in China usually has a shelf with books presenting 'collections of experiences of famous contemporary doctors': these are often the most interesting books on Chinese medicine because experienced doctors present their own views on diagnosis and treatment. These books greatly enrich our understanding of Chinese medicine and expand our therapeutic tools. It is also refreshing to see how Chinese doctors apply the theories of Chinese medicine creatively according to their clinical experience. This book (*Acupuncture in Practice*) is the first to present the clinical practice of experienced Western acupuncturists spanning a wide range of traditions, schools of thought and techniques, ranging from the treatment of acne to that of possession: I believe this makes it one of the most important acupuncture books ever published in the West. The diagnoses and treatments presented in this book show a large degree of adaptation of Oriental medicine to Western patients.

Practically ever since Oriental medicine was introduced to the Western world, at least in recent times, there has been a dynamic tension between the need to absorb, understand and preserve Oriental medicine and the need to adapt it to Western conditions. Two opposing views could be presented, the first advocating the need to swiftly adapt Oriental medicine to Western conditions, the second advocating the need to first absorb, understand and master Oriental medicine as it has been handed down in Asia. The advocates of this latter point of view, point out that one can only adapt something that has been mastered in the first place, otherwise we will spawn theories, treatment strategies and techniques that will be ultimately ineffective. At worst, if we do not master Oriental medicine, its adaptation to Western conditions may simply mask our inability to carry out a good diagnosis and treatment. As one author puts it 'In the face of such gaps (i.e. gaps in the available books on the various aspects of Chinese medical theory), claims that we are able to "adapt Chinese medicine for the West" may be an heroic expression of confidence, but are almost certainly premature. We have much work to do' (Clavey 1995). Thus, if we take this approach, it may take generations of acupuncturists before we can truly speak of adaptation of Oriental medicine to Western conditions.

However, there may be factors that would shorten the times necessary to master and adapt Oriental medicine. Perhaps one of the greatest weaknesses of Oriental medicine (or at least, Chinese medicine, with which I am more familiar) is the slavish acceptance of tradition, which is essentially a Confucian trait. In spite of the introduction of Marxism to modern China, I believe that the greatest influence on Chinese medicine is still essentially Confucian, rather than a 'state-led and bureaucratically-controlled systematisation': after all, there may have been a systematisation but all the old classics of Chinese medicine have also been reprinted in their entirety for everyone to study. The Confucian heritage is such that traditional theories are blindly accepted, the teacher is never questioned, and no theory is ever challenged. This leads to a serious lack of searching, questioning, critical appraisal which, in my opinion, is the greatest weakness of Chinese medicine, far greater than the much-criticised 'systematisation' of Chinese medicine which took place in China in the last 40 years. I will always remember asking a Chinese doctor, when I was voicing my first doubts about the Chinese view of allergic asthma, 'why is it that asthma is always due to Phlegm even when there are no signs of Phlegm (i.e. there is no expectoration of sputum, no slippery pulse, no swollen tongue, no sticky coating)?'. He confidently replied: 'Don't worry, asthma is due to Phlegm'. It is because of this Confucian attitude that Chinese medicine has developed relatively slowly over the centuries, certainly compared to Western medicine. When a Chinese doctor of Western medicine was staying at my house I noticed that the light in her bedroom was always on until very late in the small hours, whereas Chinese doctors of Chinese medicine who stayed at my house always went to bed at 9 p.m. I asked the doctor of Western medicine why she stayed up so late compared to doctors of Chinese medicine and she said: 'It is because Western medicine changes very fast and there is always something new to read and learn, whereas Chinese medicine never changes, so doctors of Chinese medicine can go to bed early!'. Thus, if we discard the Confucian attitude we can perhaps shorten the times necessary to master and adapt Oriental medicine to the West if we can strike a good balance between a slavish, uncritical acceptance of the tradition, and a hasty, superficial adaptation without first mastering the tradition itself. If something is adapted without first mastering it, this will only give rise to spurious forms of acupuncture without roots in any tradition and which will, ultimately, not help our patients at all.

The extraordinary range of diagnoses and techniques presented in this book shows the vitality of Oriental medicine in the West and it would be a mistake to use this as a criticism of any systematisation of Oriental medicine. There is no contradiction or 'dynamic tension' between a systematisation of the theories of Oriental medicine and the reverence and respect for the experience of teachers and their individual approaches: Chinese medicine has always evolved along these two pillars. If our practice is rooted in mastery of the theories of Oriental medicine, the experience of practitioners as presented in case histories is nothing but the link between the 'reality of the patient's illness and the relevant texts' as the introduction to this book says. Interestingly, many of the authors of this book cite the same texts as sources and this has not prevented them from developing original ideas and treatment strategies. A 'system' is not a straight-jacket but simply a collection of guidelines based on fundamental principles: after all, no matter how great the diversity of ideas and approaches, our diagnosis has to be 'right'. We cannot give Kidney-Yang tonics in Kidney-Yin deficiency or vice versa; or, to mention a different school of thought, we cannot treat an Earth 'CF' as a Fire 'CF'.

A systematisation of Chinese medicine is actually not a new phenomenon at all, but one that has taken place during every dynasty (if we consider the present regime as just another 'dynasty'). There has been no greater systematisation of Chinese medicine than that which occurred during the Song and Yuan dynasties at the hand of the Neo-Confucianists. After all, is the 'Yellow Emperor Classic of Internal Medicine' not a systematisation of an extraordinary range of different strands, views, theories, approaches, and techniques of acupuncture originated before 200 BC? Thus it would be a mistake to see the rich and fascinating variety of approaches described in this book as proof that there is no coherent theory of Chinese medicine and to consider every system as an aberration of Chinese medicine. In fact, no matter how great the diversity of approaches reflected in the case histories in this book, they *are* linked by common threads that are typical of the Oriental medicine methodology, i.e. the careful observation of the patient, the logical identification of patterns of disharmony, the sensitive investigation of the causes of disease in the patient's life, the unity of physical and mental-emotional disharmonies, the creative application of the teachers' instruction and the skilful application of treatment techniques.

1997   G. M.

REFERENCE

Clavey S 1995 Fluid Physiology and Pathology in Traditional Chinese Medicine, Churchill Livingstone, Edinburgh, p. xxiv.

Preface

A profound voice of encounter speaks throughout this collection of case histories. The authors of these clinical vignettes are prominent leaders and pioneers involved in the transmission of East Asian medicine to the West. These descriptions of clinical meetings between patient and practitioner provide a vibrant glimpse of the ongoing movement of Eastern medicine beyond its original geographic confines. The many narratives of this book dramatically portray Oriental medicine's new texture and the clinical diversity that has come to be included within its approach to illness and health. But, more importantly, this book demonstrates that the new Western environment has not diluted or weakened East Asian medicine's vitality and strength. On the contrary, the Western context of these clinical case histories has enabled Oriental medicine's original inspiration to shake itself from its previous cultural-bonded idiom and become sharper and richer. The authors of these true stories demonstrate that the journey to the West has given East Asian medicine an opportunity to reach a new maturity and genuine universalism.

The clinical narratives of this book provide ample evidence that East Asian medicine now takes place in a new cultural, social and even biological context. There are new disease entities: from AIDS to chronic fatigue syndrome. There are new health models to engage: from osteopathy to homeopathy. There are new life-styles: from Italian sophisticated to California casual. There are new religions: from Christian fundamentalism to Steiner's anthroposophy. There are new sensibilities of personhood: from expectations of self-fulfillment to desires for meaning. There are new moralities: from accepted premarital sexual relationships to a culture-wide absence of any discussion of virtue. There are even new physical bodies: from Mediterranean genetic disorders to bodies sustained on a fruit salad of modern pharmaceutical drugs. The patients and practitioners in these clinical stories are enveloped in an ambience very distinct from East Asian medicine's original home. The collective voice of this book is spoken in the health care language of modern Europe, North America and Australia.[1] Yet, East Asian medicine's ability to adjust and find its vision is unmistakable and evident.

The collective voice of this compendium is made up of diverse perspectives. Just as China, Japan, Korea and Vietnam have each had distinct national traditions of medicine which were further subdivided into schools, camps and even factions, the Western version of Oriental medicine has had multiple approaches, emphases and interpretations. The practitioners in this volume filter the East Asian medical tradition through different training, skills, life experiences, passions and wisdom. These practitioners are not mechanical robots applying technical skills to cardboard people. Each practitioner weighs, evaluates, considers, ponders and links each clinical and human nuance in a way that exemplifies their formal training and their unique sensibilities. Most of the patients are remarkably distinct. Together, these narratives of patients and doctors reveal a multisonorous mosaic of unique conversations and relationships engaged in distinct strains of Oriental medicine.

Yet, unexpectedly, it seems to me, the deepest tones of this book are not about the adaptation of Oriental medicine to the West or the diversity of East Asian medical practices. Rather, what comes through most clearly in this collection of histories are the consistent and ancient qualities of East Asian medicine. It is as if, by adapting to the West it is suddenly easier to hear the essential and universal method of East Asian medicine as distinct from its culture-bound voice. The deepest assumptions of most, if not all, the practitioners in this volume, seem fundamentally similar. A unified East Asian grammer and syntax of illness and health seems to abide underneath the diversity.

The collective vision of these case narratives, it seems to me, has several points of clear agreement. The most fundamental a priori assumption is the possibility of change. Things are not fixed, flux is the enduring reality in human life. Because all sensations, motivations, functions, activities and events partake of this potential transformation and transmutation, all phenomena can be considered a manifestation of an inherent tension describable as complementary opposition. This dialectical perspective is symbolically described by the principles of yin and yang, eight principles, five elements, or other emblematic systems.

A second component of the underlying unanimity in these cases is that in the dialogues of health and illness there is no sharp dichotomy between mind and body, objective and subjective. The physical, mental, emotional, behavioural, social, existential and spiritual dimensions of life interpenetrate and are emblematically described with similar vocabularies. I think that most of the authors would agree that this mutual interpenetration of all being and behaviour is possible because phenomena and its transformation share the common denominator of a dynamic quality and presence that is usually called *qi*. Phenomena transforms *qi* and *qi* transforms phenomena. Just as the flux is a given, phenomena and *qi* are inseparable.

A third component of shared vision for most of the authors would be that health is not thought to be an objective state, but a dynamic harmony and interaction of an inner world of sensations, activities, needs and intentions, with an outer world of demands, desires, requirements, symbols and meaning. One patient's restored 'health' and new found 'healing' can be what brings another patient to see the doctor.

A fourth aspect of the coherence in this text is that for most of these case histories, change and healing is not primarily the outcome of an external mechanical stimulus-response nexus. Rather, healing comes from what the ancient tradition calls *resonance*, an eliciting of inner potential to recreate balance.[2] Change is evoked from what already in-dwells. The human being already has the potential within for harmony. The microcosm has all the ingredients of the macrocosm. The healer evokes the potential.

A fifth point of unified approach is that for most of these clinical encounters, sensory observation — looking, listening, smelling, asking and touching — is thought to be sufficient to allow the healer to obtain an understanding, gestalt and feel of another human being. Few 'objective' tests or measurements 'untainted' with human subjectivity and perceptions are required in this medicine. This is a medicine where human sensibilities are central.

A sixth aspect of coherence in these cases is that a synthetic logic, as opposed to an analytic logic, propels each one of these medical narratives. Each healer attempts to develop a composite picture which allows for a representation of what in modern times is called a diagnosis, or in older times might be called a *pattern of disharmony*. The healers are not trying to isolate a cause of disease but rather to capture a sense of energetics and wholeness. Each one of the healers in this volume is traditional in this way. Furthermore, each healer can be called 'traditional' because he or she relies on previous clinical experience and historical theoretical understanding to guide their skill, art, judgment, intuition and compassion.

Finally, in each of these case histories, even when the patient is most broken, there is always room for a healing intervention, the discovery of renewed integrity. Ultimately, the East Asian medical tradition sees the possibility of some kind of movement towards healing and intactness in all people. The strong unity of vision found in these clinical narratives is more impressive than any differences in detail and demonstrates that, despite the appearance of fragmentation in the West, Oriental medicine's original inspiration has been renewed and reaffirmed.

Peculiarly, this volume recreates a critical discussion of the East Asian medicine tradition that has generally been overlooked in the West and avoided in the modern East. This is the question of how to balance systematic knowledge and medical 'certainty' with the 'real' clinical encounter which is always idiosyncratic and nonreplicable. What is the relationship of theory and practice in East Asian medicine? Historically, case histories were the vehicle that attempted to bridge this tension and forge a resolution. In modern Asia, the case history has become 'standardised' to make it seem that this tension has been resolved. Under attack by Western medicine, the indigenous tradition has had to close ranks and appear more cohesive than was historically true. But, in fact, when one examines the historical compilations of case history literature, it is obvious that diversity and disagreement is the only common denominator in this tension. The diversity in this volume, while mild compared to the disparateness in the case histories of the Eastern tradition, demonstrates this tension.

Probably the best single source of an overview of the historic case history literature can be found in the recently produced massive four volume compilation: *Case Histories of Famous Physicians of the Song, Yuan, Ming, and Qing Dynasties (Song yuan ming qing ming yi lei an).*[3] In this vast compendium it is evident that the contention between theoretical therapeutics and clinical reality is resolved differently by each practitioner. The style of each practitioner in this compendium is often strikingly different. Sometimes each individual case of a single practitioner manages to strike a different balance between theory and practice. This encyclopedia of case histories leaves the impression that the tension between theory and practice is necessarily resolved by the absence of resolution. Only by maintaining multiple voices and avoiding any false synthesis or artificial yin-yang harmony can the actual balance of theory and practice in medicine emerge in its true form.

Many formal and stylised case histories can be found in the classical case history archives of Chinese history. In these formalised writings, the doctor seemed to want to provide the reader with certainty, finality and precision. These cases lack 'real' descriptions of patients: the important signs and symptoms are just subtracted from the human being. The case is meant to be an application of theory. These stylised cases provide a conception of medicine that is laden with the reassurance of omniscient theories and the certainty of unfaltering therapeutics. The resolution of the cleavage between theory and practice favours the theory side, the replicable bits, the 'known' side. This voice is a critical and defining one in East Asian medicine and is essential for self-definition and self-recognition. It provides ultimate coherence and substance. It also allows for the cultivation of courage and confidence when practitioners confront the vicissitudes of human life.

A totally different resolution to the tension of theory and practice also finds its expression in the classic Chinese medical case history. In these case histories, theory is a raft in an ocean of uniqueness, therapeutics a drinking cup being used to empty a river. Medicine is no longer buttressed by all knowing theory and powerful therapeutics. Here the details of personal trauma, family relationships, economic hardships, emotions, values, belief, hopes and fantasy create a different clinical terrain. These cases explicitly elicit empathy, compassion and connection. Real people are at stake here; any textbook 'correct' symptoms are epiphenomena. The case history finally dissolves into life and drama. Medicine is a meeting of two souls in empathic witness to life's frailties and verities. Replication is totally abandoned. Immediacy, intuition and even the outrageous are the currency of this type of encounter. Are we studying medicine or reading a play? Is healing so real that only a dramatic presentation will capture it? These type of cases intentionally abandon all formalism. Only the unique, immediate and 'real' is enacted.

Many of Zhang Zi-he's (1156–1228 CE) case histories are an important example of this pole. For example, in one case, after a detailed and eloquent description of a shouting, angry, destructive, and even dangerous woman he immediately sends word to two assistants to enter the patient's bedroom and pretend that they are eccentric prostitutes. The patient laughs for the first time in months. To continue the laugh therapy, Dr Zhang tells his assistants to dress as animals for the second day and so on, until the patient recovers in a matter of days.[4] He intentionally does not use any therapeutics that can be learned from books. The case itself seems to say that true healing is ultimately life itself and the doctor sometimes needs to provide it! Therapeutics are merely an expendable minor part.

Zhu Dan-xi, the 'Cinnabar Creek Master', (1280–1358 CE) obviously appreciated Dr Zhang's case histories as psychodrama and a century later recorded many of his own 'clinical performances'. The cases are again improvised living theatre. For example, in one case he stages a fraudulent seance for a daughter grieving her mother. When the daughter 'hears' that the mother is punishing her from beyond the grave, she gets angry for the first time in her life and recovers from the over-extended mourning.[5] Again, Dr Zhu seems to being saying that what was needed can never be recorded in the didactic books. Zhang Jie-bin (1569–1640 CE), the Ming dynasty general who turned practitioner, often referred to this tradition of no established therapeutics, and often employed it. For example, in one case, he decided to act like a haughty dignitary and just stared furiously at his patient until she blushed. Only then, we are told, would her energetics be ready to absorb the needed herbs.[6] These types of dramatic histories seem to be implying that everything is at risk in the clinical encounter.[7] There are no certainties or absolutes, no regular kinds of treatment. Healing is beyond theories and therapeutics and includes the entire humanity of the patient and healer.

Most of the recorded classic case histories of Chinese medicine fall somewhere between the two extremes just described above. They seem to utilise the case history as a literate medium to move theory and practice towards one another. The patient is more or less recognisable from theory and the treatment is more or less reproducible. Yet even this middle ground in the historical literature demonstrates a fluidity and dynamic concern that is still remarkable. None of the cases in the four volume collection mentioned (including the most stylised ones) has the structured format of a 20th century formal diagnosis and summary treatment plan.[8] Instead they generally free-flow from encounter to response. The patient was like this, and then was engaged this way. Even in the cases that depended on 'correct' signs, there is a sense of immediacy. There is generally a sense of the enormous value of the clinical encounter. Important details, such as dosage of herbs or acupuncture needle technique, are generally omitted, seemingly implying that these details were too situation-dependent to be worth recording. There is a striving in this middle ground to work out a compromise between replicability and uniqueness.

In this volumn of Western case histories, most narratives fall into the middle range of historic case histories, somewhere between systematic theory and absolute uniqueness. Compromise between theory and practice seems advisable. Few of these Western practitioners take either of the two extreme positions that were comparatively common in Chinese medical history. The West still has not generated enough of its own confidence to easily adopt either of these radical positions. Nonetheless, this new volume of Eastern medicine in the West demonstrates that the tension between theory and practice, and the ambiguity between therapeutics and context, is an ongoing one. Each practitioner has made his or her own unique compromise and synthesis to the perennial question of how to synthesise theory and practice.

This collection of illness narratives ultimately manages to touch what for me are some of the deepest truths of East Asian medicine. The coherent vision of this collection touches the fundamental importance of the patient-doctor relationship. Discussion of the patient-doctor relationship began in the literate Chinese medical tradition in the 13th chapter of the *Su Wen* section of the *Yellow Emperor's Classic of Internal Medicine*.[9] In this chapter, the minister Qi Bo introduced a critical discussion of what became an ongoing and central motif in East Asian medical thought. (In the modern era, in an attempt to make Asian medicine appear materialistic and not dependent on 'non-specific' factors, this discussion has often been suppressed.) In this section of the *Yellow Emperor*, Qi Bo mentioned, very unexpectedly, but with a sense of awe, his elder teacher Dai Ji and began the Oriental medicine meditation on the patient-doctor relationship. This archetypal master figure, the text tells us, was not dependent on normal diagnostic methods, nor therapeutic interventions. Rather, Dai Ji understood illness by the method of 'penetrating divine illumination' (*tong shen ming*) and treated exclusively by using something called 'incantation' (*zhu*). The ancients, Qi Bo tells us, relied on these methods alone to 'move the jing (essence) and transform the qi'. Acupuncture and herbs were unnecessary. From this textual moment onwards, the importance of the actual clinical encounter is established in Oriental medicine. By letting us glimpse his teacher, Qi Bo tells the reader there is an elusive dimension of medicine that is concerned purely with the dynamics of the actual clinical engagement.[10] Seasoned old practitioners, Qi Bo seems to be saying, are able to evoke transformation by the patient-doctor relationship itself.

This proposition became a central focus of the premodern Asian medical tradition. Wu Kun (1551–c.1620 CE), writing in his *Verified Medical Prescriptions* (*Yi fang yao*, 1584 CE) defined this aspect of healing as 'the medicine without form' and said it could only be grasped through the mysterious subtleties of experience.[11] He was not optimistic that it could be communicated and therefore resigned himself to a writing career of explaining herbal formulas. Sun Zun, the leader of the 17th century Korean medical delegation to China and senior editor of *Eastern Precious Mirror* (Dong yi bao jian, 1611 CE) said that 'by using this method the healing process begins even before the medicine reaches the mouth'.[12] Xu Shu-wei, author of *Prescriptions of Universal Benefit From My Own Practice* (Pu ji ben shi fang, 1132 CE), cautioned his reader in the same vein that 'to feel better before taking the medicine is the most direct method'.[13] Earlier famous teachers discussed the issue in similar or even more extreme ways. For example, Zhu Dan-xi, the 'Cinnabar Creek Master' (1280–1358 CE) mentioned earlier, described how he often had to abandon his acupuncture and herbs and just relied on his interaction with patients.[14] He cautioned that he could only rely on the healing engagement itself, after he had attained the 'capacity of a sage'. In a similar manner, Zhang Zhe-he (1156–1228 CE), author of the *Confucians' Duties to their Parents* (Ru men shi qin, 1228 CE), as mentioned earlier, described many cases where he relied entirely on the patient-doctor relationship instead of actual therapeutics.[15] This kind of discussion concerning the importance, subtlety and ultimate value of the patient-doctor relationship continued well into the 18th century. For example, even such rigorous systematic herbal methodologists as Wu Ju-tong (1758–1836 CE), who pioneered the theory of four levels of febrile disease, once cautioned his readers that whenever he treated 'internal and complex illness' he first treated with the 'divine' method of 'incantation' described in Chapter 13 of the *Su Wen*. Wu Ju-tong thought that this method might mean, in different circumstances, that he needed 'to inform his patient of the origin of the illness (label) so that it would not return, carefully examine their hidden sexual feelings or use tactful (gentle) words to lead (or) use imploring words (or) use shocking words . . . When the patient absorbed his (words and emotions), (only then could he speak of himself) as the Spirit doctor (mentioned in the 13th chapter of the *Su Wen*)'.[16] Well into the 19th century, East Asian healers continued to emphasise the difficult-to-capture intangible qualities of the patient-doctor relationship. Only in the 20th century, when Asian medicine needed to appear more 'scientific' and less 'placebo-like', has this dimension of the tradition been neglected.

What is truly wonderful about the collective voice of the authors of these illness narratives is that this timeless aspect of the tradition re-emerges. Ultimately, for me, these case histories make clear that the most critical dynamic of East Asian medicine, like all true healing, is the 'medicine without form'. Yet even further, for me, the deepest communication in this book is never quite verbalised. It touches on what Sun Si-miao (581–682 CE), the great physician, healer and alchemist of the Tang dynasty, wrote in the last year of his life when he was supposedly 99 years old. In his final statement on healing, Sun Si-miao made what for China was an icono-clastic and radical declaration: people have illness 'because they do not have love in their life and are not cherished'.[17] Ultimately, for me, this modern collection of case histories affirms Sun Si-miao's approach to health care: loving patients is the core of the healer's work. Nothing is more fundamental for the practitioner in this volume, for Oriental medicine and for all healers in every tradition everywhere.

---

[1]For a fuller discussion of the cultural dimensions of East Asian medicine transplantation to the West see: Kaptchuk, T J. The culture, history and discourse of Oriental medicine. *Journal of Chinese Medicine* 24 (1987) 7–17.

[2]The *Yellow Emperor's Classic of Internal Medicine* uses the word *resonance* (gan ying) to describe causality in many places. An excellent example can be found in Chapter 71 of the Ling Shu (Spiritual Axis). See: *Classic of the Spiritual Axis with Annotations* (Ling-shu-jing Jiao-shi) Hebei College of Traditional Chinese Medicine (Beijing: People's Press, 1982) page 272 as an example. The notion of resonance is rarely mentioned in the English language literature or modern Asian language discussion of causality in Oriental Medicine. Modern practitioners of Asian medicine seem to prefer to make Oriental medical causality resemble the proximal mechanical causality of classical Western science. One of the few excellent discussions in English of the Chinese notion of resonance appears in C L Blanc's *Huai Nan Tzu: Philosophical Synthesis in Early Han Thought*. Hong Kong: Hong Kong University Press, 1985.

[3]Riao Ruo-qin and Yu Heng-zhi (eds). *Case Histories of Famous Physicians on the Song, Yuan, Ming, and Qing Dynasties (Song yuan ming qing ming yi lei an)*. Shanghai: Shanghai Shudian, 1988. Vols I, II, III, IV.

[4]This case appears in Chen Meng-lei et al (eds) *Complete Medical Section: Collection of Ancient and Modern Books (Yi bu quan lu: gu jin tu shu ji cheng)*. Hong Kong: Yuguang Press, 1962, vol 7, page 1649 (first published in 1726 CE). This case also appears in Riao Ruo-qin and Yu Heng-zhi's Case Histories. Ibid. Vol 1, p.10.

[5]Chen Meng-lei et al. Ibid. p. 1610. Also see Zhu Zhen-xiang *Secrets of the Cinnabar Creek Master*. (Dan xi xin fa) Beijing: Beijing City Zhongguo Shudian, 1986.

[6]Zhang Jie-bin. *Illustrated Wing to the Classic of Categories*. (Lei jing tu yi) Beijing: People's Health Press, 1965.

[7]All the cases just cited are involved with 'benevolent deception'. Although this practice is widespread in Chinese medical history, to my knowledge, there is no scholarly discussion on the topic. Actually, the issue of 'benevolent deception' is common cross-culturally in all societies before the modern concept of 'informed consent' dominates medical ethics. Examples are easy to find. For example in Islamic medicine, see A J Arberry (trans) *The Spiritual Physick of Rhazes*. London: John Murray, 1950. For a discussion of benevolent deception in 19th century Western medicine see S J Reiser. Words as scalpels: transmitting evidence in the clinical dialogue. In: *In Search of the Modern Hippocrates*. R J Bulger (ed) Iowa City: University of Iowa Press, 1987.

[8]For a discussion on this issue in Western medical histories see: G B Risse and J H Warner. Reconstructing clinical activities: patient records in medical history. *Social History in Medicine* 4: 1992 (183–205). J D Stoeckle and J A Billings. A history of history-taking. *Journal of General Internal Medicine* 2: 1987 (119–127). S T Anning. A medical case book: Leeds, 1781–84. *Medical History* 28: 1984 (420–431). The modern case history format seems to have entered the Chinese medical literature in the late 1930s.

[9]*Translations into the Vernacular of the Inner Classic of the Yellow Emperor: Simple Questions* (*Huang di nei jing su wen yi shi*). Nanjing College of Traditional Chinese Medicine (ed). Shanghai: Shanghai Science and Technology Press, 1981. p. 109–113.

[10]This discussion in the *Su Wen* seems to have nothing to do with the modern *qi gong* movement or any of its historical antecedents. For a discussion related to this issue see K Miura. The revival of qi: qigong in contemporary China. In: *Taoist Meditation and Longevity Techniques.* L Kohn (ed) Ann Arbor: Center for Chinese Studies. The University of Michigan Press, 1989.

[11]Wu Kun. *Verified Medical Prescriptions* (Yi fang yao). Jiangsu: Jiangsu Science and Technology Press, 1985. (1584 AD)

[12]Quoted in Zhong Jian-hua and Man Ming-ren (eds). *Practical Chinese Medical Psychology.* (Shi yong zhong yi xin lin xue) Beijing: Beijing Publishers, 1987. p. 127.

[13]Xu Shu-wei. *Prescriptions of Universal Benefit from My Own Practice.* (Pu ji ben shi fang) Shanghai: Shanghai Science and Technology Press, 1978 (first published 1132 CE).

[14]A discussion of what Zhu Dan-xi (Zhu Zhen-xiang) called the 'living noose' (*huo tao*) is presented in the *Complete Medical Section: Collection of Ancient and Modern Books* (*Yi bu quan lu: gu jin tu shu ji cheng*) collected under imperial order by Chen Meng-lei et al. Volume 7 Hong Kong: Yuguang Press, 1962, p. 1610 (first published in 1726 AD, and this discussion was in Vol. 295 of the original edition). Also see Zhu Zhen-xiang. *Secrets of the Cinnabar Creek Master* (Dan xi xin fa). Beijing: Beijing City Zhongguo Shudian, 1986.

[15]Zhang Zhe-he (Zhang Cong-zheng). *Annotated Confucian's Duties to their Parents* (Ru men shi quin jiao zhu). Zhang Hai-cen et al (eds). Henan: Henan Science and Technology Press, 1984 (first published 1228 CE).

[16]Quoted in Wang Ke-zhong. *Spirit Dimensions in Chinese Medicine* (Zhongyi shen ju sue sho) Beijing: Zhongyi Guji, 1988. p. 132.

[17]Sun Si-miao. *Supplemental Wings to the Thousand Ducat Prescriptions.* (Qian jin yi fang). Beijing: People's Press, 1982 (682 CE) Vol. 15. p. 166. Love is not usually thought of as a positive feeling, cognitive state or passion in Chinese thought with the exception of Moist idea of 'universal love' (bo ai). The Confucian idea of 'human-heartedness' (ren) is much more critical in medical ethics. Sun-Si miao is remarkable in his positive use of the word love. See Fung Yu-lan's *A History of Chinese Philosophy* for a discussion of the Moist idea of love. (Bodde D trans. Princeton: Princeton University Press, 1983.) To my knowledge, a systematic discussion of this aspect of Son Si-miao's thought has never appeared in any language.

Acknowledgements

Many people have helped bring this book to fruition. Both Ted and I have been delighted with the support, cooperation and constructive advice of each of the 40 practitioners who contributed a case. Individually and collectively, they have provided many useful insights about the state of acupuncture in the West and how best to present it to the world in all its richness and diversity. We also appreciate what a significant role has been played by the patients whose case histories make up this book. By agreeing to have their 'stories' included, they have provided interesting perspectives on their experiences and validated the work of the practitioners.

I would personally like to acknowledge people who have helped in very specific ways: Jenny McNamara, for providing the reflective space from which creative projects such as this book emerge; Yarrow Cleaves, for her steady confidence in the value of the work and for her feedback and practical skills towards improving the copy; Randall Barolet, for some helpful conversations in the early stages, when the book was taking shape; Oran Kivity, for his translation of Yves Requena's case, and François de Menthon, for his translation of Eric Marié's case; Michael Burgess, for providing practical and editorial help when energy for the project was flagging; Geoff Wall, for engaging discussions on tradition and texts in a manuscript culture, and the implications for diversity in practice; Alison Gould, for her quiet enthusiasm in the face of what seemed at times like an uphill struggle; and Mike Fitter, for his insights on the value of the case study method.

At the Northern College of Acupuncture, many of the staff have pitched in and helped out in all sorts of ways. In particular, I would like to acknowledge Pam Simpson for her brilliant administrating; Tracey Homer for wonderful efficiency with no fuss; Anne Beresford, for her unstinting willingness to lend a helping hand; and Angela Hudson, for her desire always to do the best. At the Ch'ien Clinic, Doris Beavis has supported this project with her warmth and sense of humour.

I would also like to acknowledge Giovanni Maciocia for his role in sowing seeds for this book. He had the original idea for a book of cases, although not exactly in this form.

Finally, I would like to express my appreciation to my family — Sara, Angus and Shona — for never complaining about time I spent away from them while working on this book, and for trusting that it would all be worthwhile in the end.

1997   H. MacP.

Introduction

Hugh MacPherson <small>YORK, UK</small>

This book has brought together an extraordinary range of case histories. Not only are the patients of these case histories diverse in terms of their backgrounds, experiences, personal dramas, conditions and presenting complaints, but so too are the contributors, who bring to their work as acupuncturists their differing traditions, their clinical experiences and their own distinctive styles of practice. As each unique interaction between patient and practitioner unfolds, we see the emergence of the various practitioners themselves, in relation to their patients and in relation to the practice of acupuncture.

The ensuing diversity, in all its dimensions, is enchanting, inspiring and empowering for all who continue to be open to what acupuncture and its practice can mean. The collage of case histories provides support for practitioners to realise their own way within the tradition of Oriental medicine and its present flowering. The contributors come from many different countries and together they bring an international flavour. The editors hope their personal experiences, as leading practitioners, educators and writers in Oriental medicine, will add to the ongoing debate about the practice of this medicine and how it can continue to develop and blossom in the West.

Intentions and aspirations

The editors hope this book is timely in its aim to uncover how acupuncturists really work in practice. In the West, we have a growing library of texts in English that provide instruction on acupuncture, diagnostics, pattern differentiation, treatment strategies and protocols. A number of useful case history texts have been translated from Chinese but there has been a growing awareness that we have yet to develop our own case history tradition. Patients in the West have some uniquely Western experiences and issues to contend with, from diet and lifestyle through to the way in which we experience and deal with illness in our culture. One aim of this book is to uncover the various ways in which leading acupuncturists engage with these experiences and issues, and how they work with the complexities and uncertainties that are inherently part of an ongoing therapeutic relationship.

As editors of this book, we sought to find out what actually happens when someone consults an acupuncturist in order to receive treatment. We were interested in the process of having acupuncture as well as in the diagnosis and the treatment. We wanted to know what it was like for the practitioner, what was difficult, and how she or he rose (or not) to meet any challenges. We were not looking for sanitised cases which moved inexorably to a successful conclusion. We wanted the cases to provide opportunities for learning, insight and support. We accepted that each practitioner would present his or her own way of working, with individual interpretations and style, and we encouraged this. Readers will make their own interpretations, draw their own conclusions and, hopefully, use each case as another small contribution to their reservoirs of understanding and experience.

Our wider goal with this book is to present the diversity that currently exists within the acupuncture communities in the West. We have not succeeded in thoroughly representing every tradition of Oriental medicine; indeed, there would be considerable debate about what *would* constitute a balanced sampling of acupuncturists from the West. The sample of 40 cases presented here, drawn from leading practitioners, educationalists and authors, reflects the stimulating diversity that currently exists in the West. Nevertheless, within this diversity there are also threads of commonality, and of resemblances and themes that are part of the bedrock of Oriental medicine. These apparently contradictory trends reflect the paradoxes that have always existed in Oriental medicine but which provide an exciting dimension to the present blossoming of acupuncture in the West.

This book is aimed at practitioners, students, educationalists and patients.

For practitioners, the cases present glimpses of what can actually happen in practice — the way practitioners often wrestle with the issues involved and become discouraged because they have reached a standstill. As editors, our agenda includes the encouragement of multiple perspectives. If practitioners reach a stalemate from one perspective, what are the possibilities from another perspective? These cases should reinspire and reinvigorate practitioners because, from the range of possibilities and opportunities presented, the comprehensive referencing can be used to follow up ideas to their source.

For students, it is often the difficulties of a case, with their complexities and uncertainties, that offer the greatest opportunities for learning. The patients presented in this book do not always progress smoothly from ill health to health: setbacks abound, partial recoveries are common and not everyone survives. This is the reality of an acupuncturist's practice. The cases present the range of outcomes as it really is rather than a carefully selected group of success stories. Also, the layout of the book, with the more technical sections separated off from narrative, is designed to support ease of access for people grappling with the more fundamental aspects of Oriental medicine.

For educationalists and teachers of Oriental medicine, the book provides an important bridge between theory and practice[1]. We have encouraged contributors to provide well-organised and internally consistent case presentations while, at the same time, providing opportunities to show how the theory and practice of acupuncture are integrated. The structure of the more technical sections ensures clarity by providing significant detail in the area of pattern differentiation, in showing how the patterns interrelate with the aetiology and pathology diagrams, and in discussing the treatment procedures and the rationale for the use of key acupuncture points. The emphasis on structure, which is not at the expense of relevance, makes a useful adjunct to teaching. It cannot replace a training in a teaching clinic but instead provides a wider range of vicarious clinical experiences for students.

We have also been interested to find that people who have no background in the theory of Oriental medicine have found the sum of the cases a compelling introduction to acupuncture and have frequently said 'Yes, I'd like to try acupuncture now'.

The contributor's role

The contributors have made choices, whether deliberately or intuitively, about the nature of their role in the book. In compiling their case studies, they have had to ask themselves a variety of questions: How much do I participate in the story of my case? How much explanation and interpretation do I provide? How much importance do I give to storytelling? How much do I reveal of myself, my thoughts and my feelings? Each contributor has put her or his own emphasis on the combined roles of storyteller, teacher, advocate and interpreter.

The storytelling aspect of a case is particularly important. The elements of a good story include a situation in which a person is suffering or has a problematic condition; initial efforts are made to help but are unsuccessful and the situation worsens; the situation is transformed by a dramatic or extraordinary intervention. The case history of a patient coming for acupuncture can often fit into this mould. However, the stories told in this book are not being told for their own sake[2]. A good story engages a reader's interest sufficiently for it to be read. It then provides the reader with the sense of 'being there'. This vicarious experience gives the reader a basis for reflection, interpretation and establishing meaning. A well-told story can open a window from which to view the complexity of a case and its related dilemmas and issues.

Differences in interpretation have always existed in Oriental medicine. The practice of Oriental medicine involves a dynamic interaction between practitioner and patient which is shaped by the experiences and intentions of the practitioner as well as the unique context of the patient. No interpretation by the practitioner of what happens can be neutral and similarly few interpretations by different readers will have the same meaning. Oriental medicine is not helped by coating it in the gloss of a value-free activity[3]. If we accept that differences exist, and that diversity is inherent to Oriental medicine, then inevitably there will be advocates of particular styles and approaches. The reader should be aware of the contributor's role as advocate rather than believe the contributor to be 'neutral', and therefore delight in the possibilities and opportunities presented. Advocates do their best to convince people to follow them and to believe what they have come to believe. Advocacy has an honourable tradition within Oriental medicine and, without the incentive of an opportunity to advocate a style and approach to acupuncture, we would probably not have had so many contributors willing to submit cases for the book.

The traditions of Oriental medicine continue to develop. This is a two-way process of looking backwards, drawing upon existing sources, ideas and interpretations and looking forwards, by drawing out new meanings and interpretations. The practitioner is the agent of the interpretation[4], drawing on our existing understanding, and facilitating us to think through and develop this understanding by making new connections, developing fresh insights and gaining a richer awareness.

The role of interpreter is an important one in this book for several reasons. The practice of acupuncture inevitably involves the activity of interpretation because acupuncture is not a theory, or even a collection of theories, about disease and its treatment but is an interpretative activity that involves the practitioner, the patient and the context. The practitioner draws on her or his experience and tradition, which includes the oral tradition and the texts which are the source of the practitioner's work, and, from this perspective, develops an interpretation of what needs to happen for the patient. Because acupuncture continues to be practised in new contexts, with unique patients who are faced with new dilemmas and opportunities, and because it is part of an ever-developing tradition, it is essential that there are new interpretations. This is especially relevant to the transition that Oriental medicine is making to the West, with its particular culture, expectations and demands, and challenges and constraints[5]. Patients of acupuncture in the West seek help with different problems and look for resolutions which require different interpretations and interventions. The different approaches provided in the case studies should widen and stimulate the debate on Oriental medicine in the West.

Reflections on uniqueness

The case study is a much underrated method of investigation in the West. This attitude derives from the dichotomy between theory and practice in modern orthodox medicine[6]. When Western medicine shifted from being practice-led to being theory-led, scientific principles came to dominate. This shift was reflected in the central role that the case history once had (Hunter 1989) to the case history being used to report the unusual, problematic or rare in clinical situations. The perspective of today's biomedical researcher emphasises homogenous groups of patients, statistical significance, and generalisation but to the clinician, a perspective oriented towards relevance and significance for the patient makes more sense. While the status of clinical experience within medical science may currently be low, there is little doubt that medical knowledge and its development is dependent on the clinical contexts and the patient[7].

Farquhar (1992) argues cogently for a central role for the case history literature in the development of Chinese medicine. The written records of medical experience, with all their controversies and contradictions, remain, as Mao Zedong said, 'a vast treasurehouse' on which students of medicine and experienced doctors can draw. Practitioners of Chinese medicine forge a masterful link between the reality of the patient's illness and the relevant texts, including the case history literature from the medical archives. In so doing, they reanimate the experience of their forebears and simultaneously contribute towards practitioners acting masterfully in the future. Case histories, therefore, provide us with the opportunity to study the virtuosity and mastery of senior practitioners and contribute to our steady accumulation of experience.

In terms of the English language literature on Chinese medicine, there is a relative dearth of case history material. This reflects our Western bias towards theoretical texts and a fundamental lack of appreciation of the role case histories can play in the development of clinical practice. Chase (1992) has argued that the Chinese case history literature, little of which has been translated into English, is of 'much greater utility' than the premodern classics. He also perceives that, by the very nature of case histories, clinical utility is emphasised over purely theoretical considerations. The most valuable source of useful information on the treatment of real-life patients, argues Chase, is case histories.

The purpose of a case study is to catch the uniqueness, with its complexity and indeterminancy, in a single case. The emphasis is on the context, the subtleties and nuances, the unfolding of events and the wholeness of the individual[8]. The focus of the case study is on understanding what happens for the individual, following his or her story, seeking patterns and connections, and drawing out meanings.

Interpretation is of central importance in a case study. Practitioners present their experience in the narrative. This may include what they see, feel, hear, smell, and ordinarily pay attention to, and from this the practitioners present their interpretation of the experience. This may involve puzzling over meanings, reflecting on implications, recognising connections and patterns, evaluating interventions and moving towards conclusions. In this interpretative activity, practitioners also draw on their own experience of Oriental medicine and possibly other healing arts, including the texts and teachings which have been instrumental in their development as acupuncturists.

The case history also provides an experience, albeit vicarious, for the reader. A strong description of the patient, of the sensory experiences of the practitioner, of the dilemmas and challenges in the encounter, and of the unfolding drama of the treatment process, all add to the potency of the reader's experience. It is this experience that provides the opportunity for readers to feel the uniqueness of each case, to understand what is significant, to make their own interpretations, and to establish its meaning and value for themselves. Readers bring their own personal history, their understanding of Oriental medicine and, perhaps, the influences of seminal teachers, together with their preferences and inclinations, to this process.

Tradition and diversity

Uniqueness is one of the defining characteristics of the clinical encounter in acupuncture; the diversity which derives from the traditions of Oriental medicine is another. These traditions are rooted in texts that have evolved from a manuscript culture which had certain characteristics: modified versions of manuscripts appeared in different regions, variations in the development of these manuscripts occurred at different times, vibrant traditions were elaborated by charismatic physician-writers, and no single text or tradition had a monopoly on what constituted Oriental medicine. So, the traditions display an extraordinary diversity while at the same time retaining some threads of commonality.

The Chinese word for classic text, '*jing*', carries the connotation of lengthy warp threads, running back through time, and the repeated wefts of generations of writers conveying their experiences through the centuries

(Clavey 1995). At periods in the history of Oriental medicine, attempts have been made to create a single systematic approach, intending it to eventually dominate practice. The most recent example is the state-led and bureaucratically controlled development of Chinese medicine in the People's Republic of China, which is often labelled Traditional Chinese Medicine (TCM) in the West[9]. However, as has been argued elsewhere (Unschuld 1985), TCM is only a small part of Oriental medicine, although its current influence in the West is undeniable. The spectrum of case histories in this book bears witness to both a dominant strand of what we might loosely call TCM, in parallel with many other strands.

There has always been a dynamic tension between two trends in Oriental medicine (Scheid 1995). One trend wants to systemise Oriental medicine, more recently, for example, presenting itself as modern and scientific. Although admitting to diversity and conflict, implicit in this approach is an expectation that developments will occur in a linear and progressive manner. The other trend manifests in reverence for the personal experiences of the masters, in the case history literature, and in the value placed on flexibility and virtuosity in clinical practice. In this context, analyses of case histories provide deep insights not into medicine as a system, but into medicine as it is actually practised, with all its diversity, subtle nuances, unexpected happenings, varied interpretations and wealth of potential meanings.

With a focus on medical practice, rather than on a system of medical knowledge, it is easier to understand that the diversity in acupuncture does not need to lead to finding one approach 'right' and another approach 'wrong'. In the West, with our Cartesian logic, we may find it difficult to accept that such diverse approaches to acupuncture can potentially all have value. For example, from an Oriental perspective, the process of diagnosing a patient has less to do with trying to uncover an objective reality, as would be the case in orthodox Western medicine, and more to do with establishing a working hypothesis. The practitioner of Oriental medicine seeks to engage the patient in an unfolding process where, over time, a series of working hypotheses or interpretations are used to point the way towards the most appropriate interventions. What is important is that we assess these interventions in terms of their appropriateness in being able to undertake effectively our task of tending to the health and well-being of our patients.

Interpretations not only draw on practitioners' past experiences and traditions but are also grounded in the unique situation and condition of the patient. In this way, we can understand that diversity is inherent to Oriental medical practice. Consistency and the formal application of rules may be part of a systematic approach but we also need an awareness of the nuances of the clinical encounter, an attentiveness to subtle changes over time, a responsiveness to the unexpected, a willingness to engage with the complexity of a case, and a virtuosity in our role as practitioners. Through the case history literature, these subtle issues can be explored, diversity can flourish, the traditions of Oriental medicine can maintain their vitality, and meaningful dialogue can take place.

A flexible framework

It has been a challenge to bring together diverse contributions in a way that would draw out their commonality. We wanted to maximise the accessibility of case histories with some common themes, while at the same time allowing the uniqueness and extraordinariness of each case and each contributor's approach to shine through. As with any attempt to provide structure for life events, there has inevitably been some compromise between asking contributors to write within a narrow and possibly rigid framework or allowing them an overly free hand to construct their individual case presentation.

We decided to emphasise certain aspects in the clinical encounter, such as the initial contact with the patient, the taking of the case, the process of identifying the patterns, the analysis of the aetiology and pathology, the treatment procedures, and the ongoing treatment and outcome. Not all contributors found this structure appropriate, or wanted to work within our guidelines. This is quite acceptable and is, in fact, a healthy situation for a book which highlights the strengths of diversity.

Initial encounter and taking the case

The first encounter with a patient can be very revealing. We wanted the cases to cover questions such as: What did the patient look like? What was his or her body build? What could be seen from the facial expression and colouring? Practitioners often sense or intuit things about the patient that can take some time to understand or verbalise; the significance of first impressions carries over into the clinical encounter as a whole.

We were also interested in practitioners' early reactions to the patient, how they established rapport and built trust, and we wanted to know if any difficulties arose in the therapeutic relationship. We wanted practitioners to become more aware of any subconscious habits or expectations which filtered their perceptions and attitudes. We asked them for their reactions to patients as they discussed their main problem or complaint, their procedures for physical examinations (including tongue, pulse and body palpation) and for questions of referral and medication, and how lifestyle issues were addressed.

Identifying the patterns of disharmony

In this section, practitioners elaborate their understanding of the patterns of disharmony[10]. We encouraged a structure of syndrome differentiation (*bianzheng*), which holds a pivotal role in Chinese medicine (Farquhar 1994). To ensure a clear and unambiguous identification of patterns, these are presented in a separate box, and for each pattern a list of evidence is provided in the form of signs and symptoms pointing to the pattern. These separate boxes add to the clarity and rigour of the analysis, and allow the remaining narrative to flow in the text. However, this framework did not meet with universal approval among the contributors. For some, the processes of diagnosis and treatment are so intertwined that to separate them out would be artificial and not helpful to an understanding of what was happening. For others, the process of diagnosis is an ongoing one, where the significant pattern(s) only emerge over time. These practitioners have quite properly presented their cases in ways which are appropriate for them.

Aetiology and pathology

This section offered the case history writers an opportunity to add some depth to their analysis. In particular, we encouraged practitioners to elaborate on what they saw as the key causes or aetiological factors that had precipitated or led to the patterns of disharmony. One of the strengths of this approach is that it shows clearly what life events or lifestyle issues (such as diet or overwork) are of significance and may need to be addressed as part of the treatment process.

Another feature of this section is the discussion of the pathological processes, which includes an understanding of the way in which multiple patterns interrelate — knowing which syndrome, or Element, is feeding an imbalance elsewhere. As part of this, a discussion on the role of the *ben* (root) and *biao* (manifestation) can be relevant.

We encouraged contributors to present a summary of the aetiology and pathology in a diagram that would capture the complexity of the case. As Aristotle said, 'the soul . . . never thinks without a picture'. Diagrams have limitations but, for students of Oriental medicine, they can provide a useful stepping stone towards understanding the interrelationships of patterns and processes.

Starting treatment

We were interested in knowing how the contributors started their treatment: What treatment principles were used? Was there a treatment plan and, if so, was the patient involved in its discussion? What was the patient's reaction to the plan? Did issues of money, time or commitment arise? Did any lifestyle issues need to be addressed at the outset or later, and would this raise any dilemmas for the patient in relation to, for example, diet, work or family?

For the first treatment itself, we encouraged practitioners to spell out their rationale on a point-by-point basis. We also wanted to include the level of explanation given to the patient, the patient's experience of needling, the practitioner's expectations of the first treatment, and any discussions between practitioner and patient that were particularly relevant. Technical information on the needles, needling depth and technique and any auxiliary treatments, such as moxa, herbs and massage, were also requested.

Our goal here was to obtain a snapshot of this first treatment session. However, for some practitioners this may give undue attention to the first treatment because, for them, the first treatment involves a clearing process and the underlying patterns, which may only emerge over time, are addressed at subsequent sessions.

Ongoing treatment and outcome

Treating a patient with acupuncture is a process that unfolds over time. Clinical manifestations, such as the signs of the tongue and the pulse, may shift subtly; new patterns may emerge; the patient may improve or deteriorate. Practitioners need to respond flexibly to the moment so this section provides an opportunity for them to present the patient's ongoing situation, to give details of subsequent interventions, to summarise the outcome, and to pull together the threads of the case.

We were interested in conveying any problematic issues which arose, for instance, around the issues of ethics, sexual feelings, or compliance. We wanted to know what challenges there were for the practitioner when improvements did not materialise as expected, or when a patient had a setback, or when his or her condition steadily deteriorated. Also, if appropriate, how did the practitioner address issues of death and dying? These are important issues for all practitioners and, by intentionally seeking to be explicit about these difficulties and dilemmas, we can learn from the contributor's experience.

Many contributors summarised their experience with an overview which looked at what patients had learned about their illnesses, what changes the patients might have made to the way in which they cared for themselves, and what the practitioners had learned about acupuncture and about themselves.

In this last section, practitioners had an opportunity to identify clearly their individual approach to their work.

Acknowledging sources

It was not easy for many practitioners to provide sources for their work because often they did not have sources that they could easily reference. Many were taught at a time when few English texts were available in the West. Others were taught in a doctrinaire or dogmatic way, at schools and colleges where Oriental medicine was handed down as a self-evident and incontestable truth. As practitioners, however, we can benefit from knowing that particular traditions evolved at certain times, and that these traditions were strongly promoted by individuals or groups of physicians. Oriental medicine in the West is moving beyond dogma and doctrine so we are now ready to engage with our traditions. This involves interpreting the texts that make up our tradition and, when discussing what we do and why, giving our sources by referencing. In this way, we not only honour our traditions but also, through addressing the contestable notions that imbue Oriental medical practice, we contribute to the generation of new insights and knowledge.

Labels and themes

In ordering the cases for this book, we had to make some difficult choices. We could have categorised the cases in groups according to the different styles of acupuncture practised by contributors, but an individual's style cannot always be labelled in an unambiguous way. Also, within each tradition there can be extraordinary variations in approach which could render the original distinction almost meaningless. For example, the group of practitioners in this book who use a predominantly Japanese style of acupuncture might be very technique-oriented, or might have a strong psychological emphasis, and these differences could be of greater significance than the uniting factor of the Japanese style of acupuncture.

Another obvious way to divide up the cases is according to the disease label or category. However, a simplistic categorisation could act like a straightjacket for the cases, limiting the depth and richness of the patient's experiences which generally transcend labelling. Furthermore, one of the aims of this book is to draw out the uniqueness of every clinical encounter and to demonstrate the possibilities inherent within a holistic medical practice to match the diagnosis and treatment to the patient, both at the outset of treatment and over time as the patient's condition unfolds.

We therefore chose to present the cases in a single group of 40 without any overt subdivisions or subcategories, but, to give some sense of continuity, we ordered them around themes. The first theme includes cases dealing with the most problematic conditions a practising acupuncturist is likely to encounter. In these cases, the contributors write of their experiences of treating people who have AIDS or who are HIV positive, who have degenerating and progressive illnesses, such as diabetic neuropathy, ankylosing spondylitis and motor neurone disease, and where the chances of complete recovery are low. The second theme focuses on gynaecological problems, from difficulty in conceiving, through morning sickness and postpartum depression, to difficulties with the menstrual cycle or with the menopause. The third theme revolves around issues of chronic tiredness and fatigue. The fourth theme is concerned with digestive disorders and, as this group of cases illustrates clearly, a great strength of Oriental medicine is that it provides a framework for healing the mindbody split. The fifth theme looks at the area of chronic pain, an area in which acupuncture gained an early reputation in the West yet, as these cases show, the complexity of the approaches goes well beyond the simple formulae or explanations once used to describe treatment of pain by acupuncture. The final theme focuses on patients who have emotional and mental difficultes, including those where there is some psychic or spiritual dimension.

The case as a work of art

As the case histories in this book illustrate, the practice of Oriental medicine is a complex activity. The descriptions in the cases are interpretations of what happened, filtered by the framework of this book and the focus of the practitioner. As Lawrence Durrell wrote, 'Truth disappears with the telling of it'. Much in the way that the *dao* that can be described is not the real *dao*[11] so it is with these cases. Given this limitation, what can we learn from this collection of case studies? What insights can we perceive, what meanings have value for us, and what conclusions can we draw? As with any activity, the context is important, and each of us will draw on our own experiences and traditions in answering these questions.

As coeditor, I offer some final thoughts on this book and its meaning for me. Firstly, the book has opened up a much wider view of acupuncture than the one I had developed from within the confines of what is called Traditional Chinese Medicine. I had been taught, and sincerely believed, that there was a 'right' way to practise acupuncture based on a 'systematic' and 'coherent' theory of Chinese medicine. This is not the place to elaborate on why this 'system' has come to dominate our perception of Chinese medicine, it has been well analysed elsewhere (Scheid 1994), but I do recognise that Oriental medicine is a far richer and more diverse tapestry than I had previously acknowledged.

Secondly, I have learned that this diversity, even if it can be problematic, is evidence of a vitality and resilience that has survived, and will continue to survive, all attempts to impose an orthodoxy on it. Essentially pluralist in character, Oriental medicine can adapt and change to new situations and contexts, much in the way that a practitioner can be flexible and responsive to the ever-changing subtleties of the clinical encounter.

Thirdly, I see an interpretative activity as central to the practice of Chinese medicine, built not only on the practitioner's experience, tradition and intention, but also on the patient's situation and expectation. It is a multifaceted activity: no two practitioners will respond identically. Our work involves levels of complexity and uncertainty that necessarily require more of the artist than the technician from within us.

Finally, I see every case study in this book as a work of art. Each study provides an opportunity for us as readers to see and experience a clinical encounter and, through this vicarious experience, reflect on what happened, engage our interpretative powers, and derive meanings of value for ourselves. I hope that, in some small way, this will help each of us find our own unique way of being creative in the world.

NOTES

1   An important distinction between Western and Oriental medicine is in the way they link theory and practice. Within the biomedical system, theory is seen as the cutting edge in the development of practice, with theory separate from, but dominating, practice. As a consequence, practitioners in medical practice are concerned to overcome this division and such tools as case study research and reflective practice are designed to assist in building bridges between theory and practice (Schon 1983). Detailed studies from an anthropological perspective demonstrate that no such split between theory and practice exists in Chinese medicine (Farquhar 1992). A consequence of this close link between theory and practice, where theory does not dominate practice, is the continued existence of diversity within the Oriental medical traditions (Scheid 1993).

2   A valuable discussion of the role of storytelling in Western medicine is presented by Hunter (1986). 'Medicine is filled with stories' she writes, and she goes on to identify the crucial role that stories play in closing the 'epistemological gap' between the general theories of disease and the particular reality of illness. Hunter sees the story not as a collection of facts but as an exploration of individual variation and its relation to the whole of human experience. Stories remind us of medicine's ineradicable uncertainty.

3   An important issue evolving from this profusion of interpretations is the realisation that the value of interpretations vary. It is not necessary or helpful to assume that all interpretations are of equal value. Quite simply, some interpretations are better than others. We need to assess their value in terms of appropriateness, relevance, credibility and utility.

4 Many contemporary advocates of professional practice as an interpretative activity nourish the belief that knowledge is constructed rather than discovered. We construct our understandings from our experiences. In this context, a case study can provide the reader with the raw material for the understanding or interpretation to be constructed (Stake 1995).

5 The issues raised by the transmission of Oriental medicine to the West are discussed in some detail by Kaptchuk (Wiseman & Ellis 1985). As Western practitioners, students and scholars, our responsibilities include becoming 'poignantly aware of how culture and history demand from us different answers than those presently fixed in the tradition as it is variously understood in different Asian countries'. As part of this process, the case histories in this book present a broader clinical dialogue and a wider range of options for Oriental medicine than would normally be part of everyday practice in the East.

6 The familiar dichotomy in the West between 'hard' science, with its dogmatic insistence on cognitive knowledge, and the 'soft' knowing of professional practice, with its artful competence, has been elegantly identified by Schon (1983). He shows clearly how scientific and professional knowledge are so often mismatched to situations in professional practice which are characterised by uniqueness, uncertainty, disorder and indeterminacy. Along with his support for the development of 'reflective practice', a tool to help to reconnect a divided theory and practice, he also strongly promotes the value of the case method based on an analysis of innumerable cases drawn from the 'real' world.

7 In a study of the case in Western medicine, Hunter (1989) describes the variables in the clinical encounter as infinite and goes on to argue for the crucial role played by case histories in bridging the gap between the general principles of medicine and the individual experience of illness. She also stresses how often a doctor's understanding depends on the chronology of the illness and its development over time.

8 In the field of case study research (Yin 1994), it is recognised that a single case study allows an investigation to retain the holistic and meaningful aspects of real-life events.

9 It should be noted that while what we know as Traditional Chinese Medicine (TCM) has dominated much of what is published in books and articles in the West in recent years, the Chinese medicine that is currently practised in China is considerably more varied. Scheid (1994) discusses in some depth his experience of modern Chinese medicine and describes the diversity as 'endless'. Contributing to this includes the lack of institutional or ideological pressure for systematic coherence between theory and practice or between different modes of practice, the values placed on referring to original sources and the case history literature, the recognition of flexibility as one of the strengths of Chinese medicine, the veneration of living masters and the high regard paid to doctors developing their own personal style and virtuosity (*ling*) through accumulated experience (*jingyan*).

10 Patterns are basically archetypes (Chase 1992) which were never intended to mirror exactly the idiosyncracies of the individual patient. If we see patterns as emblematic, then we do not have to expect them to be complete or exact representations of an objective reality.

11 From Lao Tsu's Tao Te Ching (Gia-Fu & English 1973).

REFERENCES

Chase C 1992 Fleshing out the bones: case histories in the practice of Chinese medicine. Blue Poppy, Boulder

Clavey S 1995 Fluid physiology and pathology in traditional Chinese medicine. Churchill Livingstone, Edinburgh

Farquhar J 1992 Time and text: approaching Chinese medical practice through analysis of a published case. In: Leslie C & Young A (eds): Paths to Asian medical knowledge. University of California, Berkeley pp 62–71

Farquhar J 1994 Knowing practice. Westview Press, Boulder

Gia-Fu Feng & English J 1973 Lao Tsu: Tao Te Ching. Wildwood House, Aldershot

Hunter K M 1986 'There was this one guy . . .': the use of anecdotes in medicine. Perspective in Biology and Medicine 29(4): 619–630

Hunter K M 1989 A science of individuals: medicine and casuistry. Journal of Medicine and Philosophy 14: 193–212

Scheid V 1993 Orientalism revisited. European Journal of Oriental Medicine 1(2): 22–33

Scheid V 1994 Home and away: in search of Chinese medicine. European Journal of Chinese Medicine 1(4): 14–19

Scheid V 1995 The great *qi*: Zhang Xichuan's reflections on the nature, pathology and treatment of the *da qi*. Journal of Chinese Medicine 49: 5–16

Schon D A 1983 The reflective practitioner: how professionals think in action. Basic Books

Stake R 1995 The art of case study research. Sage, Thousand Oaks

Unschuld P 1985 Medicine in China: a history of ideas. University of California, Berkeley

Wiseman N, Ellis A 1985 Fundamentals of Chinese medicine. Paradigm, Brookline

Yin R K 1994 Case study research: design and methods. 2nd edn. Sage, Thousand Oaks

The cruel virus: a case of HIV and AIDS

Nguyen Tinh Thong LONDON, UK

A serious condition

One busy afternoon, a colleague knocked at the door and whispered in my ear: 'Do you want to see this man?' 'Who is he?' I asked. Excusing myself to the patient lying on the couch, I followed my colleague to his room next door.

A very thin man sat against the couch with four needles in the upper part of his back. Both arms were half bent and were resting on the surface of the treatment couch, with one hand holding a pad of white tissues, while the other lay palm upward. He could hardly say hello to me because of his shortness of breath. I gave him a smile and asked him to be at ease with his position. In one glance, I realised that this man was in a serious condition:

He had shiny, tired eyes, deep red, dry cheeks and a shadowy complexion. There was a dark grey colour under and around his eyes. His short, dry and withered hair could not cover the raised dark brown patches around the hairline and down the neck. These patches I was later told were 'Kaposi's sarcoma'. His spasmodic coughing caused his dry dark skin to perceptibly move up and down — his body was very skinny, especially around the hypochondriac region.

Gently touching his forehead then pressing his wrist pulse, I asked: 'Are you tired?' 'Yes!' he replied with a short rough voice. At the same time, he tried to clear his throat by coughing into the tissue in his hand, saying, 'Excuse me'.

'Can I have a look at your tongue please? Thanks!'

After examining the pulse and tongue I said goodbye softly to my colleague and the patient and walked out of the room, a 'sticky sour-sweet' smell just fading away with my quick steps. Back in my room, I washed my hands and removed the needles from my patient, offering her an apology for my 5-minute absence during her treatment.

My colleague knocked and came in. He tapped me gently on my shoulder and thanked me for seeing the patient.

"What do you think of that man?" he asked.

"He seems very sick. Has he a bad Dryness in the Lungs?"

"Yes, he has been diagnosed as having pneumonia and AIDS! You know, it's a new internal disease . . . I've seen him just a couple of times, I would like you to help and give him some Chinese herbs. Acupuncture is not really enough for him, I think . . . ! Can I book him to see you sometime next week?"

AIDS . . . ! I was in a little shock and did not know how to react for a short while apart from saying "Yes . . . yes . . . But you should help me to treat him as well!"

My colleague nodded his head with an understanding smile, and walked out to the reception area. I could hear a little voice outside saying goodbye between his spasmodic coughs.

It was the first time I had seen an AIDS patient. I felt quite nervous. Dryness in the Lungs, chronic *yin xu* with empty Fire and Damp-heat are common conditions which I used to treat almost everyday in my home country, Vietnam. However, now I felt quite nervous! Strange . . . ! AIDS, the 'new cruel virus' which had been recently defined by the medical profession and highlighted by the media. I sat quietly near the open window and took a deep breath to start my meditation before beginning the next treatment. I have the habit of contemplating my breath to start my relaxation. It is really helpful for my hard life as I am a refugee from a war-torn country.

A hard life

At 9.30 am, the first patient of the new day was Juan, the AIDS patient, the one I had seen 5 days earlier with my colleague. Looking at his file I discovered that he was a 34-year-old Argentinian and gay. At 15 he had come to the UK and had settled here. He had not been a happy child. He came from an engineering family and had two sisters whom he had not contacted for the past 18 years. His life had been hard, his parents having separated when he was 10. He had contracted bronchitis twice when he was 7, and glandular fever when he was 12.

Although he was a writer by profession, he had worked hard at different jobs to earn his living. He was living 'hand to mouth' and used drugs, heroin and hashish, from time to time. 'Drugs somehow help my writing, but now I'm paying for it,' he said.

His main signs and symptoms had been described in the file as:

- Night sweats.
- Bad headaches.

- Pain in the body as if having worked hard all day!
- Desire for cool drinks, but cannot drink lots.
- Constipation.
- Bad thrush affecting the mouth, sexual organ and anus.
- Scanty and dark urine.
- Large appetite.
- Feels lonely and fearful, especially during the night, when he wakes.

The patient had to take several drugs from the hospital to control his fungal infection and pneumonia and the Kaposi's sarcoma was developing fast. He visited the hospital once a month for injections. He had also received homeopathic treatment.

"How are you today?" I asked.

"Not much change thanks." Answering with a weak voice still.

"How is your headache and pain now?"

"Headache is much better but pain more or less the same! Around the ribcage, shoulder blades and chest is bad still . . . It is worse when I cough. After a coughing fit I have a buzz in my ears and head and if anyone is talking, his voice seems far away!"

"Any more night sweating?"

"It used to be a lot more, I used to wake up with wet sheets!"

"Any changes to your appetite?"

"Yes! My appetite lately is lower than normal. About a year ago, I used to get hungry quickly and eat a lot. I am a hot type of person but I don't know why I cannot eat as much now as I used to! It is quite worrying! Look . . . I'm quite skinny now!"

"What is your diet?"

"Well, I used to eat anything available, and my eating habits used to be bad."

"What do you mean by bad?"

"Well, I used to eat irregularly, eating on the bus or train and late at night. My lifestyle hasn't been clean with drug abuse and sex, but now I've changed. I eat regularly, and many more vegetables. I like to have a Chinese takeaway sometimes! . . . The sweet-sour taste from Chinese fried vegetables makes me eat more!"

"Do you have Chinese foods very often?"

"No, just occasionally. If I have more, I have indigestion!"

"Do you cook for yourself?"

"Yes! But recently, I have had friends who have come and helped! I'm getting weaker . . . !"

"Are your constipation and passing of water better with acupuncture?"

"Yes, but not much. I have to take linseed to make it better. Passing water is painful still . . . I think, because of the fungus around there

causing problems! I've been taking an anti-fungal treatment . . . It worked quite well at first, but not much recently!"

"How long have you been diagnosed as having AIDS?"

"It is about 3 years now. Maybe I've had it a long time. But recently I've been diagnosed as having pneumonia. I started with a long and repeated flu infection with strange signs of profuse sweating and exhaustion. I was prescribed a few strong antibiotics but they didn't work and I got worse and worse. At the hospital the blood test said that I've got AIDS. My consultant recently told me that I've got only 8 weeks to live according to his experience with other Aids patients." He spoke with tears in his eyes.

"Have you had Chinese herbs and acupuncture before?"

"No. I've seen your colleague three times for acupuncture now, but no herbs. I find acupuncture is helpful, but it does not last long! I have also had some homeopathic remedies for 3 months which I still take sometimes. They are said to be for my tiredness and cough. Coughing is bad, especially from afternoon till midnight, and it disturbs my sleep."

"A lot of mucus with your cough?"

"Yes, sticky yellow green, recently with blood in it!"

"What is the colour of the blood?"

"Light strings of blood in the mucus, but sometimes also thick dark lumps. I have also had a bad dry throat in the afternoons."

During the dialogue, his voice was weak and he made a rough noise from his throat to clear it. He hadn't been coughing much in the mornings. I took his pulse and looked at his tongue twice. The tongue was swollen, deep red, dry and quite shiny with tiny purple spots on the sides and tip of the tongue. There was also some thick dirty yellowish but unrooted coating at the back of the tongue. His pulse was hasty, floating and weak.

Summary of main clinical manifestations

- The patient is HIV positive and suffering from AIDS with pneumonia.
- Coughing is bad from afternoon until midnight and disturbs sleep.
- Spasmodic coughing with profuse and sticky yellow mucus and blood.
- Shortness of breath.
- Bad dry throat in the afternoons.
- Eyes look tired.
- Deep red and dry cheeks with a shadowy complexion.
- Dry and withered hair.
- Kaposi's sarcoma in the neck and body.
- Skinny body with dry and dark skin.
- Short and weak voice, with rough noise to clear throat.
- Night sweats; hot and damp palms and chest.
- Pain in the body as though having done a hard day's work.
- Tired.
- Thirst, desire for cold drinks but cannot drink a lot; sometimes nauseous after drinking.

- Used to have a large appetite, but now much reduced; sour/sweet taste increases appetite; indigestion from rich and greasy food.
- Thrush affecting mouth, sexual organ and anus.
- Constipation with small and dry stools; has to take linseed for improvement.

- Scanty and dark urine; pain passing water sometimes due to fungus around the sexual organ.
- Fearful and lonely.
- Tongue: deep red, shiny, swollen and withered tongue with some unrooted dirty yellowish coating at the back, tiny purple spots on the sides and the tip of the tongue.
- Pulse: hasty, floating and weak.

Patterns of disharmony

The most vigorous disharmony involves the Lungs. The AIDS virus is killing the patient's upright *(zheng) qi* rapidly.

Patterns of disharmony

Dryness in Lung, Lung *yin* deficiency, Lung *qi* deficiency

- Coughing worse from afternoon to midnight.
- Coughing blood.
- Shortness of breath.
- Thirst, dry throat in the afternoons.
- Rough and weak voice.
- Desires cool drinks.
- Tongue: dry.

Blood *xu*

- Skinny body.
- Dry, rough and dark skin.
- Dry, withered hair.
- Exhaustion.
- Eyes look tired.

Damp-heat in middle *jiao*

- Coughing profusely with sticky yellow mucus.
- Tired.

- Thrush affecting mouth, sexual organ, anus.
- Urine painful to pass due to thrush around sexual organ.

Kidney *yin xu* with empty Heat flaring

- Hot and damp palms and chest.
- Night sweats.
- Deep red and dry cheeks with shadowy complexion.
- Pains in the body as though having done a hard day's work.
- Desire for cold drinks, but cannot drink a lot; sometimes nauseous after drinking.
- Constipation, small and dry stools.
- Scanty dark urine.
- Feeling lonely and fearful.
- Tongue: deep red, shiny, dry tongue.
- Pulse: hasty with floating and weak quality.

Aetiology and pathology

The bronchitis, glandular fever and unhappiness in childhood have combined with leaving home early and working hard to create the Kidney disharmony. The bronchitis also weakened the Lungs leading to weak *wei qi* and susceptibility to infection. Additional factors affecting the Kidney include fear and the AIDS infection contracted through sex. The drug and alcohol abuse, which he used to mask his unhappiness, has combined with irregular eating habits and consumption of junk food to cause Damp-heat in the middle *jiao*.

The diagram in Figure 1.1 presents these aetiological factors and shows how the patterns of disharmony interrelate. The Kidney *yin xu*, Blood *xu* and Damp-heat in the middle *jiao* all contribute to the patient's present condition which is primarily one of Lung disharmony.

Treatment

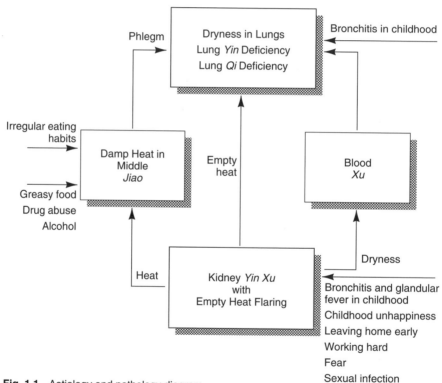

Fig. 1.1 Aetiology and pathology diagram.

The man was at a critical stage. He had a short time to live. Mindful of my breath, I talked to myself: 'Do the best you can. What is death and what is life? Nature will take care of everything.' It was strange that I had to talk to myself like this because I was in a bit of panic! As I mentioned earlier, Damp-heat with *yin xu* are common patterns, but with this patient I was quite nervous because of the new AIDS virus. This was the first case of its kind in my practice. However, I introduced a classical first treatment.

First treatment procedures

POINT PRESCRIPTIONS

For this first treatment I stimulated two different sets of points:

First set of points

- BL13 *feishu*, the back *shu* of the Lungs, and LU1 *zhongfu,* the Alarm point of the Lungs. Back *shu* points combined with the alarm front *mu* point of the Lungs were used to strengthen the Lung *qi* as well as descend the rebellious *qi* to help the patient's shortness of breath and cough. This combination — back *shu* points and alarm *mu* points — has been used in my family for a long time.

- BL23 *shenshu*, the back *shu* of the Kidneys, was added to harmonise the *qi* of both Lungs and Kidneys. In Five Elements theory, tonifying the Metal Lungs and Kidney Water at the same time creates water, and Juan has a severe *yin xu.*

  I inserted 25 mm, 32 gauge needles to BL13 *feishu* and BL23 *shenshu*. After *qi* had been obtained, I tonified BL13 *feishu* first and then BL23 *shenshu*. Three tonifying stimulations were repeated within 9 minutes before taking a 15 mm needle to use an even method on LU1 *zhongfu* for 5 minutes. Juan's pulse had changed and now had a slower and less floating quality.

Second set of points

- LU9 *taiyuan*, the Source *yuan* point of the Lung.
- LI6 *pianli*, the Connecting *luo* point of the Large Intestine.

  This combination is known as the Host and Guest treatment[1]. I inserted a 15 mm needle into LU9 *taiyuan* first, obtained the *qi* and undertook tonifying stimulations twice within 5 minutes, before needling and tonifying LI6 *pianli*. Juan's pulse felt less hasty, but he had to cough immediately after this treatment.

HERBS

I prescribed raw herbs which were based on the formula Six Ingredients Pill with Rehmannia *mai wei di huang wan* (Bensky & Barolet 1990), plus Radix Achyranthis Bidentatae *niu xi* to strengthen the *yin* of the Kidneys and Lungs and to descend empty Heat. This formula is quite cold so I also included Rhizoma Atractylodis Macrocephalae *bai zhu* powder, to protect and strengthen the middle *jiao*. Preparation of the herbs was quite complicated, especially for the patient, so I gave instructions to my own family to prepare them for him.

Hope and attachment

A week later, Juan came back with a big smile on his face! The major signs such as coughing, exhaustion, headaches, body pain, thirst, stools and urine were much better. 'The first time in 3 years I feel myself', he said with tears in his eyes. On re-examining him I found that the tongue was less swollen and not so deep red. It was wet and still looked withered. The pulse had changed from hasty floating weak to hasty full and quite tight! The pulse showed that the body's Upright (*zheng*) *qi* was still in deep conflict with the pathogenic factor.

I realised that Juan had more hope and that his attachment to Chinese medicine and to myself was greater than before. This was understandable but made me feel rather nervous as well as a little sad. It was nearly

Christmas and 12 weeks since the patient had first presented! Juan was still alive and had been to visit the hospital. His consultant was happy and very suprised. He told Juan, 'Well, I'm happy for you. But I must say that I'm still not convinced that Chinese medicine works!' The consultant was right. Although Juan had improved greatly from taking the Chinese herbs, his pulse and tongue showed that his condition had not changed at a deep level yet and could relapse at any time.

Acupuncture treatments were now given twice weekly. The main points I used were the Wood points and Water points on the channels of the Lungs, Heart, Liver, and Kidneys: LU5 *chize* and HE3 *shaohai*, combined with LU11 *shaoshang* and HE9 *shaochong*. I inserted 25 mm needles into LU5 *chize* and HE3 *shaohai* first. I twice applied tonifying stimulations with a 5-minute interval before using a sharp tip instrument to stimulate LU11 *shaoshang* and HE9 *shaochong* for 3–5 minutes. After these treatments, Juan's pulse was much calmer and less floating!

I applied a similar technique to the following points: LIV1 *dadun*, LIV8 *ququan*, KID1 *yongquan* and KID10 *yingu*. These points were used on the right (*yin*/Blood) side to stimulate re-growth of young *yang* within *yin* whilst strengthening the *yin* and the *qi* at the same time. (This method has been used in my family for long time).

I also used the Back *shu* points of the Lungs, Spleen and Kidneys BL13 *feishu*, BL20 *pishu* and BL23 *shenshu*. In addition to these I added some other assistant points such as REN12 *zhongwan*, REN4 *guanyuan* and ST36 *zusanli*.

I prepared the following new herbal decoction for Juan:

- Radix Ginseng *ren shen* 25 gm.
- Radix Angelicae Sinensis *dang gui* 20 gm.
- Radix Astragali *huang qi* 30 gm.
- Radix Polygoni Multiflori *he shou wu* 15 gm.
- Fructus Amomi *sha ren* 10 gm.
- Tuber Ophiopogonis Japonici *mai men dong* 15 gm.
- Fructus Schisandrae Chinensis *wu wei zi* 15 gm.
- (Baked) Radix Glycyrrhizae Uralensis *zhi gan cao* 6 gm.
- Pericarpium Citri Reticulatae *chen pi* 6 gm.

Boiled with water and concentrated down to a jelly form, this decoction was taken with the following powder:

- Rhizoma Atractylodis Macrocephalae *bai zhu* 40%
- (Grey) Rhizoma Atractylodis *cang zhu* 40%
- Radix Ledebouriellae Divaricatae *fang feng* 20%.

The main action of these herbs was to strengthen the Blood and the *qi* and strongly increase the appetite.

Improvement and decline

My colleague and I visited Juan in his flat because we wanted to take precautions for our other patients and we wanted to protect Juan from external pathogenic factors. AIDS in 1986/87 was still relatively new for Chinese medicine practitioners in the UK. It was a very cold winter. We wanted to protect his *qi*. Apart from advising him to eat the right foods and to do some gentle *qi gong* exercises we asked him to stay indoors as much as he could until the spring. Each time I saw him, his condition improved slowly.

Juan had to go to his bank on a windy and cold day in mid-March. He caught a cold. Acupuncture and herbs did not help him much, nor did antibiotics from the hospital. His *qi* started to decline. I started to do more counselling with him, introducing him to the concepts of Impermanence and Nonself and encouraging him to practise mindfulness breathing and to face whatever might happen to his physical body.

I was busy and my colleague had a cold, so we could not see the patient for 2 weeks. During a mild day at the beginning of April, I had news that the patient had moved to his friend's house because he was very weak, and he wanted to see me. I went to see him after my last patient of that day. It was a great shock. Only a fortnight had passed but the man looked so different: pale, dry, skinny, some cold sweats sticking on his forehead. His breath was nearly collapsed! He tried to look up and say hello to me. I told him to relax and tried to be mindful of what was going on within him.

His friend told me that he had had an attack of shortness of breath and wheezing 8 days earlier, and had been taken into the hospital. The hospital had diagnosed water in the lungs and this had been removed. Pointing to a small table, his friend showed me three different bottles of pain-killers, and said 'He seems to be in less pain with these tablets!'

Clear and peaceful

The patient held my hand and gently put it on his chest saying,

> *"I'm having difficulty breathing, Thong . . . My chest's very stiff and . . . it's very difficult for me to turn around . . . But I feel that I'm very clear . . . and peaceful . . . I'm very grateful . . . that you came. . . !". I gently touched his chest and back and said, "I will give you a herbal rescue remedy for your tiredness tomorrow, but right now, please relax as much as you can . . . ".*

I made his pillows higher to support his neck and held up my A–Z[2] book to his eye level saying

Juan, look at this book. Before this book appeared in the world, it came from nowhere . . . because it is made up of water, wood, labour and so on . . . to become a 'Book'. Supposing we burn this book, it will not go anywhere or be dead, like our ordinary mind commonly thinks, because it will turn into ash and become a rich fertiliser for the flourishing of trees and flowers . . . Then perhaps, a book again!

Please look deeply at all things and understand them this way . . . to me, understanding this way will help us to become liberated from the fear of death, and we will suffer less from the idea of Birth and Death . . . ! If you find it difficult to understand now, don't worry, just contemplate on your breath and recite Jesus Christ deep within yourself . . . It is a matter of peace and relaxation . . . I have to leave very soon, because I came straight from work. Juan, close your eyes and please do this . . .

The man gave me a little smile as well as some tears and closed his eyes . . . I walked out of the room . . . His friend asked how long he would last. I replied: . . . "I don't know" and asked him to let me know the following day if anything happened. I prepared Ginseng Rescue Remedy for him and took it with me to work. But by the end of my working day I had news of his last breath! I took a deep breath and said some prayers for him! I felt quite sad for the rest of that evening and did more meditation that night!

I did my best! However, I could not fulfil the hope that the man had extended to me! The only thing I wished for him was that the Impermanent and Nonself aspects of nature might have helped him to die peacefully. I still do not know whether it was Chinese medicine that had kept him alive for another 6 months or his strong will to live with something new to focus upon.

NOTES

1   For details of the Host and Guest treatment, see Ellis et al, 1988, page 445.

2   A–Z London Street Atlas 1992 Geographers' A–Z Map Company, Sevenoaks.

REFERENCES

Bensky D, Barolet R 1990 Chinese herbal medicine: formulae and strategies. Eastland Press, Seattle

Ellis A, Wiseman N, Boss K 1988 Fundamentals of Chinese acupuncture. Eastland Press, Seattle

FURTHER READING

Bensky D, Gamble A, Kaptchuk T 1986 Chinese herbal medicine: materia medica. Eastland Press, Seattle

■ Nguyen Tinh Thong, MAc, CHM (Saigon)

Nguyen Tinh Thong was born in South Viet Nam, to a family of healers. His grandfather specialised in treating psychological and spiritual disorders while his father focused on the treatment of physical problems. Both used acupuncture and herbs. As a young child he helped to grow, harvest and prepare the herbs for his father's clinic before being apprenticed as a novice monk in the *Mahayana* Buddhist tradition under the tutelage of the Most Venerable Thich Tu Van, Master of *qi gong, kung fu* and herbal medicine.

Thong formally studied Vietnamese traditional medicine for 6 years and received his Diploma in 1968 before supervising his father's clinic for 2 years. He attained his Master in traditional medicine and acupuncture in 1971 at Duoc Su Tinh Xa from Master Thich Tam An, a venerated monk and highly respected practitioner of Japanese acupuncture. Further study with other masters, from whom he learned advanced techniques of pulse reading and *qi* projection, prepared the foundations for his own clinic which opened in 1974 in Binh-Dinh.

The Vietnam conflict created a deep trauma in the psyche of the Vietnamese people. Folk culture and traditional pursuits were discouraged and many monks were forced to disrobe. This was an attempt to subdue the spirit of the masses in 1975 when the Communists took over the south of the country. The authorities were suspicious of Thong's influence in the community because he had established a wide reputation as a gifted doctor and healer. He was eventually imprisoned on dubious charges.

Thong arrived in Great Britain as a political refugee in 1979 and began learning the English language and prevalent practices of Chinese medicine. In 1988, he founded the London Academy of Oriental Medicine based in London. He is a cofounder of the Lotus Healing Centre, and runs a busy practice in the centre of London. He teaches meditation and *qi gong* and lectures in Buddhist Dharma.

Harry

Sandra Hill LONDON, UK

Warning: possibly HIV positive

When I saw Harry for the first time I did not take a case history. He came to me having more or less done the rounds of the group practice in which I worked at the time. I found a set of notes with the words written in the corner, 'Warning; possibly HIV positive!'. The picture I had of him therefore fell into place during the first few sessions we spent together.

Harry was gay. An ex-junkie, disturbed by compulsive sexual behaviour, an occasional frequenter of certain public lavatories. My first impression of him was one of a caged animal. His eyes moved quickly, taking in his surroundings. He didn't actually pace about, although perhaps that was what he wanted to do, instead he sat still, like a coiled spring. At other times, later, I saw him limp as a rag, silent, spent. I had noticed that his birth date was the same as mine and had sympathy for his excess of fiery Arian energy trapped within a tight Wood-type body.

The first time I saw him he had pains in the lower back, accompanied by trembling. He felt fearful and shocked. A few days earlier he had seen his parents for the first time in 2 years and was now experiencing a mixture of euphoria and rage: euphoric that he had managed to stand up to his father, dazed and confused at the feelings this had released. It was certainly not until later that he talked about his childhood: his mother's sexual projections, his father's anger and jealousy, his own fear and confusion. Since the episode with his parents, he had been unable to sleep.

Harry was in constant pain. His lower back ached. He had pains in his testicles radiating into the inner thighs. Occasionally, the pains went up the sides of his body, and at times he had rushes of energy into his head. His neck felt rigid, his temples throbbed, his eyes felt sore and dry and sometimes misty. At times his scalp itched and formed a red rash. It was always dry. Harry's head was that of a typical Arian ram, almost triangular, with a wide forehead. His brow was often hot and pounding with such an excess of energy that I imagined he might easily grow horns. He suffered from severe headaches, and was aware that these often accompanied outbursts of frustration and anger.

Caught in an energetic web

The visit to his parents and the following rage had thrown him into a cycle of compulsive sexual behaviour, the first for quite a few months. These episodes no longer held any pleasure for Harry, but were full of fear, shame and self punishment. He was caught in an energetic web; battered by his own emotions which he experienced as movements of energy. He understood the concept of fear descending in the body and anger rushing upwards and he seemed to be constantly searching for ways to fill the emptiness left in the centre.

Despite these severe symptoms and his emotional instability, Harry had managed to keep up his job as a community welfare worker, helping in old people's homes and caring for the aged in his community. It was a kind of penance.

On that first visit he seemed nervous of being touched, and lay on the couch pretty much fully dressed. His pulses were wiry and superficial in all positions, though at other times they were crowded into the middle *jiao*, leaving the upper *jiao* empty and the lower *jiao* empty on the left, and tight and thin on the right. He was reluctant to show his tongue, which was small and slightly crooked with a red tip.

I would usually feel the abdomen, but as Harry obviously did not want to undress I did not do so at this initial consultation. I could tell from looking at him that it would be tight. As he gradually relaxed, massage and touch became one of the most important aspects of treatment for him.

The details of his case fell into place over the following weeks and months, depending on Harry's insights . . . what he would allow me to hear . . . what he would allow himself to express. It took a while to build complete confidence. Maybe he needed to know that I would not judge.

Summary of clinical manifestations

- Lower back pains, occasional, accompanied by trembling.
- Lower back ache, constant.
- Pains in testicles radiating along inner thigh, sometimes to inner knee.
- Neck felt rigid, temples throbbed.
- Eyes sore, dry and sometimes misty.
- Pains in the sides, shoulders, neck, head and eyes.
- Dry scalp, occasional red spots.
- Sits like a coiled spring.
- Generally fearful or angry.
- Occasional outbursts of rage, accompanied by a rush of energy up to the head; feels as if the head will burst; head hot, pounding with energy.
- Severe headaches accompanied by frustration and anger.
- Mouth ulcers.
- As rage recedes he becomes hopeless, despairing and suicidal.
- Emotional instability, lack of will.
- Lack of sleep, always thinking.
- Exhaustion, limp as a rag, spent.

- Pulse: Changeable depending on energy cycles. At times, all positions full wiry, superficial, lack of root. At other times, middle *jiao* full and wiry, lower *jiao*, left side empty, right side tight.
- Tongue: Small, red tip and sides, slightly crooked.

- Body: Tight, nervous of being touched. Muscles rigid, especially along spine, neck, jaw.
- Abdomen: Lower abdomen slack, hollow, upper abdomen tight with palpable aorta. Some tightness and discomfort under right rib-cage.

Identifying patterns of disharmony

Harry lacked fluid. He needed watering, cooling, calming, earthing, centring, grounding. His Kidney *yin* was exhausted. As a result his Kidney *yang* energy was fuelled by an empty fire which raged intermittently, causing periods of excessive sexual energy and insomnia followed by exhaustion and impotence.

Constant depletion of the fire of the gate of destiny, the fire of *ming men*, caused a lack of will, which led eventually to the lack of will to live. Fear and fright injured the spirits by attacking the relationship between the Heart and the Kidneys, the *jing* and the *shen*, preventing free communication between the sexual centre and the Heart centre.

Depletion of Liver *yin* and Blood (the Kidney and Liver having a common source, *gan shen tong yuan*) and the false fire in *ming men* caused an intermittent flare up of Liver *yang*, giving rise to symptoms in the flanks, head and eyes. Lack of Blood in the Liver also caused tightness and stiffness in the muscles. Though symptoms of heat and excess were intense, they were occasional and obviously caused by false *yang* and false heat due to deficient *yin*. After any excessive episode he was always exhausted.

Harry didn't like himself, didn't trust himself and felt no sense of peace in coming home to himself. His dependence on the 12-step plan, a method developed by Alcoholics Anonymous that had successfully helped him over his heroin addiction, seemed to be failing for his present crisis, though he regularly attended his group. There was just too much guilt involved. He could find nowhere to hide, no place of peace. Just the constant round of anger, acting out, shame, grief, exhaustion and pain.

Patterns of disharmony

Deficiency of Kidney *yin* and Kidney *jing*
- Lower back pains and aches.
- Pains in testicles, inner thigh, inner knee.

- Generally fearful.
- Excessive sexual energy followed by exhaustion and impotence.
- Emotional instability, lack of will.

- Pulse: superficial, lack of root.
- Tongue: small, red tip.

Flare up of Liver *yang*

- Pains in the sides, shoulders, head, eyes.
- Outbursts of rage accompanied by an up-rush of energy to head; feels as if the head will burst.
- Head hot, pounding with energy.
- Severe headaches accompanied by anger and frustration.
- Neck felt rigid, temples throbbed.
- Eyes sore, dry and sometimes misty.
- Sits like a coiled spring.
- Abdomen tight, body tight, muscles rigid, especially spine, neck, jaw.
- Pulse: full wiry, changeable.
- Tongue: red sides.

Heart not communicating with the Kidneys

- Insomnia followed by exhaustion and impotence.
- Lack of sleep, always thinking.
- Loss of self control.
- Sexual centre and heart centre disconnected.
- Jumpiness, starting with fright.
- No sense of peace.
- Broken heart and spirit.
- Mouth ulcers.
- Tongue: small, red tip.

Deficiency of Liver and Heart Blood

- Tightness and stiffness in the muscles.
- Emotional instability.
- *Shen* and *hun* not housed.
- Dreamlife invades waking reality.
- Easy access to other dimensional reality.

Aetiology and pathology

As a child Harry had suffered various types of abuse. He had lived in fear and shame and confusion. As a teenager he became a drug addict as this helped to numb his pain. Kidney energy depleted from childhood would have affected his willpower, making addiction an even more likely route. Drug and alcohol abuse further depleted his Kidneys and Liver, creating a false fire in *ming men*. Sexual excess later drained his Kidney essence.

Emotionally, the anger he had experienced since childhood depleted not only the *yin* of the Liver, but the *yin* of the Kidneys as both have the same source, an example of the son, the Liver, stealing from the mother, the Kidneys. He had also experienced fear leading to 'unrestrained collapse' (Larre & Rochat de la Vallée 1992), and jumpiness, indicating a separation of *yin* and *yang* and a breakdown of communication between the Heart and Kidneys.

These problems were of such long standing, that to differentiate between root and manifestation was no longer clear. Each phase of the pattern was feeding the next in unrelenting cycles. Kidney *yin* depletion was the key issue in treatment, but whether anger and fear caused the depletion or the depletion caused the anger and fear was no longer an issue. Each mutually drained and fuelled the other (Fig. 2.1).

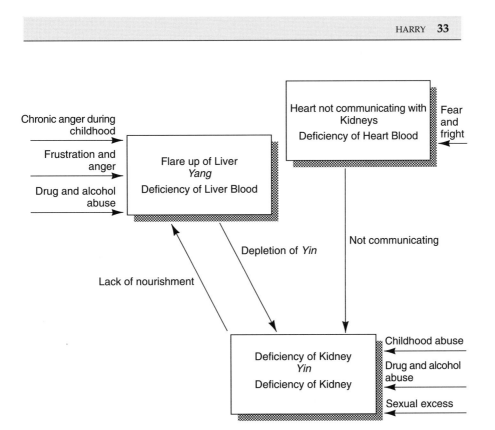

Fig. 2.1 Aetiology and pathology diagram

Breaking the patterns

Although Harry had an array of symptoms they all came back to the same root, the lack of Kidney *yin*. This would form the basis for all treatments whether with acupuncture, herbal remedies, massage or exercise. Secondary acupuncture points would be selected to ease specific symptoms.

We both knew that progress would be slow. There is no quick cure for a lifetime of abuse and *jing* depletion. We needed to gradually bring these energetic outbursts under control, to break the patterns and give him some peace. He needed to feel in control of his own destiny rather than battered around by constantly shifting tides of emotional and physical energy.

One of the difficulties was that he no longer trusted his body. He no longer felt connected with his own inner wisdom, the spiritual aspect of the Kidneys. The 12-step plan had given him strength through belief in an external power, but the very nature of addiction and the nature of its cure is one of self denial: denial which can ultimately fuel an already energetically explosive situation. Repression leads to blockage, which eventually has to find an outlet.

What Harry had to do was to learn to stand back a little and observe. To strengthen his detachment until he was able to observe the patterns without judgement, without becoming emotionally involved. Only in this way would the patterns eventually lose their strength.

Harry had been through enough therapy, groupwork and 12-step programmes to know what he was doing. Intellectually he was completely aware of his situation. He would decide when to come for treatment and, as he learned more of the jargon, would sometimes tell me what needed to be done. I knew that we had to move at his pace or not at all. It was important that he did not become dependent.

A complete ease with needles

During the first treatment it was clear that Harry was one of those rare patients who is completely at ease with needles. He could feel energy move and change and could describe the course of the meridians. He intuitively understood what I was doing and why. He found the framework given to him by a Chinese medical diagnosis very helpful. It gave him a key to make sense of his obscure feelings and sensations, and to verbalise his inner confusion.

In the early days we talked a lot about the Kidneys and the Liver, about fear and anger, about wisdom and human kindness. Though he did not seem to want to talk about his heart. In the same way I did not treat his Heart, knowing that only when the body is at peace can the *shen* return to the Heart. In volatile cases of Liver and Heart fire it is often safer to treat the Kidneys. There are warnings in many classical texts that when nourishing or relaxing the Liver you must take care not to release anger (Larre & Rochat de la Vallée 1994).

While the needles were in place I applied gentle pressure to KID1 *yongquan*, the bubbling spring, to stimulate water and literally to help to keep him on the ground. Then to the head, tracing the *du mai* and Bladder meridians from above the eyes to the top of the head and applying pressure at the base of the skull to release and relax the head. I encouraged him to breathe deeply, to release and relax the diaphragm.

We talked about exercise and Harry mentioned that at times of anger he would often find release in using a punch bag. I showed him simple *qi gong* exercises to balance the Liver and suggested he paid attention to his breathing, trying to make it deeper and more even, imagining a rise and fall of breath between the centre of the chest, the upper sea of *qi*, and the point below the navel, the lower sea of *qi*.

First treatment procedures

POINT PRESCRIPTION

- REN4 *guanyuan,* the gate to the origin, affects the primal source of *ren mai, du mai* and *chong mai*, the origin of being. It is the meeting point of the Liver, Kidney and Spleen meridians with *ren mai*, affecting the genitals and inner thighs. It nourishes Blood and *yin*, regulates *yang*, strengthens the Kidneys, especially in cases of long term or constitutional deficiency. Nourishing *yin* and Blood, it also helps to calm the spirit and to house the *hun* and *shen*.
- KID2 *rangu*, blazing valley, or long *yuan,* also means dragon in the abyss. Fire within water, the fire dragon rising up from the depths of the water, balancing fire and water within the Kidneys; clearing heat.
- GB39 *xuanzhong*, suspended bell, clears Gallbladder heat and strengthens Kidney essence. The Gallbladder, as an extraordinary *fu*, stores clear essence. It is the *fu* of central essences. If the essence stored in the Gallbladder is empty, the Gallbladder lacks the ability to move forward, to make progress, to break out of repetitive cycles.
- KID16 *huangshu*, treatment point for the *huang*, the vital space between the diaphragm and the Heart where vital essence is stored. Harmonises the Heart and the Kidneys when Kidney *yin* is deficient and fails to nourish the Heart. Being located at the centre of the body between REN8 *shenque*, spirit watch tower, and

ST25 *tianshu*, heavenly pillar, it regulates the upper and lower, the link between the spirit and the essence.

These points were chosen for the first treatment as they are all nourishing, cooling and calming. I chose not to treat the Liver or Heart directly, though I did so in later treatments. I used gentle massage on the dispersing points.

Needles: I used 25 mm Japanese needles, size 0, inserted with a guide tube. I used even method in needling to a depth of 3 mm. Needles were retained for 30 minutes.

MASSAGE

1 KID1 *yongquan* to clear Kidney heat, bring down Kidney fire, stabilise the spirit and aid grounding.
2 Massage to Bladder, *du mai* and Gallbladder meridians on the head to help clear heat and excess.
3 Shoulder and neck massage.

HERBS

1 Six Flavour Tea *liu wei di huang wan,* was prescribed to nourish Kidney *yin* and Liver *yin* initially in tablet form. Later it was prescribed as the K'an herbal tincture 'Quiet Contemplative', an adaptation of *liu wei di huang wan*.
2 Another K'an herbal, 'Temper Fire' *zhi bai di huang wan*, was also prescribed for acute episodes.

Of love and wisdom

I have seen Harry now for about 3 years though his visits become less frequent. He is still alive. He is still fighting with the council to be re-housed, still working with his old ladies. Still in pain. At times of optimism, I believe that he has come through and that the odd moments of relapse are mere shadows of his former addictions, working their way out.

He is certainly more stable. Less a victim, more detached. His detachment has allowed him insight and he has experienced happiness in a relationship for the first time in years. He is able to talk about his heart; able to understand the energetics of Heart and Kidney, of *jing* and *shen*, of love and discriminating wisdom. He has learnt that 'reflective thought prevails over fear' (Larre & Rochat de la Vallée 1990) and that by strengthening the action of this emotion on the centre he can help to link the Kidneys and the Heart.

As with so many victims of child abuse, the feelings of guilt and shame are the hardest to remove. To abuse others, or to allow yourself to be sexually abused, and continue the old pattern are often the easiest routes. Harry is aware that his most important task is to change the pattern, to make sure that the family *karma* goes no further, but stops with him.

At times when Harry was particularly low we would talk about the possibility that he had chosen this body and these parents to put an end to this perpetual round of abuse and suffering; and that if he had made this choice he must somewhere have the strength to see it through. I don't doubt that he has. Maybe, through his increasing awareness and detachment he has already done it.

A power to create change

Over the years I have developed immense respect for Harry. As a practitioner he has helped me to redefine my ideas of treatment and cure, success and failure; to understand that we sometimes need to stand back and look at the larger context. He has strengthened my appreciation of the philosophy underlying the medicine that we practise and its power to create change.

We live in a time and a society in which many people are looking for more than an alleviation of symptoms. They need to have some understanding of how and why, and be empowered to help themselves. Chinese medicine can provide much wisdom and guidance.

With its roots in a time when the earth was revered, when the rhythm of the seasons was seen to be reflected in the rhythms of the body, and the balance between heaven and earth to mirror that of body and mind, the teachings of Chinese medicine may prove to be particularly valuable. Especially at this time in our history, when unless we regain some of our ancient earth wisdom, we may not have a future.

REFERENCES

Larre C, Rochat de la Vallée E 1990 The Spleen and Stomach. Monkey Press, Cambridge (Extract from Su Wen Chapter 5)

Larre C, Rochat de la Vallée E 1992 The Kidneys. Monkey Press, Cambridge (From Ling Shu Chapter 8)

Larre C, Rochat de la Vallée E 1994 The Liver. Monkey Press, Cambridge

■ Sandra Hill

After obtaining an MA in Fine Art, Sandra travelled extensively in Asia. She settled in Japan and spent 4 years studying martial arts, meditation and shiatsu. For the final 2 years she studied with Dr Hiroshi Motoyama and worked in the international department of his Institute of Human Science, assisting with the publication of the English language newsletters and journals. On her return to England she attended the International College of Oriental Medicine, graduating as an acupuncturist in 1983. For the past 12 years she has run an acupuncture practice in London.

Sandra Hill was the founding editor of the International Register of Oriental Medicine Review, and is currently on the editorial board of the European Journal of Oriental Medicine. She is a partner in Monkey Press and coauthor with Peter Firebrace of 'A Guide to Acupuncture'.

Diabetic neuropathy in the lower extremities

3

Kiiko Matsumoto and David Euler NATICK,
MA, USA

A diabetic since childhood

Cynthia is a good-spirited, 65-year-old Caucasian woman. She is a relatively round and fair person, about 1.6 m tall, and looks about 10 years younger than her real age. As a diabetic since childhood, she has injected insulin regularly.

Cynthia came to our office complaining of pain, numbness and lack of feeling in her lower limbs which had been diagnosed as diabetic neuropathy in the lower extremities. The numbness in her legs and feet had started about 1 year before she came to see us. The reason she was troubled and seeking help was that the numbness seemed to have progressed from the foot to the ankles and, just recently, she had felt the numbness climbing to her calf.

The neuropathy in the lower extremities was constant and did not seem to react to massage, heat or cold therapy. Cynthia was relatively calm when she told us about its progression and showed no sign of fear or anxiety, even though diabetic neuropathy can result in the loss of feet or legs. She did not seem stressed.

Cynthia also had suffered from mid-back spasms and calf cramps for many years. The mid-back spasms were worse after eating sweets and fruits. Her calves cramped, usually in the morning, with occasional episodes in the evening; during the rest of the day she did not seem to suffer from cramps.

Physical examination

The physical examination included palpation of the abdomen, back and legs. In the abdomen we found what we call a 'sugar lump' or 'sugar caterpillar'[1]. This is a soft, oval-shaped lump at the left side of the abdomen between KID16 *huangshu* and the area around ST25 *tianshu* and ST26 *wailing*. On her back we found hyper-sensitivity in the area around BL20 *pishu* and BL21 *weishu* on the left, and pressure pain between the thoracic vertebrae of T11 to T12. Also, the intravertebral space between the thoracic vertebrae T11 and T12 seemed to be less than that between other thoracic intravertebral spaces. Our patient experienced cramping in the gastrocnemius muscles when these were grabbed.

All these palpatory findings corresponded with a condition that we call a 'sugar imbalance' (Nagano 1986, Kawai 1986). The palpatory process to detect this condition is not very pleasant for the patient but we keep it brief and explain to the patient our findings and their meaning.

Dietary issues

Cynthia liked to eat and told us that she especially loved all kind of sweets. She did not smoke and only drank alcoholic beverages (sweet cocktails) on social occasions. Cynthia found it relatively easy to gain weight and had tried many times in the past to lose it. However, this was especially hard for her since she found it difficult to resist rich meals and sweets. Nevertheless, given her condition, she was willing to reduce her sugar consumption, stop all alcoholic beverages, and work on changing her diet with the help of a nutritionist. We mentioned the importance of a correct diet and the role that blood sugar played in her condition. She was well aware of these facts and was very willing to cooperate, although she suspected that it might be difficult for her to do so. Cynthia's positive attitude and willingness to discuss her difficulties in resisting sweet foods, made us confident that, in time, and with acupuncture treatment, Cynthia would maintain a healthy diet designed for her needs.

Summary of clinical manifestations

- Numbness and pains from the bottom of both feet to the inferior portion of the gastrocnemius muscle; no reaction to massage, heat or cold.
- Mid-back spasms.
- Cramping of the calves.
- Craving of sweets.
- Fatigue, especially after meals.
- No sign of stress or emotional reactions.

Palpatory examination

- A soft, oval-shaped lump at the left side between KID16 *huangshu* and the area around ST25 *tianshu* and ST26 *wailing*.
- Hypersensitivity on the left, in the area around BL20 *pishu* and BL21 *weishu*.
- Pressure pain between the thoracic vertebrae T11 to T12.
- Reduced intravertebral space between the thoracic vertebrae T11 and T12.
- Cramping in the gastrocnemius muscles when they were grabbed.

Diagnostic procedure

Our diagnostic procedure is mainly based upon the palpatory findings and the patient's dietary intake. The differential diagnosis of a condition is made by a cross-examination procedure where different possible acupuncture points are palpated and the reflex areas are checked. If a point releases a particular reflex area, we know the possible path or cause of pathology. In this case, for example, the cramps in the calf disappeared when points at the lumbar eye were palpated. The lumbar eye is just above the sacroiliac joint and sometimes looks like two dimples on either side of the lower back where the sacrum and the ileum join. This corresponds to a condition we call 'sugar imbalance' and the treatment for this condition is then chosen.

We use Western terms to name most of our pathological conditions (e.g. 'sugar imbalance'). However, our diagnostic procedures, whilst including orthodox medical examination results, rely heavily upon palpation of the body at key reflex areas and the acupuncture points that relieve the pressure pain on these reflex areas[2]. Mostly Japanese, this style of diagnosis and treatment yields very quick responses and results.

Aetiology and pathology

A diabetic patient since childhood, Cynthia has been injecting insulin regularly according to her physicians' instructions and the blood sugar levels that she measures. Unfortunately, her eating habits are not regular and there are many episodes of in-between snacks and sweets. These raise her blood sugar to a level that is higher than normal, until the next scheduled meal, after which she again measures her blood sugar levels. These prolonged episodes of elevated blood sugar are contributing to the pathological pattern we call 'sugar imbalance'. The hereditary aspect of the diabetes explains her constitutional sugar imbalance whilst her lifestyle might explain the occurrence of her symptoms and signs. Cynthia's irregular diet and regular consumption of sweets and alcoholic beverages, together with her lack of physical exercise, are very important issues to deal with and will determine the overall outcome of the treatment.

Approach to treatment

We usually address the constitutional problem of the patient first, and then treat the signs and symptoms. Since Cynthia is a diabetic patient and the palpatory findings clearly show a 'sugar imbalance', we administer the needles to treat this condition first. The 'sugar imbalance' treatment is not going to cure the insulin-dependent diabetes mellitus, but we expect the blood sugar levels to decrease and to remain lower and more stable than before. This will prevent deterioration of the neuropathy, stabilise the symptoms and reduce the dosage of insulin required during the day.

We explain to Cynthia what we are about to do and, in simple terms, why. She is excited about the idea of receiving a very different kind of acupuncture procedure. The treatment procedures for the first treatment are exactly as described below.

First treatment procedures

POINTS PRESCRIPTION: SUGAR IMBALANCE

First of all, needles are inserted in the front of the body with the patient in the supine position.

- 'Sugar lump': palpate the region between KID16 *huangshu* (left) and the ST25 *tianshu* (left) and ST26 *wailing* (left) area to find the soft lump which we call 'sugar lump' or 'sugar caterpillar'. We insert a Japanese #2 needle into the lump vertically.
- Above SP10 *xuehai*: on the left side only, insert the needle vertically into the most sensitive point, three fingers above the SP10 *xuehai* area[3].
- *Huatuo jiaji*: at the thoracic vertebrae T11 to T12, needle into the most 'gummy' point at a 45° angle toward the *du* channel line (see Fig. 3.1A). Gummy means that your fingers feel some extra soft tissue at a location which is expected to be bony. Alternatively, it might be where there is an accumulation of soft tissue which feels like chewing gum under the skin.
- *DU6 jizhong*: we call this point the sugar imbalance point of the spine. It is relevant because it has proven helpful in regulating sugar metabolism in patients diagnosed with sugar imbalance. We burned thread-sized direct moxa on this point so that the patient felt the heat stimulation at least eight times.

Needling technique: It is not required to reach *de qi*. It is more important to insert the needle into the 'gummyness' or tightness at a point. The objective regarding the 'sugar lump' is to reduce its size and, regarding the *huatuo jiaji* points of the thoracic vertebrae, to loosen the tightness. The needles are retained for 20 minutes.

POINTS PRESCRIPTION: NEUROPATHY AND MUSCULAR SPASMS

This is done next while the patient is lying on her abdomen. For convenience we have divided the treatment into three steps.

Step 1: Treatment points for the main neuropathy

- 'Lumbar eyes':[4] needled bilaterally (see Fig. 3.1B).
- *Junction points*: on both legs. This is the exact point at the junction between the normal and abnormal feeling of the skin of the lower limb bilaterally (see Fig. 3.1C). It is very common to find an extremely painful or sensitive point at this area. The rationale of using this point is to try to push back the area affected by the neuropathy.

Step 2: Using triple ion-pumping cords and sparking

For the stimulation of these points we used a triple ion-pumping cord and a sparker[5]. We attached the black clips to the needles on the *huatuo jiaji*. Then, on the left, we attached a red clip to the lumbar eye and a green clip on the lower limb; on the right, we attached a green clip to the lumbar eye and a red clip to the lower limb. We detached the black clip from the needle at the *huatuo jiaji* point on one side and attached it to the metal pin at the back of the sparker. By bringing the sparker close to the needle where the black clip had been, we sparked that needle very briefly. We let the spark connect to the needle so that the patient felt the static electricity for just a second. We then detached the black clip from the sparker and re-attached it to the needle at the *huatuo jiaji*. We repeated this procedure for the black clip on the other *huatuo jiaji*, and then repeated the whole procedure four times at 5-minute intervals. The needles were retained for a total of 20 minutes.

Step 3: Adding supporting points

- *BL42 pohu*: a lumpy feeling at this point indicates a state of lack of oxygen according to the teachings of Master Nagano (1986). It is needled towards the scapula. By breaking the gummyness or nodule attached to the medial border of the scapulae, we achieve a better oxygenation, thereby helping to reduce the neuropathy and improve the metabolism of sugar.

- *Neuropathy points*: by palpating the sole of the foot around the heads of the metatarsal bones and around a half *cun* below the web line of the toes, these points are located at spots which stay white and do not return to their normal red colour after pressure has been applied to them (see Fig. 3.1D). These neuropathy points stimulate the circulation, the paucity of which is indicated by the red colour not returning (Nagano 1986).

- *LU4 xiabai*: this is an 'oxygen point' which is found while the patient lies on her back and brings her arm towards her nose, her head remaining straight. The point is where the Lung meridian and the nose meet. Direct moxa on this point helps to increase the patient's oxygen[6] and is very useful for the treatment of fatigue resulting from sugar imbalance.

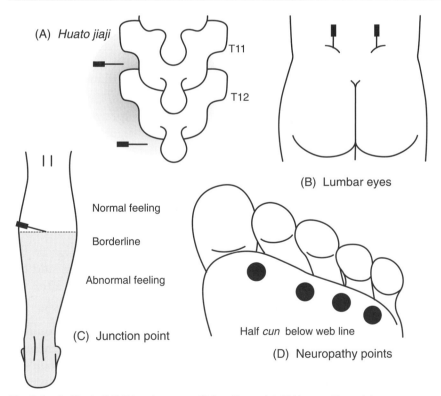

(A) *Huato jiaji*

T11

T12

(B) Lumbar eyes

Normal feeling

Borderline

Abnormal feeling

(C) Junction point

Half *cun* below web line

(D) Neuropathy points

Fig. 3.1 A *Huato jiaji*. B Lumbar eyes. C Junction point. D Neuropathy points.

Immediate changes

At the end of the first treatment, Cynthia did not suffer from any discomfort when we again grabbed her calf muscles, and there were no mid-back spasms, no lower limb neuropathy pains, and the border between the normal-feeling skin and the numbness was lowered by at least 25 mm on both legs.

Since Cynthia was responding to the treatment we explained to her that the prognosis was good and that we would try to reduce the area of neuropathy in her legs to the very minimum, if not make it disappear completely.

The importance of point location and needle angle

Cynthia came for acupuncture treatments once weekly. The treatment protocol was the same every time although, on each occasion, the correct location and angle of needle insertion was chosen. Finding the exact location of a treatment point and insertion angle to release the reflex areas is the most important aspect of this approach.

Each time Cynthia came to our office the following areas were examined:

1 The 'sugar lump' was palpated for size and shape.
2 The gastrocnemius muscles were grabbed to see how much pain remained.
3 The mid-back erectus spinalis muscle group was palpated to see how reactive it was (the left side especially indicates a 'sugar imbalance').
4 The *huatuo jiaji* points at T11 to T12 were palpated for 'gummyness'.
5 The location of the numbness in the lower extremity was checked and the location between the normal and abnormal feeling was marked.

Cynthia responded very well to the acupuncture treatment. This was expecially clear after two treatments, when the calf muscle spasms completely disappeared. After three treatments, the neuropathy pain in the legs also disappeared. The area between the 'normal skin feeling' and the numb area moved more inferiorly after each treatment until, after ten sessions, only the area around KID1 *yongquan* remained a little numb.

Cynthia also saw a holistic nutritionist and tried as much as she could to stay away from sweets. This contributed to the dramatic improvement of her condition. She also reported that she needed much less insulin than she used to need, something she attributed to the 'sugar treatment', especially the regular needling into the 'sugar lump'.

Support and maintenance

After 10 weekly treatments Cynthia came once monthly for supportive treatments and evaluation. Today, 1 year later, she attends once every 2 months for maintenance and, occasionally, when she has a spell of the 'sweet tooth' (as she puts it), 3 or 4-weekly treatments are performed.

This case is one of about 10 lower limb neuropathy cases that we encounter on a yearly basis. With no effective conventional treatment, it is always fascinating to see how the areas affected by the neuropathy slowly and steadily reduce with acupuncture treatment to a small dot around the KID1 *yongquan* area or else completely disappear.

NOTES

1. The palpatory diagnosis is a tool for determining the reflex areas that are active beyond Western findings such as radiographs, blood analyses, etc. The 'sugar lump' is a nickname that Master Nagano (personal communication, 1986) gave to this type of lump, at the left side of the umbilicus, which is related to sugar imbalances in the body. Kiiko Matsumoto added the nickname 'sugar caterpillar' because it feels as if there is a caterpillar under the skin. Much of the diagnostic procedure is in the palpation of the body, mainly developed by blind Japanese acupuncturists who still make up around half of the acupuncturists practising in Japan (Kawai 1986). For this reason, names were needed to describe palpatory findings.

2. Most of our diagnostic and treatment techniques are a combination of the teachings of various prominent Japanese masters of acupuncture and moxibustion. In this particular case, the most relevant masters from which we learn are Master Nagano, Master Hukaya, and Master Kawai. Like most of the information provided in this case, there are no written sources in English, with the exception of Kawai (1986).

3. The point SP10 *xuehai* is an important point for the treatment of 'sugar imbalance' according to the clinical experience of Master Nagano (personal communication, 1986). It is also considered by him to be a Kidney-supporting point.

4. It is essential to find the correct angle and location at the 'lumbar eye' which reduces the pressure pain at the gastrocnemius muscles. In order to do so you must first, gently, grab the calf with one hand and search for the location that hurts the most. Mark this location and release your grab. Then, with the other hand, press into the lumbar eye downwards in the direction of the painful gastrocnemius. While you are pressing into the lumbar eye, grab the calf muscle again at the same, most painful location and evaluate whether this reduces the pains in the calf muscle. If it does, insert a needle in the exact location and angle that you have palpated. If you find no change in the sensitivity of the gastrocnemius muscle, find a different angle until you do produce a change.

5. The triple cord is an ion-pumping cord, like the ones used in Dr Manaka's ion-pumping cord treatments (Manaka Yoshio, personal communication, 1985), with three alligator clips and two diodes that allow circulation of the ions in one direction. If you hook up the three clips (red, green and black) to the

needles, you create a flow of ions in the circuit in one direction between the needles. The sparker is a device similar to a hand-held, electronic lighting device used with a gas stove. It sparks static electricity at a rate of about 2 to 3 Hertz.

6   Master Isaburo Hukaya's approach was taught by his assistant Ms Osawa (personal communication, 1978).

REFERENCE

Kawai Yoshihiro1986 My acupuncture treatment: acupuncture topology, 1st edn. Kyoto, Japan

■ Kiiko Matsumoto

Kiiko first trained in nutrition at Tokyo Kasei University and then in acupuncture, moxibustion and massage therapy at the Japan Central Acupuncture and Moxibustion College of Tokyo. She subsequently studied with Dr Yoshio Manaka, Master Kawai, Master Hukaya, Master Nasako and many others, and continues to study with Master Nagano of Oita, Japan.

In 1980 she moved to the United States where she has taught at the New England School of Acupuncture in Boston and the Tri-State Institute of Traditional Chinese Acupuncture in New York. She is well known as the author of a number of texts on acupuncture and she conducts seminars and workshops for acupuncturists, shiatsu practitioners and doctors in North America, Europe, Israel and Australia.

■ David Euler

David studied acupuncture at the Israeli College of Naturopathy in Tel Aviv, and cofounded the Israeli Team of Integrated Medicine, also in Tel Aviv. He practised acupuncture and shiatsu and taught at both the Israeli College of Naturopathy and the Israeli Team of Integrated Medicine.

After marrying Kiiko Matsumoto in 1992 he moved to the United States and, since then, has had a practice with Kiiko in Natick and Newton, Massachusetts. He also teaches at both the New England School of Acupuncture and the Boston Shiatsu School.

Ockham's razor and a case of ankylosing spondylitis

Volker Scheid EASTBOURNE, UK

From antiquity to the present time each generation had its own physicians. Divine sages and enlightened [persons] do not [all] divide and measure [things] in the same way. Yet, [even they] must use compass, square and plumb line to get [their] squares and circles straight. Hence, in order to treat illness, one must first understand it. [Only once] one has understood an illness can one discuss its treatment. [Admittedly,] medicines are that which conquers illness. Understanding an illness, [however,] allows one to select out of the thousand and one treatments [those] one or two which, when used, produce divine [results]. If one does not understand an illness, then the discrepancies [between medicines and illness] are many and treatment is confused. (Yu Chang 1643)

The above are the opening sentences of Yu Chang's 'Reflections on medicines' (1643), a collection of case histories published in the Qing Dynasty. Case histories occupy a place of special importance in Chinese medical history. Yu Chang's remarks, whose multiple layers of meaning unfortunately diminish in the process of translation, afford valuable insights into why that should be so. In Chinese the term *yi* refers to both 'medicine' as a practice and 'physicians' as those who practise it. The term *guilü* signifies 'compass and square', from whence comes its extended meaning of 'rules' and 'tradition'.

If I interpret Yu Chang correctly, then he establishes here a dynamic view of medical practice that differs substantially from the description of medical systems so prevalent in the West. Medicine is not merely a set of theories about health and disease, but something that is embodied in what physicians do. Hence medical practice changes. Not all practices are equal, however. Yu Chang's reference to sages and enlightened beings brings into play the distinction between various levels of medical practice that already existed within the oldest texts of the medical canon. The best physicians are those who understand correctly the ever changing manifestations of illness and respond to it in an appropriate, that is, timely manner. Such virtuosity is not the product of a romantically perceived artistry based on intuition, but consists of the skilful use of tools that are, as Heidegger would say, already 'at hand'. These tools *are* the medical tradition. It is through the sharing of these tools, the adaptations they demand and the freedoms they bestow, and not through the possession of some timeless theory, that Chinese medicine reproduces itself.

It is in understanding illness and selecting treatments that a physician's skill manifests itself. Yu Chang's description of these stages of the therapeutic process links efficacy with a specific aesthetics in the carrying out of one's craft. Like Cook Ting in the famous story by Zhuang Zi (Graham 1986), the sagely physician cuts illness to the bone in a few fell swoops that are simple because they are clear and efficacious. As one of my modern teachers emphasised, a good physician should be able to move a mountain with a feather.

The following case history reflects my personal attempt to move towards that practice of Chinese medicine of which Yu Chang and many other teachers, past and present, seem to be speaking.

Paul's ankylosing spondylitis

Paul is a 26-year-old bricklayer. He is slim and muscular, but moves slightly less easily then one would expect. He seems relaxed, though not quite at ease, and his voice is not as firm as his body suggests. His cheeks are slightly flushed and his eyes a little sunken and dull.

Paul was diagnosed about 12 months ago as suffering from ankylosing spondylitis which is a chronic inflammatory arthritis affecting predominantly the sacroiliac joints and spine. It results in progressive stiffening and fusion of the axial skeleton. Current biomedical concepts about the aetiology of the disorder assume an abnormal response to infection in genetically predisposed persons carrying the HLA-B27 antigen. The disease usually starts in the second or third decade of life and has a male to female ratio of 4 : 1. At present biomedicine can not offer curative treatment and is therefore limited to palliative response. This attempts to maintain maximal skeletal motility and to relieve pain and stiffness with the help of physiotherapy, nonsteroidal anti-inflammatory drugs (NSAIDs) and, occasionally, steroid injections and radiotherapy. In a small but significant number of sufferers, chronic inflammatory changes result in incapacitating fusion, rigidity and kyphosis of the dorsal and cervical spine as well as hip disease (Edwards & Bouchier 1991).

Paul is well aware of these facts. During our first meeting I gained the impression that he considered himself the unfortunate victim of a hereditary disease whose possible outcome he grudgingly accepted. He consulted me against all hope, following the suggestion of a friend.

Paul had begun to suffer from backache several years earlier when working on building sites in Germany. In those days he had put in 12–18 hour days, often doing nothing else but work, eat and sleep. Increasingly, the pain and stiffness in his back had started to interfere with his work. He saw his GP, and then an orthopaedic consultant. Finally, Paul was given the diagnosis with which he presented to me now. Drug treatment (NSAIDs) had been unsuccessful in ameliorating Paul's symptoms. Physiotherapy, too, had not provided any significant relief. Paul had therefore been advised to give up work, but otherwise had been left much to his own devices. He had grudgingly accepted this advice and was now living on invalidity benefit. He planned to start training for a new occupation, which would be less physically demanding, in the next few months.

On his first visit to my clinic Paul presented with the following symptoms:

Symptoms

- Pain and stiffness in the lower back.
- Pain and stiffness between the shoulder blades, extending to both shoulders but worse on the right.
- Pain and stiffness of the cervical spine.
- Occipital headaches.
- Severe tiredness and lethargy.
- Insomnia and restlessness.
- Lack of appetite, especially in the mornings.
- An occasional tight feeling in the Stomach, described as 'butterflies'; this sensation originates in the lower abdomen, but gradually moves upwards and is associated with a physical feeling of anxiety, without obvious cause.
- Occasional light-headedness.
- Recent tremor of the right hand which is now assuming worrying proportions; sometimes unable to hold a cup of tea.
- Thirst.
- Occasional night sweats.
- Extremely cold hands and feet, although he had always been a very hot person.

Most symptoms were considerably worse in the mornings. The pain and stiffness were aggravated by cold and alleviated by movement. The joint pain and stiffness had been increasing in severity gradually over the preceding 11 months. Paul now sometimes felt unable to do anything. In the mornings he would take at least 1 hour to loosen up. Sometimes the pain would wake him up during the night. He was feeling increasingly tired and often needed to lie down during the day.

My own examination elicited the following additional signs.

Signs

- A pronounced odour which I would classify as both sweet and putrid.
- A bluish hue beneath his eyes and a greenish hue around his mouth.
- Flushed cheeks.
- A low voice and a distinct lack of aggression, i.e., a mismatch between his considerable

- frustration and the manner of its expression.
- Very cold hands and feet; this frigidity extended to the lower one third of his calves and forearms.
- Tenderness over the entire spine and shoulder area.

- Pulse: wiry (*xian*) and slightly slow (*chi*); weak (*ruo*) in the left *cun* and right *chi* positions; slippery (*hua*) and strong in both *guan* positions.
- Tongue: body red, slightly swollen with a distinct Stomach crack; thick, yellow and dry fur extending over the posterior two thirds of the tongue.

Paul's life history

Paul considered himself to be a very good craftsman and took great pride in what he did. He admitted that he probably had worked too hard and that this, as well as the heavy lifting associated with his work, might have contributed to the onset of his disease. For long periods of time, work had been the only institution that had provided a consistent pattern to Paul's life. He had moved about a lot and there also had been periods of heavy drinking. Only in the last 2 years had his life become more stable when he had moved in with a girlfriend in Germany. He had become engaged, but then the relationship had broken down 1 year ago, once it had become clear that Paul would have to give up work. Unable to support himself, Paul had moved back in with his parents. At the age of 26 he was now back to where he had started 10 years earlier, with nothing much to show for his endeavours.

Paul continuously emphasised the hereditary aspect of his illness. He gave the impression that he had learned to accept this as stoically as he had accepted many other aspects of his illness. He said he sometimes felt angry and bitter, but that there was nothing much he could do. In my opinion, the hereditary aspect of Paul's illness had become an idiom around which he had organised his illness experience. It provided both an explanation and a prescription for how to proceed. Ankylosing spondylitis was an irrevocable happening, but also a challenge and, at times, an excuse.

A differentiation of patterns

When diagnosing any patient my emphasis is on discovering what is happening to the patient's *qi*. I know from experience that by understanding process I invariably will be led to pattern, but not vice versa. In the following discussion I shall follow this rule. The patterns I label are less important than the disharmonies I try to unravel. My first approach to Paul's case was to think of a complex disharmony with two, possibly three, different roots.

Root 1: Kidneys, *Mingmen*–Water

Whatever method of analysis one follows, one will be led eventually to the Lower Burner, the Kidneys and the Gate of Vitality (*mingmen*) as the primary root of Paul's problems. Internal cold, tiredness, a desire to lie down, lack of appetite, pain and stiffness made worse by cold, a low voice and a generally slow pulse which is weak in the right *chi* position, all reflect a failure of the Fire of the Gate of Vitality (*mingmen*) to rise and mobilise *yangqi*. From a *zangfu* perspective this might be identified as Kidney *yang* vacuity.

The weak pulse in the left *cun* position can be read as insufficient Ministerial Fire of the Pericardium or chest centre (*danzhong*). Some Chinese authors correlate the chest centre with the 'upper sea of *qi*' (*shang qihai*) and the function of *zongqi* (gathering or ancestral *qi*). *Zongqi* accumulates from *yuanqi* made available by the right Kidney (Kidney *yang*). The right Kidney is also known as the Gate of Vitality (*mingmen*). This is how the Pericardium relates to the Ministerial Fire (*xiang huo*) of the Gate of Vitality. This Fire is the engine distributing the influences of the Heart associated with Sovereign Fire (*jun huo*) throughout the body (Fisch 1991).

The condition thus understood reflects and exacerbates a general weakness in the distribution of *yangqi*. Although it might be labelled Heart *qi* vacuity, relating it to the function of the Pericardium and its connection to the Gate of Life, (*mingmen*) seems more accurate here. In any case, it results from the primary Kidney problem and helps to explain the failure of constructive (*ying*) *qi*, associated with Blood, the channels and thereby the Heart, to circulate.

The location of the pain in the lower back and along the course of the foot *taiyang* Bladder channel and/or the Governing Vessel (*dumai*) confirms the diagnosis so far. According to 'Difficult Issue 16' of the Nanjing, Kidney disorders are associated with countercurrent (*ni*) *qi*. According to Yu Shu, a commentator of the Nanjing, this corresponds to Running Piglet Disorder (*bentun qi*) (Unschuld 1986). This interpretation explains the rising of *qi* from the abdomen to the chest (the 'butterflies').

Other signs pointing to a lack of *mingmen* Fire are the blue hue below Paul's eyes, the putrid odour and Paul's rather subdued, introverted response to his illness. Due to a lack of *yangqi* (*weiqi*), external Wind, Damp and Cold would have found it easier to penetrate into the channels. Not only, however, is the *weiqi* weak, the circulation of *yingqi* is, as we have seen, also impeded. The channels are therefore relatively empty. This is often referred to as constructive and defensive *qi* not harmonised (*ying wei bu he*). The consequence of these problems is painful obstruction (*bi*), not only in the Kidney, Bladder and governing channels, but also in all other *yang* channels passing through the neck and shoulder and particularly the hand *taiyang* Small Intestine channel. At the same time, any existing invasion will have exacerbated the already sluggish circulation of defensive (*wei*) and constructive (*ying*) *qi*.

Root 2: Stomach–Earth

A second set of symptoms, however, is difficult to explain by the above. These are the restlessness, insomnia, thirst, occasional night sweats, the red, dry and cracked tongue, yellow fur and the red complexion of Paul's cheeks. Paul's drinking and lifestyle must have put enormous strains on his available resources. Heat will have accumulated in the Middle Burner, particularly the Stomach, leading to a gradual depletion of Stomach *yin* and the Stomach's descending function. Stomach disharmonies also often cause insomnia and restlessness (*wei bu he ze wo bu an*). Whether or not this deficiency had by now also affected Kidney *yin* was unclear to me.

Root/Branch 3: Liver–Wood

A third group of symptoms resonate, in terms of the Five Phases, with the Wood phase: tremor, a wiry pulse, lack of aggression, stiffness of the sinews, and a green hue around the mouth. External invasion of Wind into the channels and internally generated Wind can produce similar symptoms. The strong pulse in the *guan* position points to the excessive (*shi*) nature of this condition, while the very recent onset of the tremor would suggest a more internal causation. It could follow from either internal Heat and/or the floating upward of *yangqi* due to weakness of *mingmen* Fire and internal Cold. In Five Phases terms, one could simply think here of a Wood vacuity (*xu*) pattern (i.e. Water affecting Wood). It may also be a pattern in its own right, with external Wind entering the channel and eventually penetrating to the organ level.

One can also interpret many of the Liver/Stomach-associated symptoms mentioned above as originating in countercurrent *qi* rushing upwards along the *chong* and *ren* channels. This latter explanation certainly resonates with the pronounced vacuity of the Lower Burner, and the signs of repletion in the upper body. It is a disease mechanism to which some Chinese physicians pay much attention and which they associate both with the foot *jueyin* Liver and the foot *yangming* Stomach channels (Han Guangzhu 1993, Zhang Xichun 1991).

Aetiological considerations

A number of mixed causes will have contributed to the onset of Paul's illness. Using the above categorisation as a guide we could conceive of an aetiology in the following way, keeping in mind that (in Chinese medicine, at least) the significance of such schemes is predominantly heuristic (concerning explanation) and not representational (concerning truth).

Kidneys–Water

Genetic problems (ankylosing spondylitis is a hereditary disease) are often reflected in Kidney disharmonies, because the Kidneys are the root of our prenatal constitution (*qiantian zhi ben*). Cold and Damp, external pathogens to which Paul will have been exposed at work, are *yin* pathogens and tend to attack the Lower Burner where the Kidneys are located. The Kidneys also are the root of *qi* (*qi zhi ben*). Cold and Damp encumbering the Kidneys will therefore lead to debilitation of Kidney *qi*, particularly Kidney *yang*. According to Five Phases theory, Cold resonates with the Water phase and the Kidneys. Some texts, such as the Nanjing, however, associate Damp with the Kidneys (Unschuld 1986). The back is the dwelling place of the Kidneys (*shen zhi fu*) and heavy lifting associated with Paul's work as a bricklayer, may have weakened his Kidney *qi*.

Stomach–Earth

The Stomach and Spleen are the root of our postnatal constitution (*houtian zhi ben*). Overwork for a long period of time, irregular eating and drinking and a general lack of pattern to Paul's life will have taxed his postnatal constitution and thereby the Stomach and Spleen. Bouts of heavy drinking will have contributed to the retention of Heat (alcohol is hot in nature) in Paul's Middle Burner. As there are very few signs of Spleen disharmony, we must assume that, in Paul's case, the Stomach was more affected by these factors than the Spleen. This may be due to constitutional factors or ramifications of the Kidney disharmony (the Kidneys are the gate of the Stomach, *wei zhi guan*).

Liver–Wood

Wind is the pathogen relating to Liver and Wood. There is the possibility, here, of external invasion of Wind, first into the channels and, then, deeper into the Liver. Heat, the causes of which were outlined above, facilitates the stirring of Liver Wind.

In reality, the various aetiological factors are less neatly separated from each other as may appear from my scheme. Overwork and fatigue not only tax the postnatal constitution, but also prenatal *yuanqi*. Heat can damage the Stomach and the Liver, but also the Kidneys. The Kidneys are averse to dryness (*wu zao*), which must invariably result from the consummation of Water by Heat. Painful obstruction (*bizheng*) results from the intermingling of Wind, Damp and Cold.

Questions therefore remain

Outlining the aetiology and pathology of Paul's illness in this way explains, in a reasonably satisfactory manner, possible disease mechanisms. However, it still contains a number of ambiguous statements. I have outlined two, possibly three, roots, each producing several branches. I also have expressed uncertainty concerning the exact relationship between a number of variables: Where exactly did the Wind come from? And what produced the Heat above? Furthermore, some statements are nothing more than plausible conjectures. According to the famous Qing physician Ye Tianshi, for instance, the Neijing definition of painful obstruction being caused by external invasion of Wind, Damp, Cold or Heat into the channels, is too limited. He lists 13 additional disease mechanisms of which at least three provide possible alternative explanations for the present case:

1 Liver and Stomach vacuity and stagnation.
2 Invasion of Wind, Damp and Cold directly into the Lower Burner.
3 Liver Wind. (Ye Tianshi 1959).

These ambiguities become most obvious (and annoying) once one begins to translate the above diagnosis into treatment. Which root should one treat first? Should one treat the branches as well? If so, which ones? And how does one decide exactly between possible alternative explanations and, by implication, treatment strategies?

All this leaves me feeling slightly uneasy. Whatever treatment I choose, some loose ends remain. I might take refuge in 'experience' to decide between alternative explanations, but who am I fooling? I might even get results, but would I really know why? Clearly, I have not yet understood Paul's illness. Yu Chang, whom I quoted in the introduction, demands more: to understand any disorder so well that its treatment becomes not a choice between possible alternatives, but the sure selection of one or two options out of a thousand. Let me quote Yu Chang (1658) once more, this time from his famous 'Precepts for physicians':

> [T]he [foundation] for all treatment of illness is that one must seek out its root . . . If one does not know how to seek out the root, then one's [treatments are as] vague as if one was gazing at the wide sea and would not know how to ask for water. Alas, [the physicians] in today's world . . . all rush to agree that in acute [conditions] one should treat manifestations [and only] in chronic conditions the root. Such understanding of acute and chronic is all upside down. [It commits the same] error as if one was failing to correctly recognise people because one has raised one's hands [in front of one's eyes]. These mistakes are all caused by not learning from and researching into [the work] of enlightened teachers (Yu Chang 1658).

Finally, some clarity

Yu Chang here speaks of one root, not two or three. Some more research thus seemed necessary. At the time of Paul's first visit I had been investigating for some time the use of the Eight Extraordinary Channels in herbal medicine. This research helped me now to understand Paul's problem unambiguously as one problem, a *dumai* disharmony.

The *dumai* is the 'sea of all *yang* channels'[1]. It connects the lower back with the head, neck and brain and also penetrates to the Kidneys. It distributes *yuanqi* from the Kidneys and the lower 'sea of *qi*' (*qihai*) outwards and into the periphery. Having been dispersed to the extreme periphery through the foot *taiyang* Bladder channel, *yuanqi* returns to the interior by way of the hand *taiyang* Small Intestine channel (Porkert & Hempen 1986). The *dumai* furthermore connects with both the *ren* and *chongmai*. Indeed, influential commentators such as Zhang Jiebin state that these three channels should not be conceived of as separate entities: '[T]he *du*, *ren* and *chong[mai]* originally have one body. The *du[mai]* is the source of the *ren* and *chong[mai]*. The *ren* and *chong[mai]* are other names of the *dumai*' (Zhang Jiebin 1624).

From these physiological functions the pathology of the *dumai* can be deduced. If the *yuanqi* in the *dumai* does not spread, it causes stiffness of the back and frigidity of the limbs.[2] Zhang Jiebin explains: 'The *dumai* penetrates along the middle of the spine. Therefore, [its disharmony] causes back rigidity, opisthotonos and difficulty in flexing and stretching [the spine]' (Zhang Jiebin 1624). If the *yangqi* does not return from the periphery, this will lead to fullness and congestion of the *yang* channels in the head and neck area causing symptoms we would classify as Wind: tremors, convulsions, 'child fright wind', neck rigidity, etc. These symptoms can resemble those of external Wind in the foot *taiyang* channel and, through the hand *taiyang* channel, can penetrate into the chest, where they cause agitation and restlessness.[3]

As stated above, *dumai* disharmonies can also manifest in the *chong* and *renmai* where they will cause inverse ascending of *qi*. This is clearly described in the Suwen:

> *Thus generated illness [is characterised by qi] rushing from the lower abdomen [to the] Heart and [by] pain. This is neither [specifically] at the front or the back and is called 'surging shan' (chong shan). [Other symptoms are] female infertility, urinary retention, piles, enuresis and dry throat. [All these are] medical disorders generated in the dumai. Therefore treat the dumai (Huangdi Neijing: Suwen 60 1992).*

The disorder described here, more commonly known as 'running piglet *qi*' (*bentun qi*), is one where the *qi* in the Lower Burner becomes unstable

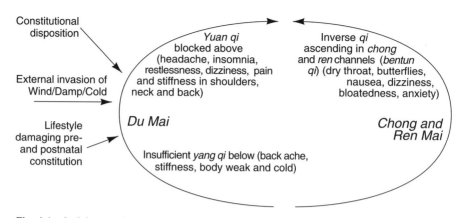

Fig. 4.1 Aetiology and pathology diagram.

because of fright, constraint or vacuity and then rushes upwards causing a sensation of something moving upwards from the lower abdomen.

Almost all of Paul's symptoms can thus be explained by one disharmony, disordered *qi* distribution in the *dumai*, which is accounted for by the aetiological factors previously outlined (see Fig. 4.1). This interpretation can also assimilate the biomedical understanding of ankylosing spondylitis. All extraordinary channels, but particularly the *du*, *ren* and *chongmai*, circulate prenatal *yuanqi*. The quality of this function is directly dependent upon our constitution, that is, our genetic inheritance. Paul's ankylosing spondylitis might then be hypothetically interpreted as a constitutional (or genetic) predisposition towards blocked and/or insufficient circulation of *yuanqi* in the *dumai* triggered by an appropriate insult (in biomedical terms: a bacterial infection; in Chinese medical terms: an invasion of Wind-Damp-Cold).

First treatment procedures

The first two points:

- *SI3 houxi*. This is the opening point of the *dumai*. As such it frees (*tong*) the flow of *qi* in the entire vessel, particularly leading the stagnant *qi* in the upper part of the body downwards and inwards. Some of its traditional indications which are explained by this action are headache, stiff neck, heat diseases, night sweats, tension and pain in the chest, gastric reflux and nausea (Porkert & Hempen 1985, Ellis et al 1988).

- *BL62 shenmai*. This is the point of origin of the *yang qiaomai* (yang motility vessel) which is often used as the associated point, in conjunction with SI3 *houxi*, to free the *dumai*. The *yang qiaomai* is responsible for distributing and coordinating the distribution of those aspects of *yuanqi* available for immediate use (Porkert & Hempen 1985). As such it complements the function of SI3 *houxi* by guiding *yuanqi* upwards and outwards from its root in the Lower Burner. It treats Wind and strengthens the *yangqi* of both Liver and Kidneys. Hence its indications for back pain, headache, dizziness, weak hips and knees, and palpitations, all of which apply to the present case (Porkert & Hempen 1985, Ellis et al 1988).

Needling techniques: Both points were needled with 25 mm stainless steel needles. *Deqi* was obtained and the needles were retained without further manipulation for approximately 2–3 minutes. Once I was sure the pulse had changed in a positive manner (it became deep and even on all six positions), both needles were removed. I would have liked to have sent Paul home at this point, but felt that he expected more, particularly some treatment of his back.

Treatment of the back

- *Three ah shi points* on the back and right shoulder. These points were selected mainly for psychological reasons, i.e. to give Paul the feeling that I was doing something *for* his back by choosing points *on* his back.

Needling techniques: 25 mm stainless steel needles were used and the needles retained without manipulation for 20 minutes. This also increased the duration of the treatment which I often feel is necessary to give patients the feeling (especially on their first visit) that they are getting their money's worth.

Results and further treatments

Paul's second appointment was scheduled 1 week later. By that time, all symptoms had considerably eased: the tremor had disappeared; the stiffness and pain of the back and neck had reduced by about 50%; the feeling of coldness had subsided; the 'butterflies' had vanished but the stomach still felt a little tight; the thirst had almost gone; sleep was more or less back to normal; Paul's energy was returning. He had been getting up most mornings without too much difficulty and did not have to sleep during the day. The pulse was stronger in the right *chi* and left *cun* positions, the tongue was slightly more moist.

Paul had two more treatments at weekly intervals. These were aimed at consolidating the effects of the first treatment by strengthening the Kidneys, as root of the prenatal constitution, and the Stomach, as root of the postnatal constitution. During each treatment I also needled various points on the right side of the back. Manipulation was as above, i.e. minimal retention of the needles used to treat the root and retention, with even technique on the needles on local points on the back.

The exact points for the second treatment were as follows:

- KID3 *taixi*, the source *yuan* point of the Kidneys, was chosen to support the prenatal constitution.
- BL23 *shenshu*, the back *shu* point of the Kidneys, was chosen to augment the effect of KID3 *taixi*.
- SI11 *tianzong* and SI12 *bingfeng* were chosen as local points to disperse

stagnation of pathogens in the hand *taiyang* Small Intestine channel on the back, where pain and stiffness seemed most acute.

- DU10 *lingtai* systemically supports the *qi* of the Middle Burner, thus the postnatal constitution, and locally treats pain and stiffness of the neck and back through activating the *qi* of the *dumai*.

For the third treatment, the points used were:

- ST36 *zusanli*, the Earth point of the Stomach vessel, which was chosen to strengthen *qi*, particularly the postnatal constitution.
- KID4 *dazhong*, the *luo* connecting point of the Kidney vessel, which was chosen to support the prenatal constitution and to free the *qi* in the foot *taiyang* Bladder vessel.
- SI12 *bingfeng*, SI13 *quyuan* and SJ15 *tianliao* were chosen as local points to disperse stagnation of pathogens in the hand *taiyang* Small Intestine and the hand *xiaoyang* Triple Burner channels on the back, where pain and stiffness seemed most acute.

In both treatments, the points chosen mainly for their systemic action (KID3 *taixi*, KID4 *dazhong*, ST36 *zusanli*, and BL23 *shenshu*) were needled sequentially in the order outlined above. After *deqi* had been obtained, the needles were withdrawn. In my experience, selecting the correct point is more important than manipulating the needle. I am aware, however, that this reflects my lack of skill in needle manipulation. The needles in local points were retained for 20 minutes without manipulation.

By the fourth visit Paul was virtually symptom-free. He then maintained this state for a period of 4 weeks, without treatment. He is currently seeing me at monthly intervals and it will be interesting to see whether his improvement can be maintained in the long term. Nine months after his first visit he has, so far, not had any relapse. Paul has decided to train as a welder and will commence a course in the next few months. He is learning German at night school and is on the way to building a new life. He still is rather shy, but that is his nature. I hope that he will realise, through the effects of this treatment, that fate is not hereditary, even though that which we inherit constrains us.

So what about Ockham's razor?

The reason I chose this particular case when asked to contribute to this book was not to flaunt my diagnostic skills. Most of the time I practise like the physicians Yu Chang describes — with hands clasped firmly in front of my eyes. However, I have observed similar effects with sufficient frequency in my own clinic [but more often in the work of living masters, with whom I have had the honour to study, and also in the classical literature] to see them as revealing to us something about the essence of Chinese medicine.

In the introduction I wrote about Chinese medicine as a craft. The skilful exercise of that craft, its art if you like, expresses itself in understanding illness in such a manner that there remain no doubts, no unwarranted conjectures, no ifs or maybes, no ad-hoc hypotheses. One of the expressions of such skill seems to be simplicity: the ability to select from a thousand and one herbs or acupuncture points the one or two that are right. Interestingly enough, philosophers, mathematicians, physicists and many others seem to share with Chinese physicians this sense of aesthetic efficacy.

Ockham's razor is a principle of ontological economy introduced to Western philosophy by William von Ockham (1285–1349). It states that ontological entities are not to be multiplied beyond necessity. In plain English this means that the best explanations are also the most simple ones. Paul's case makes a good argument for adding Ockham's razor to the toolbox of Chinese medicine. Being able to use it, of course, is another matter.

NOTES

1   For reference, see Maijing: Ping jijing ba mai bing (Chen Yannan 1993) and Huangdi zhenjiu. Jiayijing: Jijing ba mai (1990).

2   For reference, see Huangdi Neijing: Suwen 60, Gu kong lun (1992) or Nanjing 29 (Unschuld 1986).

3   For reference see Yixue gangmu: Zhi ouhan (Deng Liangyue 1993, p 754).

REFERENCES

Edwards C R W, Bouchier I A D (eds) 1991 Davidson's principles and practice of medicine, 16th edn. Churchill Livingstone, Edinburgh

Ellis A, Wiseman N, Boss K 1988 Fundamentals of Chinese acupuncture. Paradigm Publications, Brookline

Fisch G 1991 Der Herzmeistermeridian. Verlag für Traditionelle Orientalische Medizin, Jouxtens

Graham A C 1986 Chuang-tzu: the inner chapters. Unwin, London

Han Guangzhu 1993. Zhongyi neike zhi yan (Chinese internal medicine [based on] therapeutic experience). Guizhou keji chubanshe, Guiyang

Huangdi Neijing: (The inner classic of the yellow Lord simple questions) 1992 Renmin weisheng chubanshe, Beijing

Porkert M, Hempen K.-H 1986 Systematische Akupunktur. Urban & Schwarzenberg, München

Unschuld P U 1986 Nan Ching: The classic of difficult issues. University of California Press, Berkeley

Ye Tianshi (Chu Lingtai, ed.) 1766 (1959). Lin zheng zhinan yi'an (A case history guide to clinical patterns). Shanghai kexue jishu chubanshe, Shanghai

Yixue gangmu (Web of medicine) quoted in Deng Liangyue (ed) Zhongguo

jingluowenzai tongjian (Categorised Collection of Literatures on Chinese
   Meridians and Collaterals) 1993 Qingdao chubanshe, Qingdao
Yu Chang 1643 (1991) Yuyi Cao (Reflections on medicines) Shanghai guji
   chubanshe, Shanghai
Yu Chang 1658 (1991) Yimen falü: (Precepts for physicians) Shanghai guji
   chubanshe, Shanghai
Zhang Jiebin 1624 (1957) Leijing: (Classified classic) Renmin weisheng chubanshe,
   Beijing
Zhang Xichun. 1918–33 (1991) Yixue zhong zhong can xi lu. Hebei kexue jishu
   chubanshi, Shijiazhuang

FURTHER READING

Huangdi neijing lingshu jiaozhu yuyi (The spiritual pivot of the inner cannon of
   the yellow Lord with collated annotations and translations (into modern
   Chinese). 1989 Tianjin kexue jishu chubanshe, Tianjin
Huangdi zhenjiu jiayijing (The yellow Lord's AB classic of acumoxa therapy.) 1990
   Zhongguo yiyao kexue chubanshe, Beijing
Maijing yuyi (Pulse classic with annotations and translation) Chen Yannan (ed)
   1993 Renmin weisheng chubanshe, Beijing

■ Volker Scheid

I began my journey towards medicine by working on a herb farm during
my school holidays, whence comes a particular love of herbs. By a
tortuous path I came to J R Worsley's Leamington College from Germany.
There I learned much about treating patients, but little about Chinese
medicine. I also studied Western and Chinese herbal medicine, but it
was the publication of Unschuld's Nanjing translation in 1986 which
provided the key to more profound encounters. Three trips to China
had to be cancelled at the last minute, and it was not until 1992 that I
managed to travel there for the first time. Meanwhile, I had practised
much, learned Chinese, studied with different teachers and gone back
to university, where I stumbled across medical anthropology and the
sociology of knowledge. I have since tried to combine these varied
interests in the pursuit of a common goal: to understand how one
becomes a good practitioner of Chinese medicine. That quest made me
return to Beijing in 1994 for 1 year to conduct fieldwork for a doctoral
dissertation at the University of Cambridge. There have been many and
varied influences on my clinical work: living physicians who have shared
with me their art, the ever challenging work of past masters and the critical
encouragement of friends and colleagues. I am grateful to all of them.

Africa, malaria and a 'virus'

Friedrich Staebler LONDON, UK

From relative health to utter debility

Anna, a 35-year-old student of furniture design, came to me with a 1 month history of pressure in the eyes, blurred vision and photophobia which was accompanied by headaches and giddiness. The latter two symptoms occurred only at night. She also experienced 'flashing lights when moving or closing the eyes' and reported an occasional 'feeling of blindspots'.

She was very weak and managed to negotiate the short walk from the waiting room up one flight of stairs to my consulting room only with the help of two friends supporting her on either side.

She also reported 'spasms under the feet when walking', aching bones, 'hot pains in the thighs and shins' (front), soreness in the thighs (sides) and a tingling sensation in the hands and feet. She mentioned 'soreness of the underarms' and a 'fluttering in the legs when (they were) not hurting'. Furthermore, Anna reported 'constant sleepiness', anxiety, palpitations, nightmares, 'panic rising through the chest from the stomach', 'increasing incidents of epileptic aura' and a feeling of 'walking outside of the body'. When the symptoms began, she reported her blood pressure was low but now more recently it had turned high. She also mentioned feeling cold, 'hungry or nauseous' with a dry mouth, but was not thirsty. Urine and stools were apparently unaffected.

All symptoms were worse from the slightest exertion. In Anna's words: 'I am unable to watch TV, read or write without feeling ill'. Lying down with the curtains drawn was the only thing that brought some relief. Most of these details are in Anna's own words and were taken, roughly in the above order, from a written report she had prepared prior to her first visit.

Anna had been in Ghana for several months to research African furniture design when she fell ill with the above symptoms. This was significant for a number of reasons. It was her first visit to the continent of her father's ancestors and this meant a lot to her. She had been epileptic from the age of 18 but had come off the anticonvulsant drug Tegretol in her 20's after successful treatment with acupuncture. She had not had any fits since then. Her GP decided to put her on phenytoin, another anticonvulsant drug, prior to departure for Africa because Anna, who is claustrophobic, was terrified of flying and the GP felt that the emotional upheaval could bring back her epilepsy.

Contracting malaria

To make matters worse Anna contracted malaria when she was in Africa and this was treated with Plaquenil (hydroxychloroquine sulphate). She relapsed 3 weeks later and was prescribed chloroquine which, in Anna's words, 'sorted the problem out'. However, she relapsed a second time and was given a 24-hour course of Halfan (halofantrine hydrochloride). Plaquenil and chloroquine are known to impair liver and kidney function and can in some cases cause blurred vision and damage to the cornea and retina. Halfan, which is mainly used for chloroquine and multi-drug resistant malaria strains, is also known to be liver toxic and should be used with great care where there is a history of heart disease.

After 2 months, Halfan finally abolished the symptoms of malaria. However, shortly afterwards the above mentioned condition appeared. One week later Anna returned to London. When she arrived back home the full picture had developed. She was seen at the Hospital for Tropical Diseases, University College Hospital, and it was found that she had no deep tendon reflexes and that both pupils were dilated and reacted slowly to light reflexes. She was diagnosed with Holmes Adie Syndrome[1]. A second diagnosis was given, to use again Anna's words: 'A virus condition, which might last for 5 to 6 months'. As far as I am aware no connection was made with the previous malaria episode and the subsequent anti-malarial drugs. She was given supplements (vitamin B complex, calcium, iron) and was told to rest and wear dark glasses.

Anna's eyes had healthy sparkle

Anna, who was tall and athletically built, appeared tired and weary. The face was dull and pale yet the eyes showed a healthy sparkle. She acted calmly and spoke in a firm voice which was somewhat in contrast to her visibly weakened state. Her pulse was full and driving except for both rear (proximal) positions which were deep, thready and deficient. The tongue was pale and slightly swollen, large yet with few teeth marks, and without a central crack. The tip was red. The tongue coating was slightly thick, sticky and yellowish-white.

Further enquiry revealed that Anna also had a history of painful periods with a mild degree of endometriosis confirmed by laparoscopy. Her menses were more or less regular with considerable premenstrual tension dominated by fluid retention and distended crampy pains which would reach their crescendo on the first day of the flow with subsequent relief as the flow continued. She would lose a considerable amount of dark clotted blood yet feel better when the period was over. Since being in Africa her menses had become lighter and more erratic. There was also a history of atopic asthma and eczema. The latter had been absent for several years. For the asthma she occasionally needed a Ventolin inhaler.

A basic neurological examination showed no obvious abnormalities except the above mentioned deep tendon reflexes, which were completely missing on both legs, and the discussed changes of the pupils and their responses to light reflexes. Her BP was 110/80.

Anna was accustomed to a balanced wholefood diet, didn't smoke and, although she liked the occasional drink of alcohol on social occasions, hadn't touched any since falling ill with malaria. She had tried alcohol on one occasion since, and felt rather ill afterwards.

Summary of clinical manifestations

- Pressure in the eyes.
- Blurred vision, photophobia.
- 'Flashing lights when moving or closing the eyes'.
- 'Feeling of blindspots'.
- Headaches and giddiness only at night.
- All symptoms worse with slightest exertion.
- Very tired, weak and debilitated, better from lying down.
- Constant sleepiness.
- Feeling cold.
- Dry mouth, but not thirsty.
- Very hungry or nauseous.
- Spasms under the feet when walking.
- Fluttering sensations in the legs.
- Aching and hot pains in the thighs and shins (front).
- Soreness in thighs (side) and underarms.
- Tingling in hands and feet.
- Incidents of epileptic aura, nightmares.
- Claustrophobia, terrified of flying.
- Out of body experiences.
- Anxiety, episodes of panic rising through the chest from the stomach.
- Palpitations.
- High and low blood pressure.
- Premenstrual tension, with fluid retention and distended crampy pains.
- History of heavy painful menses (endometriosis) recently becoming lighter and erratic.
- History of epilepsy, atopic asthma and eczema.
- Recent episode of malaria.
- Appeared tired and weary.
- Face dull and pale; eyes showed a healthy sparkle.
- Pulse: full (slippery-wiry) except for deep deficient, rear (proximal) positions.
- Tongue: pale, slightly swollen, large yet few teeth marks, red tip. Tongue coating moderately thick, sticky and yellowish-white.

Physical examination

- Abdominal palpation showed slight tenderness in the hypogastric area: REN3 *zhongji*, REN4 *guanyuan*, ST29 *guilai*.
- The liver and spleen were not significantly enlarged.
- Channel palpation revealed tenderness most noticeably over the following points: SP4 *gongsun*, KI2 *rangu*, KI6 *zhaohai*, SP6 *sanyinjiao*, SP9 *yinlingquan*, GB34 *yanglingquan* and LIV8 *ququan*.
- The back *shu* points were tender for: Blood (BL17 *geshu*), Liver (BL18 *ganshu*), Spleen (BL20 *pishu*) and Kidney (BL23 *shenshu*).

Hospital examination

- Dilated pupils slowly reacting to light.
- Missing deep tendon reflexes in the legs.

Patterns of disharmony

This unusual case presented me with a few problems as to the order of pathology present. Four symptom complexes appeared dominant (in the following order of importance):

1 *Eyes:* (tender, sensitive to light, visual field disturbances, dilated pupils).
2 *Exhaustion:* (debilitated, sleepy, cold, all symptoms worse from the slightest exertion).
3 *Extremities:* (aching bones, 'hot pains', 'fluttering in the legs', 'tingling in the hands and feet', missing deep tendon reflexes, 'spasms under the feet when walking').
4 *Mental-emotional:* (anxiety, nightmares, palpitations, 'panic rising through the chest from the stomach', feeling of epilepsy aura, out of body experiences).

The disharmony pattern likely to account for most of these symptoms was in my mind Liver Blood *xu* with underlying Liver and Kidney *yin xu* and Kidney *yang xu*. Both the eye and extremity symptoms suggested Liver and Kidney *yin xu* leading to Liver Blood *xu*. The exhaustion could have arisen from the same pathology but had an altogether more *qi* and *yang xu* flavour. The mental-emotional symptoms also agreed with a diagnosis of Blood *xu* (Heart and Liver).

The fact that these symptoms were of relatively recent onset and had arisen after an episode of malaria suggested the possibility of a pathogenic factor (Damp-heat or Phlegm-heat) that had not been eliminated completely. Evidence for the latter could be seen from both pulse and tongue (full pulse and sticky yellowish-white tongue coating). This also fitted with my first impression of Anna's overall appearance: utterly debilitated and worse from the slightest exertion, yet there was a strength and togetherness about her which suggested that her *qi* resources had been battered and obstructed but not been chronically consumed. Further evidence for the presence of Phlegm-heat were 'constant hunger or nausea', 'panic rising through the chest from the stomach' and dry mouth with no desire to drink.

I therefore concluded that the major pattern was Liver Blood *xu* with the simultaneous presence of Stomach Phlegm-heat from an earlier invasion of external Damp-heat. The secondary patterns in my estimation were Liver and Kidney *yin xu* and Kidney *yang xu* and Spleen *qi xu* with Heart Blood *xu* (Maciocia 1989, 1994).

Patterns of disharmony

MAJOR PATTERNS

Liver Blood *xu*

- Pressure in the eyes, blurred vision, photophobia.
- Flashing lights, blindspots.
- Dilated pupils (Holmes Adie Syndrome).
- 'Spasms under the feet when walking'.
- 'Fluttering sensations in legs'.
- Tingling in hands and feet.
- Missing deep tendon reflexes (Holmes Adie Syndrome).
- Epilepsy aura.
- Out of body experiences.
- Headaches and giddiness only at night.
- Debility, better from lying down.
- Appeared tired and weary.
- All symptoms worse from exertion.

Stomach Phlegm-heat

- 'Constant hunger or nausea'.
- Dry mouth, but not thirsty.

- Nightmares, anxiety, palpitations.
- Panic (oppression) 'rising through the chest from stomach'.
- Pulse: full (slippery-wiry).
- Tongue: coating sticky yellowish-white.

SECONDARY PATTERNS

Liver and Kidney *yin xu* and Kidney *yang xu*

- Eye symptoms.
- Aching bones and hot pains.
- Soreness in legs and underarms.
- Coldness and heat sensations simultaneously.
- Pulse: deep deficient in both rear (Kidney) positions.
- Tongue: red tip.

Spleen *qi xu* and Heart Blood *xu*

- Face dull and pale.
- Tiredness, sleepiness, anxiety, palpitations.
- Tongue: pale and slightly swollen, large yet few teethmarks.

Aetiology and pathology

Given the history of the onset of symptoms and the events leading up to it, I concluded the following scenario of aetiological factors to be of importance in this case:

Anna suffered from atopic asthma and eczema early in life and was epileptic from the age of 18 which suggests the presence of fetal heat and constitutionally weakened Kidney *qi* (Kidney *yin* and Kidney *yang*). This would have been further weakened by anticonvulsant and more recently antimalarial drugs.

However, the fact that she had overcome epilepsy with acupuncture treatment in the past showed that she had plenty of reserves left and that her constitutional Kidney *qi* was not exhausted. Anna didn't smoke or abuse her body and was accustomed to a balanced diet. It was conceivable that she took her studies quite seriously, and a little too much to heart, which could have weakened her Spleen. The emotional upheaval surrounding her trip to Africa could also have contributed to weakening the Spleen *qi* and Heart Blood.

The pivotal factor, however, clearly seemed to be the episode of malaria, its treatment, relapse and further treatment. The invading pathogenic factors of Wind-cold, Damp, Summer-heat and the pestilential factor, malaria (Chen Xinnong 1987), and their presence in the *shao yang* and other channels and organs, led to a consumption of *qi* and *yin*. This propelled the pre-existing weaknesses (Liver and Kidney *yin xu*, Spleen *qi xu*) to progress acutely into the picture of Liver Blood *xu*, greatly accelerated by the use of antimalarial drugs.

The Damp-heat, as can be the case in serious malaria, was never completely eliminated and was converted into Phlegm-heat. It resided primarily in the Stomach where it caused constant hunger, nausea and dry mouth without desire to drink. It might also have contributed to symptoms such as nightmares, and panic rising through the chest from the stomach.

The diagram shown in Figure 5.1 illustrates how the pre-existing syndromes (Liver and Kidney *yin xu*, Kidney *yang xu*, Spleen *qi xu* and Heart Blood *xu)* became converted into Liver Blood *xu* through the presence of an external pathogenic factor, Damp-heat, which itself converted to Stomach Phlegm-heat.

The treatment plan

As main treatment principles I identified nourishing the Liver Blood and clearing Stomach Phlegm-heat. This I planned to do simultaneously, somewhat contradicting the rule of first clearing the excess and then tonifying the deficiency. My reason for proceeding in this way was the fact that, despite the pulse and tongue readings, the picture was dominated by deficiency symptoms. In order to nourish Liver Blood I also planned to tonify Spleen *qi* and to nourish Kidney *yin*. Warming Kidney *yang* and nourishing Heart Blood I considered to be secondary treatment principles.

I explained to Anna that I believed the malaria, as well as the anticonvulsant and antimalarial drugs, had worn down her health resources

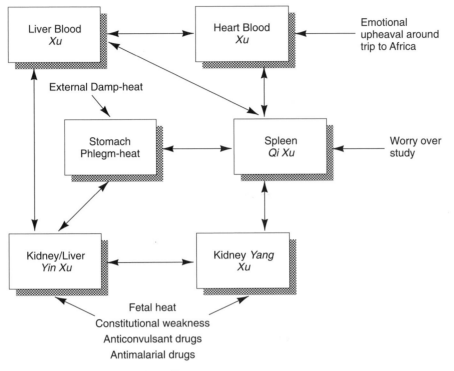

Fig. 5.1 Aetiology and pathology diagram.

and that her main symptoms were due to a deficiency of Liver Blood. I expressed concern about the degree of this Liver Blood deficiency and that I couldn't promise her a quick recovery. What I could offer was to do my best to help restore the damage. Anna, who believed in acupuncture and had come to me on the recommendation of two friends who had been my patients, accepted this explanation and was willing to persevere with treatment despite her restrained financial resources. I offered to reduce the treatment fee which I believe helped to cement a mutual sense of commitment. We arranged treatment 3 times per week for ten sessions after which we would reassess the situation.

Starting treatment

Anna was very calm before and during the first and all other subsequent sessions. She was happy to lie on the treatment bed quietly and with her eyes closed. I proceeded to insert the needles without further talking or explanations. After obtaining the needling sensations, which on most points had to be provoked through gentle lifting and thrusting and scratching of the handle, I left the needles in place for 20 minutes manipulating them with gentle lifting and thrusting, a total of three times. In the meantime I applied *qi gong* healing (Liu Lu Bang 1991) to the soles of her feet (KID1 *yongquan*), the abdomen (REN4 *guanyuan* and REN12 *zhongwan*) and the top of the head (DU20 *baihui*). At the end of the session I asked Anna to turn face down. I applied reducing method (strong rotation) to DU14 *dazhui* for 30 seconds. Anna felt somewhat refreshed after the treatment. I helped her down the stairs and I thought I detected a minimal improvement in her ability to walk.

First treatment procedures

First prescription of points (in order of insertion)

DU20 *baihui* stimulates ascending *yang*, lifts the spirits, tonifies *yang*.

SP6 *sanyinjiao* tonifies Liver Spleen and Kidney, nourishes Blood and y*in* and calms the mind.

LIV8 *ququan* nourishes Liver Blood and benefits the sinews.

GB34 *yanglingquan*, an influential point for the sinews, relaxes the sinews, promotes smooth flow of Liver *qi* and clears Damp-heat.

ST40 *fenglong* resolves Phlegm, clears Heat, opens the chest and clears the mind.

DU14 *dazhui* clears interior Heat.

The first three points of this prescription tonify the Kidney and Spleen *qi* and nourish the Liver Blood. The last three points eliminate Phlegm and Heat. LIV8 *ququan* and GB34 *yanglingquan* specifically act on the sinews. I used no specific points for the eye symptoms.

Needling technique: Insertion with guide tube. All points with reinforcing method except DU14 *dazhui* which was reduced.

Needles: For all points 40 mm needles with medium gauge (0.28 mm) were used. Needles were retained for 20 minutes except DU14 *dazhui* where the needle was withdrawn after 30 seconds.

Response to treatment

Anna's response to the first treatment went far beyond what I had dared to expect. She felt much less cold, more relaxed and more energetic. I began to understand what I had sensed when I first saw her: the strength and spark of life despite the utter debility; the clarity and spirit despite the confusion and despondency. I remembered my first thought when I saw Anna's tongue and took her pulse: 'This woman's fabric of *qi* is still intact'.

I kept to the same principle of treatment with minor changes, introducing points that affected the eyes and the *du* channel, including LI4 *hegu*, LIV3 *taichong*, GB20 *fengchi*, SI3 *houxi*, BL62 *shenmai*. I also added the herbal prescription Eight Treasure Decoction *ba zhen tang*, with Uncaria Rhynchophylla *gou teng* and Lycium Barbarum *gou qi zi*, to nourish Blood and *qi*, eyes and sinews.

Anna started to come to the treatments by herself from the third session onwards, travelling by bus which she dreaded so much. She improved steadily despite regular episodes which she described in the following words: 'Butterflies in the stomach', 'life energy drains out of me', 'I'm not here', 'very drained, especially from the right leg'.

I shifted the treatment towards nourishing Spleen *qi* and Heart and Liver Blood and away from clearing Phlegm and Heat. A typical treatment at this stage would have been: SP6 *sanyinjiao*, HE7 *shenmen*, ST36 *zusanli*, LIV8 *ququan*, DU20 *baihui*, GB34 *yanglingquan*, SI3 *houxi* and BL62 *shenmai*, or alternatively BL15 *xinshu*, BL17 *geshu*, BL18 *ganshu*, BL20 *pishu*, DU4 *mingmen*, DU20 *baihui*. The herbal prescriptions were now based on *gui pi tang* (Return the Spleen Soup) to nourish Spleen *qi* and Heart and Liver Blood.

At the seventh session I noticed a response on the right patella deep tendon reflex which filled me with some excitement. Her pulse was now wiry but no longer slippery or full. The Kidney pulse position had improved. The tongue still had a red tip but was less swollen and much less sticky.

I started Anna on a course of seven injections with Angelica Sinensis *dang gui* extract (1.5 ml) and Vitamin B1 (12.5 mg = 0.5 ml) using 24 mm (0.5 mm gauge) injection needles (Bensky & O'Connor 1984). The medicines were injected to the full length of the needle into points ST36 *zusanli* and GB39 *xuanchong* bilaterally (0.5 ml each) after obtaining a fairly strong needling sensation. The other described treatments were continued.

After 15 sessions we stopped the treatments because Anna couldn't afford any more and she had improved so much. She now 'generally coped', was 'able to swim 15 to 20 lengths', and took part in social activities (bus, gym, college). She said: 'I am beginning to venture back into life'.

I saw Anna again 5 months later. She was back to academic work, pursuing her thesis, reading, studying — all the things she was totally unable to do before. Most of the symptoms relating to Holmes Adie Syndrome had gone and this was confirmed by a neurologist. She had weak, yet more or less normal, deep tendon reflexes and her pupils reacted to light. The Liver Blood *xu* symptoms had more or less disappeared.

The interesting twist in her saga was that now the eczema had come back, covering her hands and feet in thick, very itchy eruptions with blisters and pus, bleeding when she scratched them. This I concluded was the law of cure as applied in homeopathy, where old ailments return as the patient improves. She was prescribed antibiotics by her GP and I prescribed herbal medicines based on Eliminate Wind Powder *xiao feng san* with Herba Taraxaci Mongolicci cum Radice *pu gong ying* and Herbae cum Radice Violae Yedoensitis *zi hua di ding* to clear Damp-heat and Fire Poison.

A catalyst for recovery

For me this was an unusual case. The patient had progressed from relative health to a severe state of Liver Blood *xu* with utter debility and neurological symptoms and signs following a serious episode of malaria. After 15 treatments with acupuncture (also some Chinese herbs and *qi gong*) she had vastly improved and several months later she was back to a normal active life. Other symptoms such as painful menses also had improved. I asked Anna how she felt about her recovery. She said: 'I am thrilled, I knew I would get well again'. So, in a way, for Anna the outcome was what she had expected. For me the improvement was far greater over a much shorter timespan than I would have dared to expect.

What Anna's story has taught me more than anything is to listen to one's first instinct and to ask the overall important question: 'Is the *qi* fabric of this patient basically intact or has it been eroded, has this patient got resources to fight back or are they exhausted?'. Anna did have the resources to fight back and I can only say how thrilling it was for me to contribute as a catalyst to her recovery.

Summary of outcome

- From debility back to normal active life.
- Able to engage in academic work (i.e. intensive reading).
- Able to engage socially, in leisure activities etc., which were beyond her capacity before her illness.
- Overall much more confident.
- Symptoms relating to Liver Blood *xu* (eyes, extremities, etc.) disappeared.
- Menses (which were not the focus of my treatment):

1. Before illness: considerable PMT, dysmenorrhoea.
2. During illness: scanty, erratic, painful flow.
3. After recovery: little PMT, mild pain with much more normal flow.

- Pulse: from full, slippery-wiry with Kidney *xu* signs to a much more balanced though slightly wiry pulse.
- Tongue: from a thick, sticky, yellowish-white coating to a clear, slightly sticky, almost normal coating.

NOTES

1 Holmes Adie Syndrome is considered a permanent non-progressive condition of sudden onset which affects mainly women between the age of 20 and 40. The characteristic symptoms are: blurred vision, dilated pupil (usually one-sided) with absent or markedly diminished light reflex responses and absent deep tendon reflexes. Otherwise neurological findings are normal. The aetiology is unknown. There is no known treatment (Merck 1992).

REFERENCES

Bensky D, O'Connor J (eds) 1984 Acupuncture: a comprehensive text, 3rd edn. Shanghai College of Traditional Chinese Medicine, Eastland Press, Seattle

Cheng Xinnong (ed) 1987 Chinese acupuncture and moxibustion. Foreign Languages Press, Beijing

Liu Li Bang 1991 Director of *qi gong* research, Guang Zhou College of Traditonal Chinese Medicine, China

Maciocia G 1989 Foundations of Chinese medicine. Churchill Livingstone, Edinburgh

Maciocia G 1994 The practice of Chinese medicine. Churchill Livingstone, Edinburgh

Merck 1992 Merck manual of diagnosis and therapy, 16th edn. Merck Research Department, Rahway

■ Friedrich Staebler

Friedrich Staebler qualified as a medical practitioner from Free University Medical School, Berlin, in 1976 and held several surgical Registrar posts in Berlin and Hamburg as part of his vocational training to become a GP.

He came to London in 1980 to study at the British College of Acupuncture and was awarded a degree 'Licentiate in Acupuncture' (Honours) in 1982. He joined the teaching staff at the British College of Acupuncture in 1983 and was awarded the advanced degree 'Bachelor of Acupuncture' in 1985.

In 1987 he completed a 1 month clinical course for advanced acupuncturists in Nanjing, China. In 1991 he completed a 2 year postgraduate course with the School of Chinese Herbal Medicine, followed by a 1 month advanced clinical course for Chinese herbal practitioners in Guang Zhou, China.

Besides his private practice in London, he has represented the interests of British acupuncturists at home and abroad. He is currently senior lecturer at the British College of Acupuncture, vice-chairman of the British Acupuncture Council and treasurer of the British Acupuncture Accreditation Board. He was awarded a fellowship by the British Acupuncture Association and Register in 1992.

A heartsink patient

Charles Buck CHESTER, UK

Intolerable pain and adversity

Acupuncture is seen by many in the West as a therapy of last resort. These are sometimes our 'heartsink' patients, the ones who miss their first appointment because they are in intensive care, or worse. My heart did indeed sink as Bill made his way into my clinic, supported both by his sturdy aluminium walking sticks and his more sprightly wife. There was a real possibility that he might not even survive long enough to complete the initial consultation. How, I wondered silently, could I possibly shift his 136 kg (300 lbs) of weight should the worst happen. He groaned continually from terrible pain and his plethoric dusky red complexion overlay an ashen pallor.

Bill's spirits were so poor that much of his story was told by his wife. His pain and severe breathlessness made it hard for him to concentrate or communicate, and his lowered head made it hard to establish eye contact. When someone is so unwell it is not easy to know what to say, but on seeing Bill's list of medication (see box), I risked some humour. Luckily we managed a laugh but there was no avoiding the fact that Bill was struggling with intolerable pain and adversity. Outlining realistically modest goals, I suggested that we might be able to obtain some symptomatic pain relief through twice weekly sessions for a few weeks, but little more could be hoped for. If progress was made we could look at some of the other pain and discomfort.

Medication

During the previous 4 months, Bill had been prescribed the following medication:

Atrovent nebuliser, Fibogel, Gaviscon, Salbutamol Becotide 100, Codeine phosphate, allopurinol, diazepam, Isosorbide mononitrate, temazepam, Ventolin nebules, Diltiazem hydrochloride, Omeprazole, naftidrofuryl oxalate (Oxalat), diclofenac SR, Proctosedyl (suppositories and ointment), lactulose, glycyryl trinitrate, frusemide, Co-Dydramol, E45 Cream, insulin injection, Amlodipine, oxygen cylinder.

Medical history

Bill was a 74-year-old retired electrical engineer with severe and constant pain across the whole chest, centring in particular below the left pectoral muscle and radiating into the back of the chest. He had had chest pains for many years but they had become worse during the previous 2 months or so. His pain was aggravated by breathing and walking, which he could only do with the aid of sticks. It was also worse when lying on the left side but otherwise was lessened when lying down.

In his 50s Bill had worked for some years in Yugoslavia and this work had often involved exposure to chilly weather conditions. During this time he had developed a severely painful frozen shoulder which had been treated with corticosteroid injections. A few months later he had a heart attack which he described as follows:

> *It happened one morning at work, I felt as if I had been struck a heavy blow across my chest. I fell to the floor, picked myself up and carried on at work. I didn't tell anyone what had happened . . . I went to work the next day as usual but felt so ill that I had to be brought home at lunchtime. The consultant at our local hospital diagnosed a heart attack.*

From the time of his heart attack, Bill received medication for angina chest pains. He was admitted to a hospital coronary care unit five years later with constant pains, 'travelling from my fingertips, up my arm to my shoulder and across my chest', which were only partially relieved by angina tablets. The additional diagnosis of emphysema was given and inhalers and other medication prescribed.

Throughout the following 2 years Bill developed severe pains in the mid-back and abdomen. A urology department scan found a left kidney problem, but he was judged too ill for surgery. A year later he was admitted to hospital for surgery to remove the left kidney but first spent 3 days in cardiac intensive care. Recovering in hospital after the surgery Bill complained of pains in his legs. Initially these were dismissed by hospital staff but later deep vein thrombosis was diagnosed and warfarin prescribed over the next 6 years. Whilst in hospital Bill also developed gout in both feet.

Since spending time in hospital Bill suffered increased pain in the back which was diagnosed as arthritic degeneration and spondylosis of the spine and neck. Four years later he was diagnosed as diabetic and this led to insulin dependence 2 years later. Recent problems with his stomach and bowel led to a gastroscopy which revealed some old scarring of the stomach wall suggestive of past ulceration but no active disease. A week later he was vomiting blood. Warfarin was blamed for this and his medication was stopped although Bill believes that the gastroscopy procedure triggered the bleeding.

Severe and spreading back pain

Six months ago Bill's back pains suddenly became very severe, spreading from the thoracic spine down the midline, across the trapezius area bilaterally and into the left flank and shoulder. An epidural anaesthetic injection given at a hospital pain clinic relieved the pain for some time but by the time it wore off there were additional pains in the right groin and hips. A barium enema X-ray explained this as diverticular disease and pain killers were prescribed. Bill also had swelling, tenderness and pain in the right iliac fossa which could be attributed to the diverticulosis. In the few months before he came to see me the pain had increased substantially with a shoulder pain severely affecting the chest pain. 'None of the pain killers or the angina medication seem able to reduce it. The constant pain is really getting to me now.' Later, during the course of treatment, he intimated that he had been considering suicide.

Bill had experienced intermittent epigastric pain for more than a year but this was now constant. It was unaffected by eating but was tender to pressure. The pain sensation was sometimes stabbing, at other times it was a full feeling. 'Sometimes the pain is so severe it makes me double up and fall over. At other times it is just there constantly in the background.' Cold drinks made all his pains much worse and reduced his appetite. He was also quite constipated.

Bill continues to suffer from emphysema resulting in bad breathlessness with an inability to walk more than a few yards. 'Even just having a wash and a shave takes the breath out of me.' He has no cough and does not expectorate any mucus. He has had some visual disturbances in the last few years due to a 'lump behind the eye'. When this started it 'seemed like an earwig was crossing my vision'. This is monitored every 6 months or so by an ophthalmologist. In addition he also feels dizzy and lightheaded.

Further questioning revealed that his urination was very frequent and copious — through the night he generally urinated 6 or 7 times. He had continually experienced some pain on passing water since the kidney removal. He traces his urination problems back to the war when he experienced continual pain when passing water, a sensation described as feeling 'like broken glass'. Now Bill also has pains in the legs 'due to circulation problems' and gouty arthritis affecting both feet. He cannot stand for more than a minute or so because his legs are too weak and painful. His limbs are cold and he feels generally quite chilly.

Palpation of his back revealed extreme tenderness both on the midline and paravertebrally along its whole length. Gentle pressure anywhere on the back of the chest made him wince with pain, making it harder to navigate the back accurately for point location.

Bill's pulse was slippery, full, and very choppy. It was also racing and rapid, presumably because any sort of movement was an enormous effort. His tongue was large, pale with a greasy coating and had dirty orange-purple sides showing numerous dark chocolate-coloured spots.

Bill was a big man who was also quite overweight. His pain and poor spirits meant that most of the day was spent in bed or lying on the couch. He had been a heavy smoker but had stopped after developing angina.

Summary of clinical manifestations

- Chest pains: severe and constant, especially centred below the left pectoral muscle and radiating into the back of the chest; aggravated by breathing and walking; pain worse with cold, worse when lying on left side, otherwise better with rest.
- Dark and purple complexion, with an underlying ashen pallor.
- Right iliac fossa pain, swelling and tenderness.
- Epigastric pain: constant, tender to pressure, stabbing sensation or feeling full, worse with cold drinks.
- Poor appetite, constipated.
- Breathlessness: inability to walk more than a few yards, aggravated by slight exertion, no mucus.
- Visual disturbances, sensation of a 'lump behind the eye', dizzy and lightheaded.
- Urination: painful, copious, frequent especially at night.
- Gout, leg pains, limbs weak and cold, feels chilly.
- Overweight, poor spirits.
- Palpation: extreme tenderness of back and chest.
- Pulse: rapid, slippery, full and very choppy.
- Tongue: large, pale with greasy coating and dirty orange-purple sides showing numerous chocolate-coloured spots.

Patterns of disharmony

Pain was the main concern and no doubt Bill and his wife had heard that 'acupuncture can be good for pain'. This had to be the main focus of treatment. Bill's medical history clearly showed that a lot of issues needed to be unravelled. We often have to diagnose using symptoms and signs obscured, distorted and compounded by medication and this was a case in point. Which symptoms and signs were the result of medication? To what extent was Bill's polyuria the result of frusemide diuretic use? Did the diuretics induce his diabetes? Sometimes each visit clarifies understanding a little more. Nevertheless, it was apparent during the first session that the main patterns were Heart Blood Stagnation, Heart *yang xu*, and Kidney *yang xu*. Clinical evidence for this is summarised below.

Patterns of disharmony

Heart Blood Stagnation

- Chest pains, severe and chronic, especially on the left.
- Dark and purple complexion.
- Pain worse when lying on the left side.
- Palpation: reveals extreme tenderness of chest.
- Pulse: very choppy.
- Tongue: dark chocolate-coloured spots on sides.

Heart *yang xu*

- Chest pains aggravated by breathing and walking, and better with rest.
- Breathlessness, aggravated by activity.
- Ashen pallor.
- Poor spirits (poor shen).
- Tongue: pale.

Kidney *yang xu*

- Urination copious, frequent, especially at night.
- Low back pain.
- Chilliness.
- Legs, painful, weak and cold.
- Ashen pallor.
- Tongue: pale.

Damp-heat in lower *jiao*

- Urination painful, history of chronic urinary tract infections.
- Right iliac fossa pain, swelling and tenderness.
- Gouty arthritis in feet.
- Tongue: large, greasy coating.
- Pulse: slippery, full.

Cold Obstruction (*bi*) of Chest

- Chest and flank pain.
- Chest pain worse with cold.
- History of onset at the time of exposure to cold.
- Difficulty breathing.
- Extreme tenderness of chest.

Aetiology and pathology

Here is a very strong man whose problems over the past 20 years are rooted (from the perspective of Chinese medicine) in inadequate treatment of earlier illnesses (Fig. 6.1). During the war it seems that Bill had an untreated and ongoing lower urinary tract infection. This commonly leads to a progressive weakening of Kidney *qi* and diminishing of the life gate fire *mingmen huo*. Kidney *yin* is eroded by the long-term retention of Heat in the lower *jiao* and *yang* is lowered by the chronic presence of Dampness. The proportion of these two forms of *xie qi*, or pathogenic *qi*, determines which aspect of Kidney *qi* suffers most injury (Song Lubing 1989). Eventually long-term *yang* weakness leads to poor digestive function and weakens the *qi* mechanism (*qi ji*) of the middle *jiao*. In this case it appears that Kidney *yang* was more affected.

Yang weakness made Bill more prone to external invasion of the *jingluo* in the chest by *shi* Cold as happened while he was in Yugoslavia. The

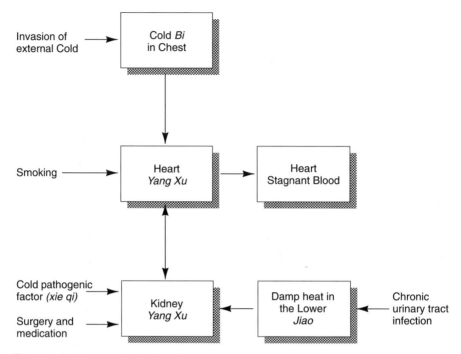

Fig. 6.1 Aetiology and pathology diagram.

corticosteroid injections moved *qi* and Blood Stagnation in the shoulder but failed to expel the Cold pathogenic factor which then progressed deeper to obstruct the chest and Heart *yang* leading to Heart Blood Stagnation. This is the Heart *bi* syndrome which is described in the Neijing:

> **Heart bi is characterised by obstruction in the blood vessels, turmoil below the Heart while feeling depressed, turmoil causing upsurging energy and asthma ... When rheumatism of various types persists for a prolonged period of time, it will move into the internal region (Lu 1978).**

It is quite common for angina sufferers to experience a frozen shoulder a year or two before the onset of their cardiac problems. In addition, deaths from myocardial infarction are more numerous during cold weather. Recently epidemiologists have confirmed the link between cold climates and heart disease (Marchant et al 1993). This has been suggested as an explanation for why northern Europeans are more prone to heart disease than those living in the south, even when dietary factors are allowed for. Throughout history, Chinese medicine has believed that coldness makes the Blood stagnate and congeal (Fu Weikang 1990).

Failure to remove the Damp and Heat *xie qi* from the Kidney water channels led eventually to organic pathology and to the point where surgery was needed to remove the damaged kidney. There was increasing Stagnation due to Dampness and Heat leading eventually to Fire Poison, Blood Stagnation, local pain and necrosis of the kidney itself.

Severe breathlessness on exertion, accompanied by weak and sore back and legs and polyuria, suggests failure of the Kidneys to grasp the *qi*. Contributing factors to Bill's breathing problems also probably included damage to Lung *qi* and *yin* by smoking and obstruction of chest *yang* by Cold and Blood Stagnation. Later, during the course of treatment, his Lung *qi* was strengthened and moved and Bill coughed up large amounts of mucus with a marked improvement in breathing. This mucus had been hidden but could have been inferred from the full slippery pulse and the appearance of the tongue.

An impossible challenge?

Initially I was not enthusiastic about treating Bill. I thought he was too far gone. I confess to slight irritation when heartsink patients appear, presenting what seem to be impossible challenges. Along with so many of the other medical professionals he had seen before, my compassion was obstructed by the difficulty of engaging with his *shen*. Also I felt anxious about the problems inherent in taking on someone in such imminent danger. Nevertheless I suggested that Bill receive a few treatments twice weekly to see if we could relieve his pain. I silently doubted the sense in planning a longer course of action.

On the first visit the worst pain was in the left flank and the thoracic spine. No electrical stimulation was used in the first session; usually it is best to use the first treatment to gauge the patient's responsiveness to milder stimulation. I explained to Bill and his wife that we would be using points on his back, hands and left leg. Bill was in terrible pain and so I asked if he would be better lying down or sitting up. He opted to sit but he groaned with pain in any position. As with all patients new to acupuncture I explained the importance of, and how to recognise, the *qi* sensation. It would have been good to use moxa because of the Cold Stagnation and *yang xu*. However, many people find this process too much of a cultural leap if used during the first visit and so I saved this for the next session.

First treatment procedures

Treatment principles

To clear Blood Stagnation from the Heart and chest.

To clear Cold *bi* from the *jingluo* in the chest and relieve pain.

To strengthen *zong qi*, Heart *yang* and *shen* and Kidney *yang*.

Points selected

GB34 *yanglingquan* and SJ5 *waiguan* on the left. The worst pain on the first visit was in the left flank, an area associated with *shao yang* channels according to *jingluo* differentiation. This combination was only needed on the first treatment.

Local points were needed for the extreme tenderness along the whole course of the back:

B17 *geshu, hui* point for Blood, a major point for Blood stagnation.

B18 *ganshu* to reinforce the action of BL17 *geshu* in regulating *qi* and Blood.

DU11 *shendao*, DU10 *lingtai*, DU9 *zhiyang*, and DU8 *jinsuo* to move *yang* in the chest and calm *shen*. Much of Bill's pain was attributable to degeneration of the vertebrae, an area controlled by the DU channel.

BL23 *shenshu* to begin the process of strengthening the root.

LI4 *hegu* on the right to regulate *qi* and reduce pain.

Needling methods

All these points were needled using 40 mm, 30 gauge needles inserted between 12–18 mm to the level at which *deqi* was obtained. On BL23 *shenshu* manipulation was stopped as soon as *qi* was obtained. The other points were given stronger stimulation for a few seconds and stimulation was repeated two or three times during the treatment. As soon as I obtained *deqi* on the points, Bill's arms started to shake and quiver. This continued for the 20 minutes duration of the treatment.

The *shen* returns

The flank pains quickly receded but it became clear that Bill's worst pains were those across his chest and in the thoracic spine. I used electrical stimulation alternately on P6 *neiguan* or P5 *jianshi* and settled on BL13 *feishu*, BL15 *xinshu*, BL17 *geshu* and BL23 *shenxu* and REN17 *shanzhong* for the next few treatments. Moxa on the needle was used on BL13 *feishu* and BL15 *xinshu*. An even method was used on the upper back *shu* points so as to both regulate Blood and *qi* and strengthen *zangfu* function. I prefer to use perpendicular insertion on the back *shu* points on the chest, taking care with the depth. I find that the *qi* sensation is more difficult to obtain when using deeper oblique insertion. Sometimes the chest pain would focus in the left shoulder in which case LI15 *jianyu* was added.

By session four Bill's pain in the upper back had reduced substantially but the chest pain was still as bad as ever. Two treatments later I was told that he had walked about for 2 hours and had pottered about in his garden. This was the first time that he had been up and about in a year. The chest pain had diminished a lot and he was sleeping better.

At the end of January, 12 weeks into treatment, Bill developed Bell's palsy on his right side with quite severe paralysis of the face, drooping mouth, and inability to close the right eye. With it came pain and tenderness over the whole side of the head which was focused on SJ17 *yifeng* and GB1 *tongziliao*. This really depressed Bill. Treatment priority shifted to dealing with this acute attack of Wind Cold to the *shaoyang* and *yangming* channels on the head. I used the above mentioned points together with GB 20 *fengchi* (needle and moxa), ST2 *sibai*, LI4 *hegu* and SJ5 *waiguan*. To maintain some effect on those points previously treated, I replaced the upper back points with DU14 *dazhui* (needle and moxa) and kept the left P6 *neiguan* and BL23 *shenshu*.

Now, gradually, treatment priorities are working more towards treating the root, or *ben,* of the disharmony. Bill is old and still not exactly well but he continues to get stronger. Previously Bill's spirits had been so low that he did not want to talk but now he is talking again. It is very satisfying to see his *shen* return so strongly. Now that we can talk I care more about what happens and I have come to know Bill's personality. I feel ashamed that my biggest concern before had been the possibility of my own inconvenience. Not for the first time I have relearned the lesson that everyone deserves our best effort even if the spirit is obscured when first we meet.

REFERENCES

Lu H 1978 (trans) Huang Di Nei Jing, Su Wen. Self-published, Vancouver, ch 23

Marchant, Ranjadayalan et al 1993 Circadian and seasonal factors in the pathogenesis of acute myocardial infarction, the influence of environmental temperature. British Heart Journal 69(5): 385–387

Fu Weikang (ed.) 1990 Zhongguo Yixue Shi. Publishing House Of Shanghai College of TCM p 272

Song Lubing (ed.) 1989 Zhongyi Bingyin Bingji Xue. People's Health Publishing Company, Beijing p 208

■ Charles Buck

Charles Buck graduated in 1977 from Bristol University Medical School with an Honours BSc in Physiology. Having had an interest in all things Oriental from his teens he went on to study acupuncture at the International College of Oriental Medicine in Sussex, graduating in 1984.

He writes, 'The time I started my Chinese medicine training was especially exciting. It coincided with a steep rise in the quality of information available in the West. Chinese medicine experienced a sudden coming of age thanks to the works of Kaptchuk, Bensky, Maciocia and other scholar-pioneers. We were no longer wallowing half-deluded in Oriental mysteries. Instead we could appreciate the tradition for what it is, namely practical, succinct and effective medicine able to relieve pain and suffering'.

Later he went on to study Chinese herbal medicine, first with Kaptchuk and Maciocia, and then in Shanghai's Shuguang Hospital and other hospitals in China. In recent years he has been tutoring in acupuncture and Chinese herbs on postgraduate courses at the Northern College of Acupuncture in York.

Treating the untreatable

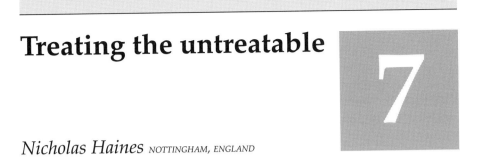

Nicholas Haines NOTTINGHAM, ENGLAND

Sometimes I hate my work. I hate seeing or experiencing things that I really don't want to, having to face up to situations in other people's lives that would be my worst nightmare, and getting to know and care about people who are already suffering or who are going to suffer horribly. I would sometimes, in my selfish, blinkered way, rather not see those things. To hell with the idea of my work being 'rewarding', 'fulfilling' and of my 'helping people to die with dignity'. Alice is such a person and I feel so guilty saying it.

Motor neurone disease

I was first asked if I would treat Alice by her best friend, who was also one of my patients. 'Alice, my friend, has been diagnosed as having motor neurone disease (amyotrophic lateral sclerosis). Can you treat it?' I said I had treated a few people and, well, they had all died, but I felt sure that things had slowed down with treatment and that the 'end' had hopefully been a little easier.

Alice came to see me 2 years ago. She was tall and was dressed in worn, casual clothes. She appeared to be quite a practical-looking person, a person who gets on with life. She had short hair, a nice smile and looked about 36–38 years old. We chatted ... she had been diagnosed with motor neurone disease 2 weeks earlier but felt that she had had the symptoms for about 6 months now.

She said:

Halfway through a telephone conversation I would have to stop talking. I know it sounds silly, but my tongue felt tired, and I would have to rest it. It got to be such hard work, and scary because I didn't know what was wrong. My left nostril went numb and dead, then so did my tongue which stuck to the roof of my mouth almost like it was made of wood.

Her right arm was numb and weaker than the left and felt really heavy and stiff in the mornings. Her symptoms were worse when she was run down or anxious, before a period or when life was emotionally difficult.

She had problems swallowing, with persistent phlegm or thick saliva in the throat.

Her stools were normal except before a period, when they were somewhat loose. Her bladder was also normal. She always felt exhausted before, during and after her period. Her period was not very heavy, but often lasted for 7–8 days with light coloured blood.

As the consultation went on, Alice became slightly harder to understand and more nasal. I also noticed that she had a lot of clear saliva which literally poured from her mouth. I decided it was partly due to her lips being very weak and not being able to contain it, and partly due to excess saliva production. She said the saliva production was always worse when she was tired or under stress.

Physical examination

I had some difficulty in looking at Alice's tongue because she could only just move it. What I could see of it was pale, swollen and wet, with a greasy, creamy coat. She was obviously quite self-conscious during this examination of her tongue because of the saliva that dribbled from her mouth. In future, I looked at her tongue less frequently than I would do normally. The same thing happened with her pulse. Her right hand had already started to contract inwards and this made it very difficult to take the pulse. What I could determine was that it was slippery but very weak.

Alice was of a reasonable build, generally carrying more weight in the lower half of the body than in the upper half. I asked her to show me where she felt numb and weak. She traced an almost perfect line along the Large Intestine channel, starting from LI4 *hegu* and running right up the arm to end at the left nostril.

She said she was also getting weak in the back of her right arm, neck and the whole of her right shoulder. This followed the Gall Bladder and *san jiao* channels in her shoulder and, at the neck, followed more the Large Intestine, Small Intestine and Bladder channels. Her left leg was also weak, but she couldn't really say where, except that her foot dropped forward, which I tend to think of as a Stomach channel. She was unsure as to the area where the symptoms had first started.

When I examined her, I could see a gentle twitching of the muscles and a definite thinning of the muscle bulk. Her neck looked very thin and wasted at the back and very fragile.

I think, in retrospect, that I became so interested in her channels that I forgot the person behind them. I realised that she was becoming quite excited about the fact that her problem followed a path known to Chinese medicine, and that she was concluding, because I appeared to understand the problem, that I must also have a cure.

Medical history and medication

Alice had very efficiently prepared a medical history. Childhood illnesses included scarlet fever, measles and glandular fever. As a teenager she had had a wheezy chest and chest infections. When she was around 10 years old, she had started to faint, usually at the start of her period. She then started to have fits and was diagnosed as a borderline epileptic. From then on she had fewer fits and 10 years ago was diagnosed as non-epileptic. There was a phase when she had suffered from an overactive thyroid, coinciding with a very difficult time emotionally. Treatment comprised a prescription of carbimazole for 2 years and there had been no recurrence of this problem, except for a slight episode during pregnancy. Alice still suffers from and catches coughs easily, usually with white or green phlegm.

In terms of medication, Alice was taking part in an extensive clinical trial in Nottingham which was evaluating the drug Riluzole, now marketed as Rilutek (MND Association News 1995). She had been told that Rilutek was supposed to delay the symptoms of motor neurone disease and might prolong life. She was not sure whether she was taking the placebo or the real thing. For the last few years she had seen a homeopath to help with her chest and the quantity of phlegm that she had.

As Alice was fairly tired at this point, I asked if she wanted to take a break and see me again in a couple of days. She said that would be good and left.

A pivotal role in the family

When I saw Alice 3 days later, I talked with her about her life. She was a community development worker and had two children, aged 4 and 7. She had been studying for an MA. Her husband was emotionally very weak and had received quite a lot of psychiatric help. He had stayed at home to look after the children but, when Alice wasn't working, she looked after him, the home and the children. She said she was exhausted most of the time. I got a real sense that she was the pivot around which the whole family turned.

I found it really difficult when she started talking about all the things she used to do, like playing the piano, walking, swimming, writing, and laughing and chatting with her friends, because I knew that she had already lost the ability to do these things,. She would be lucky if, in 18 months time, she could hold up her head. Why had I agreed to see her? She had children the same age as mine and I know how important my children's mother is to them.

Summary of clinical manifestations

- Tongue feels tired, wooden and numb.
- Weak lips.
- Left nostril numb and dead.
- Right arm numb, weak, heavy and stiff in the morning; hand contracts inwards.
- Profuse, clear saliva.
- Symptoms worse when tired, under stress and with period.
- Difficulty swallowing.
- Persistent phlegm in the throat.
- Exhausted most of the time, especially before, during and after her periods; prolonged menstruation with loose stools before periods.
- Wheezy chest, easily catches coughs with chest infections and with a lot of white and/or green phlegm.
- Muscle wasting, thinning of muscle bulk.
- Weakness of muscles in the arms, neck, shoulders and legs.
- Twitching of muscles.
- Tongue: pale, swollen and wet, with a greasy, creamy coat.
- Pulse: slippery and weak.

Identifying the pattern of disharmony

I felt sure, by the nature of this disease and the rapid destructive rate at which it progressed, that it was a clear excess condition with some underlying deficiency. The deficiency would obviously become more pronounced as things took hold, but the condition was primarily excess at this stage.

From a channel point of view, the channels had been invaded by External Damp. This had obstructed the *qi* and Blood, causing wasting of muscles and tendons. The obstructive nature of the Damp had also stagnated body fluids into Phlegm, further aggravating the condition and symptoms.

I think Alice already had *qi xu* (mainly Lung and Spleen) and Blood *xu* (mainly Liver) before the motor neurone symptoms began.

There was also evidence of Phlegm obstructing the throat, and bouts of the Lung-Phlegm-Cold and Phlegm-Heat. Although the Damp and Phlegm had combined to obstruct the channels and could be thought of as one, I have kept them in separate patterns here as their aetiologies are different.

Evidence for the patterns of disharmony

Damp obstructing the channels

- Heavy, stiff limbs.
- Numbness.
- Wasting of muscles and tendons.
- Tongue: greasy, creamy coat.
- Pulse: slippery.

Phlegm obstructing the channels and tongue

- Numb limbs, dead areas.
- Wooden tongue.
- Profuse saliva.
- Problems swallowing.
- Phlegm in the throat.

***Qi* and Blood obstructed in the muscle channels**

- Wasting of muscles and tendons.
- Weakness of muscles in the neck, arms and legs.

Lung *qi xu*

- Wheezy.

- Easily catching coughs.
- Tiredness.
- Tongue: pale.
- Pulse: weak.

Spleen *qi xu*

- Producing a lot of phlegm.
- Loose stools before periods.
- Prolonged menstruation.
- Tongue: pale and wet.
- Pulse: weak.

Liver Blood *xu* and Interior Wind

- Tired around menstruation.
- Wasting and twitching of muscles and tendons.
- Tongue: pale.
- Pulse: weak.

Phlegm-Cold/Heat invading the Lung

- Cough with white and green phlegm.
- Tongue: greasy, creamy coat.
- Pulse: slippery.

Aetiology and pathology

If I hadn't treated patients with motor neurone disease before, or if I had seen Alice at a different stage in her illness, I would have perhaps initially thought about the aetiology in a different way. However, because I know the progression of the disease is so rapid and so devastating, I know that it can't be an internally generated problem. When you very first see someone who only has a little numbness in the tongue or in a limb, with a relatively large amount of deficient symptoms, you can think that the pattern is mostly a deficient one. However, when you see your patient 18 months later, unable to talk, unable to lift her head or to feed herself, you know that it is externally generated and that it's nasty.

I also had another sense that Alice's condition was initially an external invasion. The channels that were first invaded (*tai yang, yang ming* and *shao yang)*, are similar, to some extent, to the initial channel symptoms in a six stage invasion, when the pathogen is obstructing the *yang* channels. There are obviously different pathogens at play here but the similarities can be seen in Alice's stiff neck (*tai yang*) and numb face (*yang ming*) (Hsu & Peacher 1981).

One could also think about the reverse of this, say in the case of wind-stroke, where the pathogen is clearly internally generated (Wind and Phlegm), obstructing the *yin* channel muscles first, causing contracture, numbness and stiffness, leaving the *yang* channel muscles flaccid and eventually causing them to waste (Lu 1978).

Undoubtedly, Alice's *wei qi xu* / Lung *qi xu* predisposed her to an invasion and this was aggravated by general *qi* and Blood *xu*. At the start of the disease process her Spleen *qi xu*, although fairly minimal in terms of symptoms, would have made her susceptible to increased Phlegm. Then, as she became increasingly ill and, as the *zang* as well as the channels became affected, a more internally generated aetiology added to her problems (Fig. 7.1).

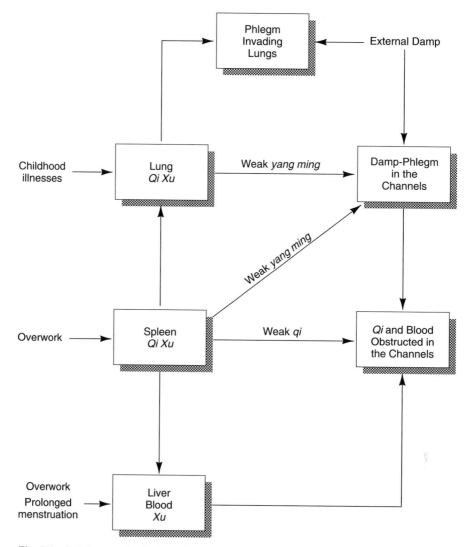

Fig. 7.1   Aetiology and pathology diagram.

Although one can clearly see how things started, stopping the process is a different matter.

Treatment issues

My primary aim was to try to clear the channels as best as possible whilst, at the same time, supporting the Lung and Spleen. I wanted to clear Damp, resolve Phlegm and move *qi* and Blood in the channels. I also wanted to support the Lung, because a chest infection would weaken Alice, thereby allowing a faster progression of the disease. In addition, I wanted to tonify the Spleen to reduce the production of Phlegm.

I planned to treat Alice twice weekly, and daily in acute episodes. I think Alice's initial reaction to the number of treatments was one of shock, especially my suggestion that she received a daily treatment when she had a chest infection. Some of it may have been the perceived cost, so we chatted about money and agreed to her paying for one treatment per week and the cost of the needles for the extra treatments.

I suggested a few dietary changes, for example asking her to remove Phlegm-forming foods such as dairy products. Other than that she needed to rest. It did cross my mind though, 'what a thing to say, telling someone to rest and do little when she has to put the remainder of her life into the next 2 years'.

First treatment procedures

POINTS PRESCRIPTION

- ST40 *fenglong*, to resolve Phlegm and Dampness and to calm asthma.
- HE5 *tongli*, because it opens into the tongue.
- SP9 *yinlingquan*, to resolve Dampness.
- LU7 *lieque*, stimulates descending and dispersing of Lung *qi*, circulates the *wei qi* and releases the exterior; opens the *ren mai* with KID6 *zhaohai*.
- KID6 *zhaohai*, coupled point of the *ren mai*, supports the *yin*.
- SP6 *sanyinjiao*, strengthens the Spleen, resolves Damp, and nourishes *yin* and Blood.

Rationale: The treatment was designed to try to clear some of the excess whilst, at the same time, supporting the deficiencies that either already existed or were developing.

Needling techniques: ST40 *fenglong*, SP9 *yinlingquan* and SP6 *sanyinjiao* were used bilaterally, LU7 *lieque* on the left, KID6 *zhaohai* on the right, and H5 *tongli* on the left (as the wrist on the right was contracted inwards somewhat). ST40 *fenglong*, SP9 *yinlingquan* and H5 *tongli* were used with reducing method. The remainder were used with even method. I used 0.30 mm × 25 mm needles on all points except SP9 *yinlingquan*, where I used 0.30 mm × 40 mm.

A wild fairground ride

Over the next 2 years, Alice's treatment was rather like being on a wild fairground ride. We had moments of calm before being plunged into an intense burst of treatment, trying to get to grips with some aspect of her deteriorating condition. The main problem area was the bouts of chest infections which she found increasingly difficult to throw off. These infections usually started with an invasion of Wind-Heat, which then turned into Lung-Phlegm-Heat. Hearing her choke with the obviously thick phlegm that she could neither swallow nor cough up, unnerved me. I felt so helpless as she struggled to breathe, choking on something that you or I would easily get rid of with a quick and powerful cough.

I tended to treat these chest infections very aggressively with daily treatments. Out of about 12 chest infections, Alice only needed antibiotics once when I really felt the situation was out of control. Even then, I think the acupuncture treatment was the main influence in her recovery. It had the advantage of being able to clear the non-infected Phlegm which would have otherwise remained, in spite of the antibiotics, only to probably thicken and re-infect.

Each chest infection, however swiftly dealt with, left some legacy. After a really bad bout over Christmas, Alice lost the ability to speak. Her speech had become difficult to understand, but I felt it was important to persevere with it. After this infection, all resemblance of understanding went. Alice started writing everything down and I have never heard her voice again. Her ability to write went 6 months later and she then used a keyboard and voice box which, whilst less personal, still allowed her to communicate.

Alice is now gradually becoming generally *yin xu* with night sweating, backache, restlessness and, probably more disturbing for her, an overactive mind with anxiety and panic attacks due to Heart *yin xu*. An interesting point is that her asthma, which was treated along with everything else, responded well to treatment and she no longer has to take any medication for this problem.

No longer a stranger

As I initially read through Alice's notes whilst writing up this case study I wondered what Alice was getting from the treatment. She had been steadily deteriorating, yet came twice weekly for treatments. When I asked her, I found her answer gave me a different dimension to her suffering. She told me that she could come for acupuncture with a sore throat, a wheezy chest, feelings of anger, sadness and heat, a whole manner of problems, and I would make them go away. Having motor neurone disease was bad enough, but being exhausted and sweating, with an inability to calm her mind, added insult to injury.

At least if those symptoms were calmer, then life, however hard, was easier. I also recognised that when we did fewer treatments, the motor neurone aspect of her illness progressed faster, with increasing loss of movement.

I have to admit that, at times, I felt pretty useless as an acupuncturist, always wondering whether Alice would have been in better health, happier, or even cured had someone else been treating her. Perhaps a better acupuncturist than I knew all the answers. When Alice first came to see me, I didn't know her. I knew nothing about her unfulfilled dreams, her hopes, and all the things in her life that she would lose. As I treated her, I learned of those things. She is no longer a stranger and her slow death has become even more painful and more agonising to watch.

Every conceivable emotion

Alice has experienced every conceivable emotion as her life has slowly dismantled around her. She has lost her job, her home, her speech, her ability to look after her children and herself, her mobility and, however caring people are, her dignity. She has lost everything except her sense of humour. I did touch on her feelings about her impending death but she was too busy making arrangements on a more practical level, like who was going to look after the kids. When we did feel there was space, she had already lost the ability to talk. So when she tried to express the emotion and terrible sadness she had inside, all that came out were heart wrenching sobs which choked her and broke my heart.

With the help of acupuncture I think Alice has lived a little longer and that her time has been a little easier. But she will still die and I will still feel that I have failed her. I loved meeting Alice and being with her but, if I'm really honest, I would rather not have seen her suffering.

REFERENCES

Hsu H, Peacher W 1981 Shang han lun. Oriental Healing Arts of the United States, Los Angeles
Lu H 1978 Spiritual axis. Academy of Oriental Heritage, Vancouver
MND Association News 1995 Rilutek: questions and answers. Private publication

FURTHER READING

Kübler-Ross E 1993 On death and dying. Routledge, London
Maciocia G 1994 The practice of Chinese medicine. Churchill Livingstone, Edinburgh

Monajem R 1989 Treatment of two cases of amyotrophic lateral sclerosis with electro-acupuncture, including patients' accounts of progress, enhanced by combining conscious manipulation of *qi*. American Journal of Acupuncture, 17(3): 205–8

Morrison J 1986 Motor neurone disease: a death sentence. An authentic case history from Australian general practice. Australian Family Physician, 15(8): 1063

■ Nicholas Haines

I often ponder about decisions and how fragile is our destiny. Obviously, some major decisions will undoubtedly send us along a certain path; others, more mundane, will probably have less influence. But what about all the thousands of in-between decisions, and which of them will alter our lives?

In 1980 I was studying Applied Biology at what is now Trent University. We had to take a year out in industry as part of our course. I remember standing with pen in hand, about to sign up for a job which involved videoing chickens and their behaviour. I remember thinking 'should I sign or not', and then, quite irresponsibly, I walked away, leaving myself without a job for the next year. Three months later I was in Los Angeles at the California Acupuncture College.

My aim was to be involved with a research project, just starting at the College, into Kirlian photography. What happened was that I discovered Chinese medicine and it changed my life.

Suddenly, I began to understand myself, and perhaps my world, a little better. I met many kind and wonderful people. Susan Wilson was my inspiration: she introduced me to herbs and Chinese culture, and made me laugh. Then, when I returned to England, I studied with Giovanni Maciocia, Peter Deadman, Julian Scott and Vivienne Brown and attended many seminars. I trained in herbs with Ted Kaptchuk and visited China. I also set up a complementary health centre in Nottingham and helped to give birth to the Northern College of Acupuncture in York. All along the way, as Ted Kaptchuk says at the beginning of his book 'The web that has no weaver', I have learned so much from my patients and my students.

Incidentally, the person who took the job videoing chickens was never quite the same again; but then again, neither was I.

Maria's children

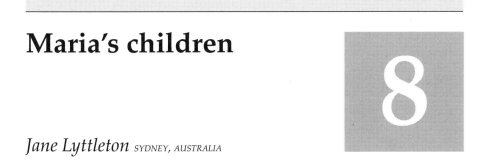

Jane Lyttleton SYDNEY, AUSTRALIA

A fortunate intervention

This is the story of one Greek woman's struggle to have children. Her personal desire to be a mother was strengthened by cultural and familial expectations.

Maria met and married her husband when she was 36 years old, and they planned to have children immediately. Her health had been excellent all her life until just 6 weeks before her wedding when she noticed a pain around her left kidney. Within a day of visiting her GP she'd had an ultrasound, had seen the specialist and was in the operating theatre. The surgeon found grapefruit-sized dermoid cysts, that is, non-malignant cysts containing teeth, skin and hair (Mackay et al 1992) in both ovaries. He proceeded to remove both the cysts and the ovaries and except for the fortunate intervention of Maria's GP, who'd popped in to watch the operation, this is exactly what would have happened. The GP knew of Maria's and her fiancee's strong desire to have a family and he exhorted the surgeon to attempt to save some ovarian tissue. And so Maria emerged from the operating theatre with one quarter of one ovary. Thenceforth she had very erratic cycles and frequent left-sided pain caused by the functional cysts which the remaining ovarian tissue continued to produce.

We can only guess as to what originally created such a blockage in Maria's pelvis to produce such cysts. She ate a good diet and at that time was not overweight. While it is true that she was not entirely content to be single and childless, she lived a busy and full life with a rewarding job and frequent overseas travel. She did not recall being particularly stressed. Perhaps, however, her subconscious distress at having neither a partner nor offspring affected the most obvious part of her anatomy, her reproductive system. Or perhaps there was some part of her childhood or upbringing which contributed to the obstruction? I was never sure.

For 6 months Maria and her husband tried to conceive. When they had no success Maria took Clomid (clomiphene citrate, a fertility drug which stimulates ovulation). When Clomid failed they tried IVF (in vitro fertilisation) many times. Time after time, however, over the next 18 months Maria would be 'cancelled' due to her 'erratic' response to the drugs; her ovarian tissue would produce cysts requiring aspiration or which would burst causing severe left-sided pain. Seldom would any follicles ripen to even close the required size and no eggs were harvested.

Dogged persistence and serendipity

Maria persisted doggedly (and perhaps misguidedly) through all the disappointment and the constant episodes of painful cysts until the month when she came to consult me. That day she had had her routine Day 12 ultrasound in a stimulated cycle to track the progress of her follicles. The news she got that day was not good. There was no response at all to the drugs — no follicles, no cysts, nothing. And she was on the highest dose possible. The specialist told her that this meant that she had run out of eggs and that was that. All that lay ahead now was the menopause. Maria, 38 years old and childless, was of course devastated by the news. Trying to comfort her, one of the IVF centre nurses mentioned that several of their patients had come to see me when they hadn't had success with IVF. Maria's husband called my clinic and in one of those moments of fortunate serendipity there was a space that very afternoon where someone had just cancelled. So they both arrived within the hour still in a state of shock and clearly distressed. Consequently getting the full story was not easy (or appropriate) through all the tears. A lot of what I have related above was told to me piecemeal over many visits. The most immediate and disturbing thought for Maria and her husband was the possibility that there might not be any more eggs left. In the face of such a dire possibility my response was to reach for a gynaecological textbook and together we consulted the section on ovarian anatomy. The information therein indicated that in one quarter of an ovary we might expect to find around 100 000 eggs. Assuming that several hundreds had been used in each of Maria's cycles over the previous 25 years we calculated that Maria probably still had in excess of 10 years worth of menstrual cycles left in that one quarter ovary.

A base from which to work

Looking back on these notes in the case history I am aware that I may have been making some rather glib assumptions; nevertheless it achieved the desired result. Maria became less despondent and we had a base from which to work. Here was a quarter of an ovary which had suffered a lot of trauma and artificial stimulation and had finally decided to stop. However, this one quarter ovary probably still had potential. What remained for us to do was to discover whether or not we could reactivate this potential.

My impression at our first meeting was of an unhappy, overweight woman. Her recent weight gain of 16 kg (35 lbs) started at the same time as the fertility programmes and may have been an effect of the drugs or else was due to an inability to exercise because of the constant, left-sided, abdominal and lower back pains caused by the cysts. Maria claimed however to be very healthy in every respect other than the problem with her ovary. She still managed her job well and never took sick days. Up until the time when she developed the first ovarian cyst her period cycle had been regular and problem free except that she had felt a little edgy before each period.

Summary of clinical manifestations

- Inability to fall pregnant.
- Pain in the lower abdomen, constant and dull but becoming sharp and debilitating with ovulation or exercise.
- Pain in the left lower back, constant, dull and heavy.
- Tendency to produce ovarian cysts.
- History of premenstrual tension.
- Abdomen has marked tenderness on the left.
- Pulse: unremarkable except for weakness in left Kidney position.
- Tongue: thick, yellowish, greasy coat.

Patterns of disharmony

Blood Stagnation: Evidently there is stagnation in the pelvis leading to the pain. Its fairly constant nature, its fixed location and the substantial nature of the cysts indicate that it could be Stagnation of Blood.

Qi **Stagnation:** I assumed some degree of *qi* stagnation concomitant with and in fact probably leading to the Blood stagnation. The early sign of this is the premenstrual edginess.

Phlegm-damp in the lower *jiao*: Her tongue clearly indicated some accumulation of Damp-heat internally. This may have been generated during the time when Maria took many fertility drugs and gained a lot of weight. The dermoid cysts, which

predate this time however, are also evidence of substantial Phlegm-damp obstruction. These cysts are encapsulated by a thick smooth skin and appear wet and shiny. (Mackay et al 1992).

Deficiency of *chong/ren* and Kidney: Since there had been so much intervention to Maria's reproductive system I wondered how damaged the *chong* and *ren* channels were and whether we could re-educate them to function on their own. Her weak Kidney pulse also made me wonder if the fertility drugs had undermined her Kidney function (of controlling the *chong* and *ren*) to the point of damaging it. The dull lower back ache also indicated Kidney weakness.

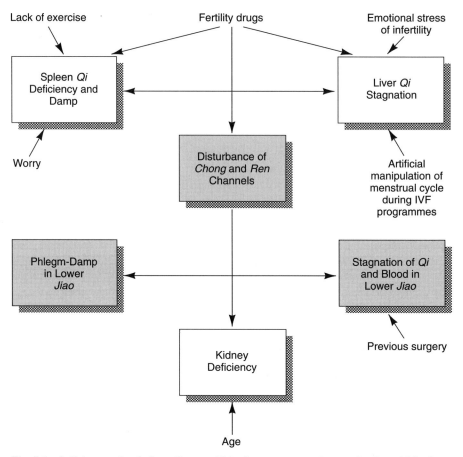

Fig. 8.1 Aetiology and pathology diagram. This diagram summarises a situation which often occurs in women taking part in multiple fertility programmes, especially those involving surgery. The three tinted boxes describe the diagnosis of Maria's infertility, cysts and abdomen pain. These three disorders interact with and generate each other. Each disorder is, in turn, affected by the dysfunction of an organ system viz Kidney, Liver and Spleen, the organs which most commonly figure in gynaecological conditions. Contributing to the imbalance in these organs are factors in Maria's life, such as age, surgery and drugs.

A therapeutic relationship takes shape

At this point I felt reasonably confident of the ability of acupuncture to circulate the *qi* and the Blood in the pelvis to the extent of relieving the pain and preventing the recurrence of future cysts, although the latter might require ongoing treatment for some time at key points in the cycle.

What I was not so sure about was the likelihood of resurrecting the *chong* and the *ren* and recovering full function of the remaining ovarian tissue. However I kept these thoughts to myself. Maria was clearly starting to feel more cheerful and perhaps beginning to place some confidence in me as our therapeutic relationship began to take shape. At this stage, and in a case such as this, establishing trust and confidence is of paramount importance to the development and outcome. As with all cases of infertility I was very careful to be honest, even brutally honest, but also where appropriate to provide some hope . . . and so we began a journey together which would span the next 4 years.

The first treatment

The first time I saw Maria was on Day 12 of her cycle and she had been taking Pergonal (FSH and LH gonadotrophin, a strong ovarian stimulant) for the previous 8 days. This had been withdrawn that very day because her ovaries had clearly not responded and a withdrawal bleed was anticipated in the near future. The first treatment attempted to encourage the movement of *qi* and Blood in the pelvis (to facilitate this bleed, and to start to address the stagnation causing the cysts), to awaken some *chong/ren* function and to soothe the distraught woman.

First treatment procedures

REN7 *yinjiao*, a meeting point of the *chong* and *ren* which regulates these two channels and a point for gathering the *yin*. This is a favourite point of mine often used in infertility cases, especially early in the cycle (Gu Ying Gao, personal communication 1986).

REN4 *guanyuan*, a meeting point of the *ren*, Spleen, Kidney and Liver channels and gate to the Original *qi*. This point strongly tonifies the *qi* of the lower heater and the Kidneys and also helps calm the mind.

SP6 *sanyinjiao*, a meeting point for the Spleen, Liver and Kidneys. This point has very many functions and is employed here to help resolve Damp, to regulate the flow of Liver *qi* in the abdomen, to relieve abdominal pain and to move the Blood and eliminate stagnation.

LI 4 *hegu*. This point was used in conjunction with SP 6 *sanyinjiao* to bring on the withdrawal bleed.

LIV3 *taichong*. This point was used to promote smooth *qi* flow but also to calm the mind, in combination with LI 4 *hegu*, the well known Four Gates.

ST29 *guilai*. This point is the main point for removing Stagnant Blood in the abdomen.

Needling methods: 30 gauge 1.5 cun needles were inserted with pressing finger method. The handle of the needle is grasped firmly in the right hand while the fingers of the left hand press the skin and help guide the needle swiftly through the skin. *Deqi* was obtained and needles were retained (even method) for 20 minutes. ST29 guilai was gently manipulated with reducing method once or twice.

Attempting to normalise the menstrual cycle

The withdrawal bleed began one day after the first treatment and we were then able to concentrate on creating a normal menstrual cycle. Maria thought this was asking a lot since she hadn't had a normal menstrual cycle for such a long time. I too wondered what it would take to resurrect/ cajole the ovary back into functioning normally. However, her abdomen and back pain were much improved already and she was prepared to commit herself for as long as it took.

In the next treatment I used the extra point *zigong* (abdomen), REN7 *yinjiao*, REN3 *zhongji*, SP10 *xuehai*, SP9 *yinlingquan* and LIV5 *ligou*. This was designed to strongly regulate *qi* and Blood and directly target the *chong* and *ren* channels (and ovary). The extra point *zigong* (abdomen) is a point I use frequently when trying to activate or regulate ovary function. Its anatomical position above the ovaries means it is well placed to move *qi* which may be obstructed there. I usually needle it quite deeply at a slightly oblique angle medially and inferiorly (Gao 1986). In addition, extra point *zigong* (abdomen) can be used to tonify and warm original *qi* (Maciocia 1989). Both REN7 *yinjiao* and REN3 *zhongji* are points where the *chong* and the *ren* intersect. Consequently they are appropriate points to use in a case like this when trying to establish a new cycle. This treatment was followed by 3 days of pain in the lower left abdomen and the lower back. It was the sort of pain Maria had experienced sometimes on ovulating.

A stunned and disbelieving Maria

I saw Maria three more times all the while using points to regulate the *qi*, Blood and Phlegm-damp obstruction in the abdomen and to strengthen the Kidneys. The Kidney pulse remained weak, but the tongue coating was gradually becoming less greasy. By now it was 34 days since her withdrawal bleed and although she had had 2 days of dark-coloured spotting there was no sign of a period. Her Kidney pulse quite suddenly felt more solid and slippery. Her tongue however remained less greasy. Something was afoot but it was too soon to say much. Maria came back a week later with still no sign of a period but this didn't surprise her at all. It was so long since she had had a natural cycle. However her pulses were slippery on several positions and I asked her to give a urine sample. We did the pregnancy test in the clinic, Maria still wondering why I was bothering. The jubilation when the positive sign appeared spread around the clinic, with receptionists and doctors all congratulating a stunned and disbelieving Maria.

I put our success down to the combined factors of stimulating a flow of *qi* and Blood through an area where it had been obstructed and calming the mind. Maria dates it back to the first talk we had whereby I convinced her (with my possibly dubious figures) that her one quarter ovary could still do the job. It is rare for me to treat infertility without the use of herbs. However, I had delayed prescribing herbs because of the effectiveness of the acupuncture in removing Maria's abdominal and back pain and also because I was feeling my way in these first few weeks until I knew where we were in the menstrual cycle.

A healthy baby and another pregnancy

Maria had a healthy baby by Caesarean section after going into labour 3 weeks prematurely. This was possibly another sign that the *chong* and *ren* were still not functioning as well as they might. At 2 months Maria stopped breastfeeding and almost immediately her ovarian pain returned. Her Kidney pulse was weak but her tongue was not greasy. Points including extra point *zigong* (abdomen), SP10 *xuehai*, SP6 *sanyinjiao* and REN4 *guanyuan* quickly improved the pain.

When the baby was 4 months old Maria's tongue started to show some very worrying signs. The thick greasy coat returned in a solid puddle in the centre of the tongue while the sides were peeled with deep craggy horizontal cracks extending to the edges. This indicated not only a return of the Damp but also profound Spleen weakness. I advised her to rest more than she was doing and to be extremely careful with her eating habits. Treatments to address this unfortunately seemed to stimulate the ovaries into activity again and Maria had a period soon afterwards. I say unfortunately because within the next month Maria was pregnant again, much to her delight. However, this time it was more difficult for me to share in her delight. I had severe misgivings, not so much for the baby as Maria's Kidney pulse was strong and confident, but for Maria's *qi*, Blood and *jing*. Pregnancy in the late 30s and 40s is particularly draining on the prenatal *jing qi* of the body and Maria was starting this pregnancy with already weakened energy and a baby not yet 6 months old! Nevertheless she survived the pregnancy with the help of some tonic herbs and delivered a healthy baby. She haemorrhaged severely after the birth and developed an infection from retained products. This indicated *ren* and particularly *chong* channel weakness.

A determined quarter ovary

She was happy but quite unwell. She had constant lower back pain, her pulse showed not only pronounced Kidney weakness but also a hollow quality on the Liver and Heart positions. This indicated Blood deficiency after the haemorrhage. Her tongue showed all the Damp and Spleen weakness as before but also damage to the *yin* as it was now darker red and even more peeled. Maria came for treatment whenever she could and we concentrated on tonifying the Kidney energy, the Blood and the *yin*. Her periods returned after 6 months although they were irregular. Her left pulse remained weak and there did not seem to be any substantial improvement to the tongue. I was not altogether surprised given the amount of damage her body had sustained over the previous years with all the surgery, drugs, two pregnancies, two difficult deliveries and two demanding small babies to care for. Maria, however, was symptom free most of the time, as long as we continued to tonify the Kidney and Spleen *qi* and regulate the *qi* in the abdomem — albeit constantly exhausted.

You can imagine my horror when she proudly told me she was pregnant again (against my firmly worded advice) just 12 months after the second baby. This time her Kidney pulse did not firm up quite so convincingly and my fears were compounded when at 24 weeks I found her pulse to be unnaturally wiry. An ultrasound the next day showed that the baby had died. A battery of tests could find no medical reason for the death but it was very clear to me after my long relationship with Maria and my knowledge of her pulse that the Kidneys and the *chong* and *ren* just had no more to give.

Maria recovered reasonably quickly and well. Her periods have just returned at the time of writing (6 months after the induced birth) and she tells me she's thinking of having another baby. 'Just joking' she adds as I waggle my finger and try to look stern. Somehow, however, I don't think we've heard the last of this determined quarter ovary.

REFERENCES

Maciocia G 1989 The foundations of Chinese medicine. Churchill Livingstone, Edinburgh
Mackay et al 1992 Illustrated textbook of gynaecology; W B Saunders, Ballière Tindall

■ Jane Lyttleton

Patients often ask me how I came to be an acupuncturist. I come from a family of scientists and was embroiled in a PhD at the University of London, doing cancer research, when I was seduced by Chinese medicine. I had no personal experience of miracle cures or even observations of such — just a chance encounter and a deep, insistent curiosity. My scepticism was held at arm's length by my intrigue, so much so that eventually I took the risky step of enrolling on a course. This entailed a move to Sydney where courses were being taught not only by 'Van Buren-trained' practitioners but also by doctors recently arrived from China. The course in those days (late 70s, early 80s) was a mish-mash of information thrown together from many disparate sources and there were no textbooks in English. Chinese herbal medicine was being taught by teachers from China who learned the necessary English vocabulary the day before!

My first real experience of acupuncture at work was in Nanjing, China, in 1982 and it was here that Dr Ni (Nanjing College of Traditional Chinese Medicine) kindled the flame that led me to explore the application of Chinese medicine to women's health. The following 4 years saw me working in women's health clinics, finding out how Dr Ni's theory worked with Western women. This was when the ground for all my future work was laid as I found ways in which to apply those unique insights of Chinese medicine to the diseases of women in modern Western society. There followed a trip to the Red Cross Hospital, Hangzhou, China, where Dr Gao pushed both my expectations and eventually my expertise to another quantum level. It was also here that my interest in fertility was kindled, Dr Gao being famous across China for her work in this area.

It was another 6 years before I would return to China, but in that time I practised and practised and practised and learned the rhythms, harmonies and counterpoints of Chinese medicine and women's bodies, minds and tides. The China I revisited was a nightmare of burgeoning capitalism, consumerism and construction. However, in the midst of all this, research in Chinese medicine was forging ahead and I was lucky enough to see at first hand some of the results in fertility clinics there. My understanding and my practice were helped to reach the next quantum level. And from here? I hope there are still many layers and levels to uncover and reach.

Pregnancy, nausea and multiple sclerosis

Bob Flaws BOULDER, CO, USA

About the patient

The patient was a 28-year-old woman whom I had been treating for multiple sclerosis (MS) for 6 months. The multiple sclerosis had started 1.5 years earlier when she had woken to find her left arm numb, her left leg difficult to move due to weakness, and her vision blurred. This initial attack lasted 2 weeks. She then went into remission for 5 months before having a second attack during which she experienced numbness and weakness from the waist down. The numbness had gone away after 3–4 months. Eight months before seeing me for the first time, she had been having problems as she put it, 'off and on'. She suffered from vertigo, which worsened with stress, and lower body numbness. An MD had diagnosed her as suffering from candidiasis and hypoglycaemia, while another MD wanted to extract four molars which she said were related to her central nervous system.

When I first saw the patient she complained of night sweats and hot flushes, nocturia, and premenstrual fibrocystic breasts which were negatively reactive to caffeine and tender before her periods. She also had a persistent abnormal vaginal discharge which had the consistency of mucus and was cloudy in colour. Her menstrual cycle was 5 weeks long with a 7-day flow. It was not clotty, only a little crampy, and was bright red in colour ending somewhat darker. Her face was pale with flushed cheeks and red lips. She said that she was either too cold or too hot. She also said that she had had sinus headaches for many years. Her tongue was red with a scant coating. Her pulses were fine and slippery in her right *cun*, deep, slippery, and forceless in her right *guan*, and deep and slippery in her right *chi*. Her left *cun* was floating and not rooted, her left *guan* was slippery and larger than the right, and her left *chi* was deep, fine, wiry, and a little slippery.

Summary of clinical manifestations	
PRIOR TO PREGNANCY • Numbness and weakness from the waist down.	• Vertigo, worse with stress. • Symptoms are 'on and off'. • Night sweats and hot flushes.

- Nocturia.
- Premenstrual fibrocystic breasts, negatively reactive to caffeine and tender before periods.
- Vaginal discharge: persistent abnormal mucous consistency and cloudy in colour.
- Menstrual cycle 5 weeks long, 7-day flow, crampy, bright red colour ending somewhat darker.
- Face pale, flushed cheeks, red lips.
- Feels either too hot or too cold.
- Sinus headaches.
- Tongue: red, scant coating.

- Pulses: fine slippery in right *cun*; deep slippery and forceless in right *guan*; deep and slippery in right *chi*; floating and not rooted in left *cun*; slippery and larger than the right in left *guan*; deep, fine wiry and a little slippery in left *chi*.

AFTER BECOMING PREGNANT

- Nausea.
- Minor period-like cramps.
- Thirsty.
- Warm and flushed.
- Tongue: bright red.

Disease diagnosis, pattern discrimination

Based on the above signs and symptoms, my disease diagnosis of this patient was *wei zheng* or atony condition and my pattern discrimination was Damp heat with Spleen *qi* vacuity, Liver/Kidney vacuity, and Liver depression. (See the box below, however; the reader is cautioned that this box gives an oversimplification of this complex case which is better understood using the Jin-Yuan Dynasty theories described below.) This combination of Damp heat associated with Spleen vacuity and Liver depression, whereby the Damp heat has damaged the Liver and Kidneys below, is known as *yin* fire. *Yin* fire (*yin huo*) is not the same as vacuity heat (*xue re*). *Yin* fire is a concept that describes a complex interaction of patterns; it is not just Damp heat with Spleen vacuity. According to Li Dong-yuan (1993), originator of the concept of *yin* fire, it can be caused by a combination of the following:

1 Damp heat (whether externally invading or internally engendered).
2 Spleen vacuity (due to overtaxation, excessive worry, thinking, anxiety, and/or improper diet).
3 Depressive heat (due to anger, jealousy, resentment, or internal damage due to the seven passions).
4 Blood vacuity (i.e. *yin* vacuity, due to bedroom taxation, insufficient natural endowment, enduring disease, excessive blood loss, or insufficient engenderment and transformation of *qi* and blood).
5 Stirring of ministerial fire (due to any combination of the above four or any excessive thought, sex, or activity); see Zhu Dan-xi (1994) for a more complete explanation of stirring (*dong*).

Although *yin* fire is created in the middle and lower burners, it may float upwards to accumulate in the Stomach, Lungs, or Heart, in which case it may cause symptoms of counterflow, evil heat, and/or damage to body fluids. In *yin* fire scenarios, counterflow commonly affects the *chong, du,* hand and foot *tai yang, shao yang,* and *yang ming* channels and vessels.

Disease diagnosis and pattern discrimination

PRE-PREGNANCY DISEASE DIAGNOSIS:

Wei zheng (atony condition)

- Numbness and weakness from the waist down.

PRE-PREGNANCY TCM[1] PATTERN DISCRIMINATION

Damp heat

- Vaginal discharge: mucous, cloudy.
- Pulse: slippery.

Spleen *qi* vacuity

- Fatigue.
- Loose stools.
- Pale face.
- Pulse: forceless in right *guan.*

Liver/Kidney vacuity (*yin* and *yang* vacuity)

- Night sweats.
- Dizziness.
- Hot flushes.
- Flushed cheeks.

- Tongue: red, scanty coating.
- Pulse: left *cun* floating and not rooted, left *chi* deep and fine, right *chi* deep, sometimes hot, sometimes cold.

Liver depression

- Premenstrual fibrocystic and tender breasts.[2]
- Pulse: wiry.

POSTNATAL DISEASE DIAGNOSIS:

Ren shen e zu

- Nausea and vomiting during pregnancy.

POSTNATAL TCM PATTERN DISCRIMINATION

Yin vacuity, floating yang

- Severe nausea.
- Scarlet red tongue with scant coating.
- Flushed face.
- Flushed warm feeling.
- Dizziness.
- Low back pain.
- Pulse: surging.

The disease causes and disease mechanisms in this case are illustrated in Figure 9.1. In my experience, *yin* fire is a common pattern associated with chronic, recalcitrant, and complex diseases such as MS, rheumatoid arthritis, myalgic encephalopathy (what in the US is referred to as chronic fatigue syndrome and fibromyalgia), polysystemic chronic candidiasis, allergies, chronic sinusitis, AIDS, and cancer. These are called difficult, knotty diseases in Chinese (*nan jie bing*). I have found a good understanding of this concept of *yin* fire to be vitally important in my diagnosis and treatment of such diseases.

Based on this diagnosis, I prescribed Chinese herbal medicine, to be taken internally, mainly based on the principles of boosting the *qi* and fortifying the Spleen, supplementing the Liver and Kidneys, and clearing

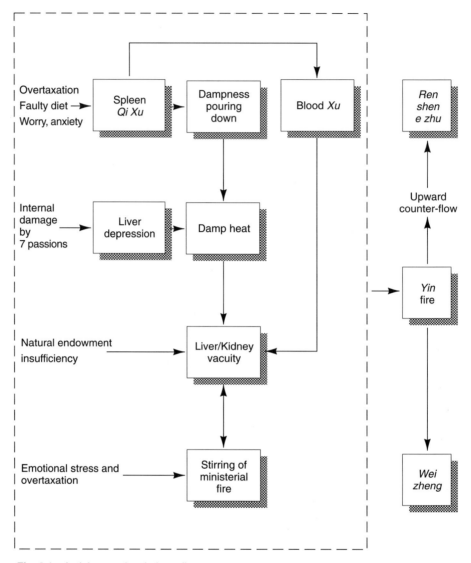

Fig. 9.1 Aetiology and pathology diagram.

heat and eliminating dampness. During the 5 months in which my patient took various combinations of medicinals based on these principles, she experienced some bouts of numbness, dizziness, fatigue, and weakness as well as loose stools and urinary hesitancy. However, these bouts did not last long and appeared to respond well to the Chinese medicinals, clearing up without any residual symptoms. In addition to taking these medicinals, I advised the patient to maintain her sugar-free diet and also to avoid foods made through fermentation (such as vinegar, alcohol, cheese, and risen bread) or which mould easily (oranges, strawberries, melons).

Acupuncture for morning sickness

After 5 months of treatment with internally administered Chinese medicinal decoctions, the patient became pregnant. As is typical of multiple sclerosis, all the signs and symptoms of that disease completely disappeared with the onset of pregnancy and the patient felt full of energy. However, she became nauseous almost immediately. Her stools were well-formed and her urination was not inhibited. According to Song & Yu (1984), *ren shen e zu* or nausea and vomiting during pregnancy can be due to any of four main mechanisms:

1 Liver *qi* upward counterflow;
2 Stomach fire upward surging (*chong*);
3 *Yin* vacuity/floating *yang*, and/or
4 Spleen/Stomach vacuity weakness.

The reader will note the close association of these four mechanisms with Li Dong-yuan's five mechanisms of *yin* fire described previously (Li Dong-yuan 1993). Upon examination of my patient for signs and symptoms of morning sickness these primarily grouped themselves into pattern number 3, i.e. *yin* vacuity/floating *yang*. These were, in order of importance to me, a scarlet red tongue with scanty coating, flushed face, a flushed warm feeling, dizziness, and low back pain.

Her pulse also accorded with this pattern discrimination, although it did not match Song & Yu's suggested pulse images. According to Song & Yu (1984), the pulse images associated with this pattern are vacuous and weak or fine and rapid. This woman's pulses were slippery, rapid, and floating, i.e. surging, especially in her inch or *cun* positions. This discrepancy highlights the fact that, in patients with *yin* fire, the pulse is often not what is given in beginners' textbooks. This is because this condition cannot simply be pigeon-holed as a single pattern.

Having diagnosed vomiting and nausea during pregnancy mainly exhibiting the pattern of *yin* vacuity, I prescribed Engender the Pulse Powder *Sheng Mai San* combined with Increase Humours Decoction *Zeng Ye Tang* with other additional medicinals to help protect the fetus (*bao tai*) since, besides the nausea, the patient was experiencing some minor, period-like cramps.

The patient was able to take these medicinals and the nausea improved for a day or so. She also reported that constant eating helped the nausea which is, in my experience, especially typical of *yin* vacuity nausea and vomiting during pregnancy. Therefore, for the next week I continued giving the patient essentially the same combination of Chinese medicinals. However, after a little more than a week, she became extremely nauseous, feeling better for a while when she drank the decoction. The patient also reported being very thirsty. Her tongue was bright red and she said she felt warm and flushed. Again I continued prescribing similar Chinese medicinals but I also suggested that she receive an acupuncture treatment solely for the morning sickness. Therefore, in order simply to harmonise the Stomach, I needled ST36 *zusanli*, REN12 *zhongwan* and P6 *neiguan*, see below. These points were each needled with passive retention for 30 minutes. I did not attempt to obtain the *qi* in a modern Chinese manner nor did I employ any specific hand techniques. The points used were chosen for their ability to rectify the *qi*, harmonise the Stomach, downbear counterflow, and stop nausea or vomiting.

Treatment procedures

FIRST PRESCRIPTION OF POINTS

The following combination of points is a standard combination for the treatment of all types of nausea and vomiting. Depending upon the root cause of the nausea, other auxiliary points are added 'following the pattern *(sui zheng)'*. In this case I used:

- ST36 *zusanli* which fortifies the Spleen, downbears counterflow, and harmonises the Spleen and Stomach.
- P6 *neiguan* which rectifies the *qi*, downbears counterflow, harmonises the Stomach, and stops vomiting.
- REN12 *zhongwan* which harmonises the Stomach *qi* and facilitates the upbearing of the clear and the downbearing of the turbid.

Needle Technique

Each point was first disinfected with a 75% solution of isopropyl alcohol. The points were located by a combination of measurement and palpation. Needles were inserted in each point using a two-handed insertion technique, no tube. ST36 *zusanli* was needled to 0.75 *cun* in depth, P6 *neiguan* was needled to 0.5 *cun* in depth, and REN12 *zhongwan* was needled to 0.75 *cun* in depth. The needles were not manipulated once in place but were left passively for 30–45 minutes per treatment.

Needles

CW Brand Korean needles, 34 gauge, 1.2 *cun* in length

Long passive retention

My long passive needle retention in the treatment of nausea and vomiting during pregnancy is based on teachings I received at the Shanghai College of TCM and on my own clinical experience. As far as I know, it is based on empirical evidence, not on TCM theory.

After the first acupuncture treatment my patient reported that she had experienced more relief from morning sickness than she had when she simply took the decocted medicinals. Although the decocted medicinals took away the nausea temporarily, it always came back but she had been less nauseous for longer with acupuncture. As a TCM gynaecology specialist, the main therapeutic modality that I use is internally administered Chinese medicinals, and this is the norm in TCM gynaecology. I only use acupuncture in conjunction with internally administered Chinese medicinals if there is a secondary condition which requires immediate treatment to relieve symptoms. In my clinic this includes severe morning sickness, severe dysmenorrhea, menstrual or menopausal migraines, acute pelvic inflammatory disease, acute ovarian cystitis, severe premenstrual breast pain, etc.

Therefore, based on my patient's positive response to the first acupuncture treatment, i.e. her nausea was relieved, I treated her with acupuncture every single day during the week and one day at weekends. My patient's condition was primarily due to a Kidney *yin* vacuity affecting Stomach fluids and, therefore, causing Stomach disharmony and counterflow. With this in mind I needled the points KID3 *taixi* and BL23 *shenshu* in addition to the three points already mentioned. Thus the total combination of points supplemented the Kidneys and enriched *yin* as well as rectifying the *qi* and harmonising the Stomach. I also changed my patient's Chinese herbal formula. Previously she had received primarily Stomach fluid-engendering medicinals and now I prescribed Kidney *yin*-supplementing and enriching medicinals augmented by Stomach fluid-engendering medicinals. Her main formula now was Six Flavour Rehmannia Pills *liu wei di huang wan* with added flavours. Since the patient experienced some lower back pain, ingredients were added to strengthen the lower back and protect the fetus.

We continued this regime for 2 months, using both Chinese medicinals in decoction and daily acupuncture or acupuncture every other day. When the daily nausea ceased, we stopped the acupuncture and relied solely on the Chinese medicinals in decoction. The patient took Chinese medicinals throughout her pregnancy and gave birth to a healthy baby girl without complications. Two months after giving birth, she again had an MS attack with weakness and numbness on the left side and fatigue. According to the patient's Western medical information, the first 3 months after delivery are the most dangerous time for an MS attack. We immediately increased the doses of her *qi*-supplementing and *yin*-enriching medicinals and her attack diminished extremely rapidly.

Outcome of acupuncture treatment

Since the case was specifically about the TCM acupuncture treatment of nausea and vomiting during pregnancy (*ren shen e zu*), there is one relevant outcome: reduced nausea during pregnancy.

Clarification of acupuncture treatment of nausea during pregnancy

Based on a review of the Chinese TCM literature, morning sickness during pregnancy can be associated with any of several patterns, including simple Stomach disharmony, Spleen vacuity, accumulation of phlegm and dampness, Liver depression/*qi* stagnation, depressive heat, Stomach *yin* vacuity, and Kidney *yin* vacuity. In my experience, those women exhibiting the Kidney *yin* vacuity pattern tend to have the most recalcitrant and difficult-to-treat type of morning sickness. I treat most cases of morning sickness without recourse to acupuncture, internally administered Chinese medicinals alone working satisfactorily. However, in *yin* vacuity cases, either there is such severe nausea that the *yin*-supplementing medicinals cannot be 'stomached' at all or else, as in this case, medicinals were not immediately potent enough.

In such cases of severe nausea during pregnancy, frequent treatment is essential. Once weekly treatment is almost useless in such persistent and recalcitrant cases. Therefore, I believe it is imperative to needle daily or even twice daily. In addition, although it is often believed that long needle retention is a draining technique, I frequently leave needles in patients suffering from severe *yin* vacuity morning sickness for up to 1 hour per treatment with excellent results.

One other point of clarification: it is also generally believed that acupuncture of ST36 *zusanli* is forbidden during pregnancy. My gynaecological experience, spanning 15 years, suggests to me that this point is only forbidden if it is not specifically needed to treat a particular condition. In such cases, it is both safe and necessary. However, the reader will note that I did not use SP6 *sanyinjiao* even though this point is typically included in formulae designed to enrich *yin*. Instead, I chose KID3 *taixi* which also enriches *yin* but without any chance of *cui chan* or hastening delivery. While recently retranslating Song & Yu, I noted that they say that 'reckless' acupuncture and moxibustion are prohibited during pregnancy. I believe that this means both unnecessary acupuncture/moxibustion in general and the reckless or unnecessary use of points traditionally described as forbidden during pregnancy in particular. In other words, if their use is indicated, they may and in some cases even must be used.

Nausea, vomiting during pregnancy and *yin* fire

Nausea and vomiting during pregnancy occur because the cessation of menstruation causes a repletion and thus temporary counterflow in the *chong mai*/sea of blood. The *chong mai*'s connection to the Spleen, Stomach, Liver and Kidneys, means that symptoms of so-called morning sickness are usually grouped into patterns associated with these viscera and bowels depending upon which signs and symptoms are most prominent. However, *yin* fire is intimately associated with the *chong mai* as Li Dong-yuan (1993) & Zhu Dan-xi (1993) explain and, in particular with counterflow affecting the *chong mai* and the channels and vessels with which it connects. Thus women with *yin* fire often have trouble with morning sickness, as did this woman. In other words, her *yin* fire scenario had already predisposed her to counterflow of the *chong mai* with floating *yang* and vacuous *yin* above.

Pregnancy, *yin* vacuity, morning sickness and MS remission

Liver/Kidney vacuity in this case is not just *yin* vacuity. There is *yang* vacuity as well. Therefore, Liver/Kidney vacuity here means Liver/Kidney *yin* and *yang* vacuity or Liver Blood/Kidney *yang* vacuity. Li Dongyuan is very clear when he says that damp heat pouring down from the middle burner to the lower burner can damage the Liver and Kidneys, resulting in *yang* losing its root in its lower origin. Thus *yang* floats upward, potentially affecting any of the viscera or bowels which participate in the larger notion of lifegate fire, i.e. the Liver, Gallbladder, Stomach, Spleen, Pericardium, and Triple Burner. At the same time, *yang* is left vacuous below. In my experience, often and maybe even typically, such *yang* vacuity signs and symptoms are obscured by the other signs and symptoms of *yin* fire. They may be reduced simply to cold feet or, as in this case, to sometimes feeling cold and sometimes feeling hot.

If we posit both *yin* and *yang* vacuity we explain both the *yin* vacuity/floating *yang* nausea and vomiting during pregnancy and, once the morning sickness has abated, the complete remission of the patient's MS symptoms. In TCM there is a saying, 'No vacuity during pregnancy, no repletion postpartum'. During pregnancy, most women experience a growth in *yang qi*. This is intimately associated with morning sickness which occurs as long as this growth and accumulation of *yang qi* causes or aggravates counterflow. The explanation of *yang* growth during pregnancy is based on the same mechanism as the rise in basal body temperature at ovulation. *Yin* is retained in the lower burner, and out of this accumulating *yin*, exuberant *yang* is transformed. I believe that this growth of *yang qi* is directly related to the typical remission of MS. This is because MS is due to a combination of Spleen vacuity, Damp heat, and Liver/Kidney vacuity (Liver/Kidney *yin* and *yang* vacuity). In addition, counterflowing heat due to damp heat below and floating *yang* often affect the Lungs, also participating in the causation of *wei zheng*. As the fetus grows, not only does *yang* grow, but *yin* accumulated in the lower burner/uterus helps to root this *yang* in its lower origin.

Thus this heat, once counterflow is reversed, does not damage the Spleen or the Lungs. Free from heat floating upward and damaging the source *qi*, the Spleen makes sufficient Blood to nourish the sinews and sufficient *qi* to empower the limbs. While the Lungs, free from heat floating upward and damaging its *qi*, diffuse the *qi* to the body. This then ensures empowerment of the limbs whilst spreading fluids and humours to moisten the joints and sinews and wash away phlegm obstruction. Hence, *wei zheng* or atony remits during pregnancy, when seemingly we might expect it to get worse, since pregnancy does place extra demands on *yin* essence. In my opinion, the key to understanding this otherwise seemingly contradictory situation is that there is *yang* vacuity hidden below the more obvious signs and symptoms of *yin* vacuity.

NOTES

1   When I use the term TCM or Traditional Chinese Medicine as in the above case history and its discussion, I am using it as the proper name of a specific style of Chinese medicine. In Chinese, the words are simply *zhong yi*, Chinese medicine. However, Chinese medicine can mean either all traditional medical practices ever practised in China or it can mean, as I am using it here, that specific style of Chinese medicine taught at the provincial colleges of Chinese medicine in the People's Republic of China which emphasises treatment on the basis of pattern discrimination (*bian zheng lun zhi*). This is a rational style of medicine which follows a step-by-step progression from information collected by the four examinations to the discrimination of patterns, to the statement of treatment principles and thence to the erection of a treatment plan based on those stated principles. This style is founded on the Confucian medical literary tradition and emphasises Chinese herbal medicine, with acupuncture/moxibustion and Chinese remedial massage (*tui na*) being adjunctive modalities.

As an extension of this, I have deliberately written my case history in the way that case histories are written and published in the People's Republic of China. In comparison to many of the other case histories appearing in this book, my case may seem devoid of the human touch. I did not say that the patient was blonde-haired and blue-eyed. I did not say that she was very pleasant nor that she was Norwegian-American and that she had married a Frenchman she had met at the University of Trondheim. This is because all this information is extraneous to making a proper TCM pattern discrimination. In a well written Chinese TCM case history, everything that is mentioned is mentioned in order to substantiate the final diagnosis and treatment. Since none of the above information is germane to making the pattern discrimination I reached in this case it is not included.

It is my experience as a practitioner and teacher of the TCM style of Chinese medicine that Western practitioners attempting to practise this style have a hard time making it work in clinical practice. This is in large part because the internal logic and step-by-step methodology is often lost in English language translation. TCM patterns are only defined by certain signs and symptoms which unfortunately are often not correctly translated. Thus, often, Western practitioners are not asking the correct questions of our patients. Further, Western patients typically present with unusual conditions or complicated conditions, the so-called difficult, knotty diseases mentioned earlier. Therefore, pattern discrimination is often quite complicated — much more complicated than beginners' textbooks suggest.

TCM as a style can describe such complicated patients and can offer great relief based on that description. However, in making such complicated pattern discriminations, it is necessary to process the patient's complaints according to TCM's step-by-step methodology. It is my experience that Westerners all too often get bogged down in collecting and thinking about extraneous information about our patients — at least extraneous from the point of view of TCM. In my own experience, the more clearly focused I am about exactly what information to use when deducing my TCM equation about the patient's pattern discrimination, the more accurate my diagnosis. As an extension of that, the more accurate my diagnosis, usually the better my treatment and its results.

This does not mean that I and my patients may not have a jolly time together or that we do not form bonds of strong friendship and empathy. However, when thinking and writing about my patients, everything I have mentioned is meant to be taken as a clue in a Sherlock Holmes mystery. Everything should tie together and there should be no loose ends. Quite frankly, for me that is the challenging and intellectually interesting thing about doing TCM as a style. What I am getting at here is that I have written my case history in a deliberately focused way. Although there is a time for right-brain intuition, precision always requires a narrowing of focus which in turn means leaving out extraneous information.

2   However, this is overly simplistic since the fibrocystic breasts in this case have to do with the *chong mai* and a wiry pulse can be associated with vacuity. In fact, coursing the Liver and rectifying the *qi* alone will not remedy this woman's breast disease but could actually aggravate it.

REFERENCES

Li Dong-yuan 1993 Treatise on the Spleen and Stomach. Translated by Yang Shou-zhong & Li Jian-yong, Blue Poppy Press, Boulder
Song Guang-ji, Yu Xiao-zhen 1984 Zhong Yi Fu Ke Shou Ce (A handbook of traditional Chinese gynaecology), 4th edn. Zhejiang Science and Technology Press, Hangzhou; English translation by Zhang Ting-liang & Bob Flaws 1995. Blue Poppy Press, Boulder
Zhu Dan-xi 1993 The Heart and essence of Dan-xi's methods of treatment, 'atony'. Translated by Yang Shou-zhong, Blue Poppy Press, Boulder pp 291–295
Zhu Dan-xi 1994 Extra treatises based on investigation and inquiry. Translated by Yang Shou-zhong, Blue Poppy Press, Boulder

FURTHER READING

Blackwell R, MacPherson H 1994 La sclerose en plaques (multiple sclerosis). Medicine Chinoise & Medicines Orientales, Vitre 9: 37–50
Cheng Xin-nong (ed) 1987 Chinese acupuncture and moxibustion, 'Wei Syndrome'. Foreign Languages Press, Beijing pp 442–445
Flaws B 1988 Filling the gaps in the Chinese literature on the diagnosis and treatment of morning sickness. Blue Poppy Press, Boulder pp 207–231
Fu Qing-zhu 1992 Fu Qing-zhu's gynaecology. Translated by Yang Shou-zhong & Liu Da-wei. Blue Poppy Press, Boulder
Flaws B 1993 Path of pregnancy, Vol. I: A handbook of traditional Chinese gestational and birthing diseases. Blue Poppy Press, Boulder

Flaws B 1994 Statements of fact in traditional Chinese medicine. Blue Poppy Press, Boulder

Flaws B 1994 Sticking to the point: a rational methodology for the step by step formulation and administration of a TCM acupuncture treatment, 2nd edn. Blue Poppy Press, Boulder

Hua Tuo 1993 Classic of the central viscera. Tranlated by Yang Shou-zhong. Blue Poppy Press, Boulder

Wiseman N, Boss K 1990 A glossary of Chinese medical terms and acupuncture points. Paradigm Publications, Brookline

■ Bob Flaws

Bob Flaws, DiplAc, DiplCH, FNAAOM, is one of the leading Western authorities on TCM gynaecology. He is author or translator of a dozen books on this subject as well as scores of articles published in professional journals all over the world. In all, since 1981, he has written, translated, or edited more than 50 books on all aspects of Chinese medicine. In the meantime, he conducts a private practice in Boulder, Colorado, USA where he has specialised in TCM gynaecology for the last 16 years. In addition, Bob is founder of Blue Poppy Press, cofounder and past president of the Acupuncture Association of Colorado, cofounder of the Council of Oriental Medical Publishers, and editor of the Journal of the National Academy of Acupuncture & Oriental Medicine. Bob teaches postgraduate certification courses in TCM gynaecology at the Anglo-Dutch Institute of Acupuncture & Oriental Medicine in Harlem, Netherlands and in Boulder, Colorado, USA through the Blue Poppy Press.

Depression and fatigue after giving birth

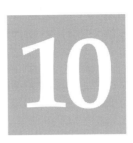

Arne Kausland TRONDHEIM, NORWAY

Mary, a single parent

Mary, who was 28 years old, came to my clinic at the end of the summer, about 7 months after she had given birth to her child. She was quite strongly built and had a pale complexion. She was not very talkative and I could sense that she was a little sceptical and suspicious of me. This lack of confidence in health professionals stemmed from some disagreement she had had with the medical establishment regarding her child. She was a single mother with one child, and the relationship with the child's father had dissolved at the time of the child's birth. Mary had been unemployed for the last 3 years and before that had worked in an office.

Mary's main complaint was depression, which had started after the birth of her child. However, the background to this problem presented a more complex story including a tough pregnancy involving feelings of hopelessness and anxiety, and a past history with a lot of depression. The pregnancy had been a difficult time for Mary, full of worry and fear, mainly because the fetus had heart failure and there was a high risk that it might not survive.

When I asked Mary to try to tell me how she experienced her depression, she said that she felt down and that everything was heavy. She had withdrawn from social relationships; she also felt some anxiety and she was thinking and worrying a lot. She had what she described as 'unclear contact with the world or society'. In addition, she was often irritable and very angry. Some of the anger was directed towards doctors in general and this stemmed from her disappointment in the treatment she had received during the birth of her child.

She felt very lonely, and she experienced the world as being grey and dull. Her vision was less clear than normal. She lacked initiative and had difficulty starting any activity. She had been extremely tired and exhausted after she gave birth and she was forgetful and often felt absent-minded. Her sleep was difficult and she dreamt a lot; these were not unpleasant dreams and were very often about houses and flats. She suffered from a light and diffuse headache, nausea, some dizziness and had a tendency to feel cold.

Bleeding after the birth

Further questioning revealed that she had bled for 5 weeks after the birth, and I began to think that this was possibly a key piece of information. Although she had a previous history of difficulties, her condition had deteriorated after giving birth to her baby.

Mary conveyed an impression of being in a difficult social and psychological situation with depression, fatigue, irritation and anger, but she also had faith in the possibility of change.

I asked her to show me her tongue. Large parts of it lacked the normal fur, especially on the front and partly on the sides, as if the fur had been peeled off. In the centre there was an area with rather too much pasty fur.

She had previously seen a reflexologist, a homeopath, a psychologist and her GP. A chiropractor was taking care of her back and pelvic pain. I advised Mary to try to improve her relationship with her GP, because she would need his help and advice in the future, especially for her child. In addition, I advised her to consult her psychologist again, once she had received some treatment by acupuncture and possibly also Chinese herbs, because I thought this would help her to benefit more from psychological counselling.

Furthermore, I advised her to increase both her activity and social relationships and to broaden her social sphere which had decreased after the birth. I felt I had gained her confidence by trying to understand her story and by explaining it to her in terms of Chinese medicine. Perhaps this made it possible for her to listen seriously to my advice.

After the consultation I felt that I had most of the information I needed in order to make a diagnosis and decide upon a treatment strategy.

Summary of clinical manifestations

- Depression after giving birth.
- Depression, both before and during the pregnancy.
- Feels low, everything is heavy.
- Withdrawing from social relations, strong feeling of loneliness.
- Thinking and worrying a lot and some anxiety.
- 'Unclear contact with the world' and unclear vision.
- World experienced as being grey and dull.
- Absent-minded and forgetful.
- Sleep difficulties and insomnia.
- Dreaming a lot; not unpleasant dreams (about houses and flats).
- Lack of initiative, difficulty in starting any activity.
- Tiredness, exhausted after the birth.
- Often irritated and often very angry.
- Some uneasiness.
- Light and diffuse headache and some dizziness.
- Tendency to feel cold.

- Backache and pelvic pain (after the birth).
- Rheumatic pain in the hands and feet.
- Nausea.

- Tongue: slightly pale, peeled patches, especially on the front and sides, with pasty, slightly yellow fur in the centre.
- Pulse: slow, wiry and slippery.

Identifying the patterns of disharmony

There are many signs and symptoms indicating that the Liver and the Blood are strongly involved in the disharmony of this patient. In Chinese medicine the emotional, psychological and existential aspects of a person are inseparable from the Fundamental Substances and the Organ systems. One of these psycho-existential aspects is called the *hun* and is commonly translated as Soul.[1] Mary has many signs and symptoms indicating that the Liver system is lacking Blood, which again makes the Soul (*hun*) unstable. It is said that only when the Liver Blood is abundant will the Soul (*hun*) be 'stored' soundly and thereby contribute fully to the person's psychological activities. For example, Mary's experience of the world as being dull and grey is a symptom of Liver Blood *xu*. Her unclear vision is a symptom of the *hun* lacking nourishment because the *hun* has a close relationship with the eyes.

Evidence for the patterns of disharmony

PRIMARY PATTERNS

Liver Blood *xu*

- Dizziness.
- The world experienced as being grey and dull.
- 'Unclear contact with the world'.
- Unclear vision.
- Light and diffuse headache.
- Insomnia.
- Dreaming a lot.
- Tongue: slightly pale (and peeled).

Heart Blood *xu*

- Forgetfulness.
- Insomnia.
- Dizziness.

SECONDARY PATTERNS

Lack of nourishment to the *hun*

- 'Unclear contact with the world'.
- Insomnia.
- Dreaming a lot.
- Absent-minded.
- The world is experienced as being grey and dull.
- Unclear vision.

Lack of nourishment to the *shen*

- Depression and mental exhaustion.
- Pale complexion.
- Insomnia.
- Mild anxiety.
- Poor memory.
- Forgetfulness.

ADDITIONAL PATTERNS

Liver *yang* rising

- Irritation.
- A lot of anger.
- Pulse: wiry.

Kidney *yin xu*

- Back ache.
- Dizziness.
- Unclear vision.
- Tongue: peeled.

Spleen *xu* with Phlegm

- Nausea.
- Tiredness.
- Pale complexion.
- Tongue: slightly pale and pasty fur in the centre.
- Pulse: slippery.

Kidney *yang xu*

- Back ache.
- Tendency to feel cold.
- Lack of initiative.
- Depression.
- Pale complexion.

Aetiology and pathology

When pregnant, a woman draws power and potential from her stored reservoirs of *qi*, Blood and *jing* in order to nourish the fetus. This, in particular, depletes the Kidneys. Mary's 5-week bleed after the birth, together with the effects of the pregnancy and the birth, directly caused Liver Blood *xu*. In addition, Mary's irritation and anger were contributing factors, causing the Liver *qi* to burst out of control and generate Liver *yang* rising. Poor eating habits also weakened the Spleen *qi* and led to the presence of Phlegm, indicated by the pasty fur in the centre of the tongue. The Phlegm, in turn, was possibly misting the Mind (*shen*) and contributing to the mental symptoms.

The diagram shown in Figure 10.1 illustrates the interrelationships of the patterns of disharmony. It demonstrates the central position of Liver Blood *xu* and the way in which the bleeding, pregnancy and birth influenced several *zang* and caused several patterns of disharmony additional to Liver Blood *xu*.

Treatment principles

After identifying the patterns of disharmonies and making an analysis and conclusion, I had now to decide which treatment principles would correct the disharmonies. I believed that the primary treatment principle was to nourish the Liver Blood. The Soul (*hun*) and the Mind (*shen*) would thus also be nourished, and the Soul (*hun*) would be stabilised.

A secondary principle was to strengthen the Kidneys and Spleen. This would reinforce the primary treatment principle, as the *jing* and the Blood

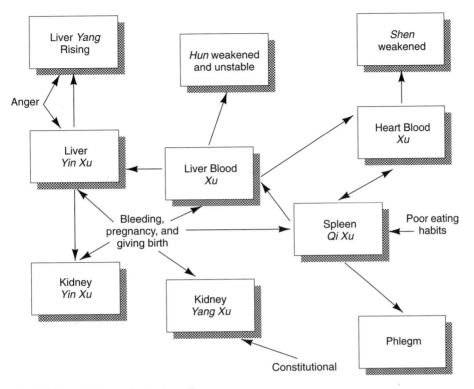

Fig. 10.1 Aetiology and pathology diagram.

have the Spleen and the Kidneys as their source. Strengthening the Spleen would dissolve the Phlegm.

Another secondary principle was to harmonise the Liver which would also help to stabilise the Soul (*hun*) and harmonise the emotions.

Treatment plan

The main purpose was to strengthen the Liver Blood. I expected some improvement after between 7–15 treatments, starting twice weekly, and then anticipated the need for further but less frequent treatment. In addition, I planned to use Chinese herbal medicine to strengthen and to nourish, and this meant that fewer acupuncture treatments would be required. Mary understood that improvement would take some time.

I told her that her psychological aspects were deprived of nourishment according to Chinese medicine, and that it was important to nourish the Soul if her condition was to improve. The treatment, when underway, would enable her to benefit more from consultations with her psychologist, whom she agreed she would consult a second time.

I suggested that she broadened her social sphere and increased her outdoor activity and that this should be done gradually, over time, as she gained strength from each treatment. After a few treatment sessions, I intended to ask Mary about her eating habits and to advise her on diet; good and regular eating habits help to strengthen the *qi* and the Blood.

The first treatment

The time came for the first needles. I would insert only two needles in the first treatment, one on the left forearm and the other on the right leg. In the first treatment I generally use very few needles and leave them in place for a shorter time than the standard 20 minutes. This procedure adjusts the patients to a new form of treatment and prevents or diminishes needle anxiety. I asked Mary to take a deep breath as I inserted the needles so that her full attention would not be on the process of needle insertion. Once the needles were in place I informed Mary that I would stimulate them and that she would feel some distension or soreness, possibly even numbness or heaviness. She was informed that the needle on the forearm was intended to provide peace of mind and that the one on the leg aimed to nourish and give strength. I told her that in the next treatment I would use an additional four needles on her back and would leave them in place for 20 minutes.

Procedures for early treatments

POINTS

- P5 *jianshi* to calm the Mind and open the orifices blocked by Phlegm.
- SP6 *sanyinjiao* and BL42 *hunmen* were used together to nourish Liver Blood and stabilise the *hun*.
- BL23 *shenshu* to nourish the Kidneys and supplement SP6 *sanyinjiao* and BL42 *hunmen*.
- BL18 *ganshu* to stabilise the *hun* and harmonise the Liver.

In the first treatment, only P5 *jianshi* and SP6 *sanyinjiao* were used, one on each side of the body. In the next treatment, BL47 *hunmen* and BL23 *shenshu* were added. Later BL18 *ganshu* was used instead of or in addition to BL23 *shenshu*, and P5

jianshi was substituted with P6 *neiguan*. After a few treatments, BL20 *pishu* was used, as was KID3 *taixi*.

Needling technique: Even method was used on P5 *jianshi*, P6 *neiguan* and BL18 *ganshu*. Reinforcing method was used on SP6 *sanyinjiao*, BL42 *hunmen*, BL23 *shenshu* and BL20 *pishu*. The rotation technique was applied on SP6 *sanyinjiao* and was combined with the lift and thrust method.

Needles: All the needles were 40 mm long and the thickness was 30–32 gauge (0.30 mm). The needles were retained for only 10 minutes in the first treatment, and 20 minutes in the following treatments.

CHINESE HERBAL MEDICINE

After a few treatments, I prescribed *dang gui wan,* a pill comprising Chinese angelica root. Later (after nine treatments), I prescribed a second herbal medicine, a decoction based on Sour Jujube Decoction *suan zao ren tang* and Eight Treasure Decoction *ba zhen tang.*

Some very good days

Mary seemed to have confidence in the treatment, but was not very informative at the beginning. She did not have a baby-sitter and so she brought her child with her, who was happy to be cared for by my secretary. I thought Mary's case was a difficult one because of the need for long-term treatment and because of her previous history. So I hoped that she would have the perseverance to stay in treatment long enough for some strength and inner calmness to manifest themselves. During the first 3 weeks (six treatments) she said that she had had several good days and that the nausea had reduced. During the next 2 weeks the nausea disappeared, although she was still tired (understandable given she was a single parent), and she was still often angry. Generally she felt better, but she tired easily. After a few more treatments she felt quite well and said that she had had some very good days. At this time I prescribed a decoction of Chinese herbal medicine, based on the same rationale as the acupuncture point prescription, i.e. to nourish and harmonise the Soul.

Nearly 2 months after the first consultation, Mary said that she was angry less often, felt some inner calmness and that she experienced headaches only when she had not had enough sleep. She had fewer problems with her sleep patterns and she had increased her social activity. I was not satisfied with the tongue which was still 'peeled', except in the centre where there was pasty fur. However, during the next 2 weeks the tongue changed quite dramatically: the pasty fur disappeared and the coat returned on the previously 'peeled' area. In the meantime, she had just started on a new Chinese medical decoction which concentrated more on strengthening the *yin* and eliminating the Phlegm.

Achieving the primary strategy

Three months and 16 treatments after the first consultation, Mary was stronger and her complexion was less dull and pale. She had increased her social activity and had agreed to ask for more help from parents and friends. She had also consulted her psychologist again and felt that she was benefiting more in this respect.

I interpreted the situation as an improvement in the *yin* and the Liver Blood, as evidenced by the improvement of the tongue and by Mary's healthier complexion. The strengthening and nourishing of her Soul and Mind also meant that she experienced less depression. Much of the primary strategy had been achieved, and I told Mary that we should now attend to the underlying condition which had existed before her pregnancy. I thought that we should consolidate her improvement at this stage and then wait for some time before undertaking further treatments.

Summary of outcome

- Better mood, less depressed.
- Nausea nearly disappeared.
- Less tired.
- Less angry.
- More inner calmness.
- Fewer headaches.
- Improved sleep.
- More glow/shine in the complexion.

- Increased outdoor activity, walking outdoors nearly every day with the child in the pram.
- Benefiting more from consultations with her psychologist than she had prior to the acupuncture treatment.
- Tongue: had improved: no longer peeled and no longer pasty in the centre.

A psycho-existential approach

This case incorporates the traditional Chinese theory of psycho-existential aspects which is important in our post-Freudian times. Perhaps one day the modern research on neuropeptides will prove the links between the emotions and the organ-systems and will establish the reliability of the theory of traditional Chinese medicine. In this case, however, where the theory matched the clinical situation, the use of needles was clearly appropriate in dealing with Mary's psychological problems.

NOTE

1   The five psycho-existential aspects are the *hun* (Soul), *po, yi, zhi, and shen* (Mind).

FURTHER READING

Maciocia G 1994 The practice of Chinese medicine. Churchill Livingstone, Edinburgh

Cheng Zhi-qing 1988 Comments on the *hun* and *po*, Blue Poppy Essays, Blue Poppy Press, Colorado

Liu Yanchi 1988 The essential book of traditional Chinese medicine. Vol. 1, Columbia University Press, New York

■ Arne Kausland

Arne Kausland BAc (England), NFKA (Norwegian Acupuncture Association), practises acupuncture and Chinese herbal medicine in Trondheim, Norway. He studied acupuncture full-time at the International College of Oriental Medicine (ICOM) in England (1978–81), and Chinese herbal medicine part-time at the Ted Kaptchuk seminars in London (1986–88). He has visited China several times for clinical training in acupuncture and Chinese medicine at the Jiangsu Provincial Hospital in Nanjing. Since 1981, he has run an acupuncture clinic in Trondheim, Norway. From 1983–85, he lectured in acupuncture at the Oslo branch of the ICOM. Since 1985 he has lectured at the Norwegian Acupuncture College (Norsk Akupunkturskole) and has been a member of the Executive Committee of the Norwegian Acupuncture Association (NFKA).

A case of postpartum complications?

Stephen Birch WALTHAM, MA, USA

Referral from a therapist

Margaret S was a 44-year-old married woman with two teenage sons. Her husband was a successful lawyer, and she, until recently, had worked as a registered nurse in the neurology department of one of the large Harvard teaching hospitals. She had had to stop working because of her health and had become a full time mother, which she thoroughly enjoyed.

Margaret had been referred to me by a therapist friend, who had painted a glowing picture of what she should expect from me, and had strongly encouraged her to see me. This, I think helped set the stage for the two of us to get along quite well right from the start. Besides, I also found Margaret to be a bright, cheery, well-spirited person who I expected would be easy to get along with under most circumstances. At our first meeting, she struck me as having the sensitivity that I have found in many bio-medical health care workers. I would have to proceed carefully, being sure not to overtreat or overstimulate her.

When patients are very 'sensitive', my interpretation is that they have a very responsive *qi* system, where even gentle stimulation can trigger broad responses. The reverse side to this, however, is that it is very easy to overstimulate a 'sensitive' patient, thereby pushing their *qi* system even further from equilibrium. For some this 'sensitivity' is part of their pathology; for most, it is an indication of their psychic make-up. Hence when I feel this 'sensitivity' in patients I always err on the side of caution, treating them even more delicately than I usually do. Only after gauging their responses to treatment, do I increase the treatment load. My teacher, Yoshio Manaka, touches on this issue when he discusses doses of stimulation in Manaka et al (1995).

Parkinson's disease

Margaret was of medium build, with slightly darkish skin colouration and signs of skin pigmentation and moles. She had also an obvious problem with her gait, appearing rigid in her upper torso, especially around the neck and head, as well as a somewhat flat affect. I had foreknowledge of Margaret's problems, but still found myself feeling very sorry for her when first we met. I also remember doubting whether I would be able to help her very much, as I did not have extensive experience of treating Parkinson's Disease. However, I also recalled my successes with sensitive patients after applying appropriate treatment, and quickly put any doubts out of my mind.

Until 2 years previously, Margaret had been very healthy with few things to complain about, but had then suddenly developed neurological symptoms which were diagnosed as Parkinson's Disease. At first, the symptoms were relatively mild. However, 4 months prior to coming for acupuncture, they had dramatically worsened following the news that her sister had tragically died in a plane accident. It was this accident, and the distress following it, that had caused Margaret to consult my therapist friend.

When she first came to my clinic her primary symptoms were:

1 Tremor of the left arm.
2 Dragging of the left leg with a lop-sided gait and problems of balance.
3 Weakness on the left side of the body.
4 Rigidity of the head and neck.

One physician had suggested that she might have been exposed to environmental or other toxins which are sometimes identified as a cause of Parkinsonism (Berkow 1982). However, neither the physician nor my patient followed up on this (though I made a note about possible referral to a homeopath if I were unable to help). Margaret reported that her symptoms remained at a constant level unless she was under a lot of stress or was upset about something, in which case all symptoms worsened. I had her hold out her arms so that I could clearly observe the tremor, and had her stand and take a few steps so that I could observe the gait and balance problems more closely. When I asked her to turn her head she had difficulty, needing to turn her upper torso to look either side.

Margaret was taking daily: 10 mg of Eldypryl, 50 µg of Sinemet, with 400 units of vitamin E and 500 mg of vitamin C for the Parkinson's Disease. She had taken these constantly for 2 years, since first being diagnosed, but appeared to have no side-effects from the medications, explaining that they were of low dosage. She had also attended a mind-body programme at one of the Boston hospitals, which she had found to be helpful.

Medical history

She had had viral meningitis 11 years previously, with no apparent complications. She tended to have low blood pressure: 6 months prior to seeing me it had been as low as 80/50 but had since improved. She reported that she occasionally experienced back pain, but nothing very bad, and that she had some minor problems with dry skin during the winter, which is typical in New England. Her children, aged 11 years and 13 years, had both been born by caesarean section. As a child she had had the usual childhood diseases: measles, mumps, chickenpox, and tonsillitis with a resultant tonsillectomy. Other than these problems, she was in good health. She reported good energy levels, good pulmonary and cardiovascular systems, a good gastrointestinal system with regular bowel movements, a normal urogenital system and an unremarkable menstrual history.

What struck me as she described herself and her medical history was the odd coincidence that as a healthy nurse with a speciality in neurological care, she had developed a nasty neurological disease. I have thought about this occasionally since, but have not penetrated its meaning if, indeed, it has any meaning. I did not pursue her emotional state regarding her sister's sudden death other than merely to note that it had happened and that she had consulted a therapist to help deal with the shock of it.

As a general rule I do not pursue deep-seated emotional issues, as I am not a qualified psychologist or psychotherapist. If I identify particular problems I will draw attention to them and refer appropriately. However, as an acupuncturist I can pursue these issues at entirely different levels by regulating *qi*, and by providing a relaxing, comfortable space in which patients can experience their feelings as they need to. In complex cases such as Margaret's, where the odds are stacked against the patient, I believe that the most important psychological help I can give is to provide hope by demonstrating how appropriate treatment can make a difference. In Margaret's case this involved showing how a diagnosis such as Parkinson's Disease was not necessarily a permanent, irreversible condition.

The physical examination

I asked Margaret to remove socks, shoes and all metal jewellery, and to then lie down on the treatment bed in a supine position with clothes loosened to give access to the abdominal region. At this stage I was fairly confident as to the primary issues involved.

The physical examination that I perform is a combination of approaches from the '*yin-yang* channel balancing' approach learned from Manaka and the *keiraku chiryo* or 'channel/meridian, therapy' approach, learned from various practitioners and schools of thought in Japan, and the *toyo hari* approaches in particular.[1] Palpation diagnosis is a feature of Japanese-style acupuncture in general and especially of these two basic approaches to treatment. In Manaka's system, palpation focuses on the abdominal and chest regions, with peripheral palpations of the upper and lower limbs and the neck region, looking especially for pressure pain, tightness or softness (Manaka et al 1995).[2] In the *keiraku chiryo* system, palpation is primarily of the radial pulses, looking at both the relative strengths of the six deep and surface positions,[3] and the overall middle pulse, or pulse quality. Secondary and confirmatory to this is palpation of the abdominal region with light touch (at the skin level) and with pressure (at the muscle level) in key reflex areas. Further palpation is applied on the channels and around the neck and shoulder region.[4]

Overall, Margaret's middle pulse was a little weak and slightly deep, indicating a general vacuity. The left deep pulses were overall weaker than the right deep pulses, with particular weakness in the second and third deep (Liver and Kidney) pulses, typical of a Liver vacuity pattern (see Fukushima 1991, Shudo 1990).

Light touch on the abdomen revealed that the skin tonus was poor: overall it was puffy, a little rough and without lustre, indicating a general vacuity. The area in front of the left anterior superior iliac spine was particularly puffy and lustreless, typical of a Liver vacuity pattern (Fukushima 1991). With pressure I found the whole abdomen to be soft and empty, with weak muscle tone, typical of a general vacuity condition (Matsumoto & Birch 1988), and a *yin qiao-ren mai* pattern in particular (Manaka et al 1995). With further pressure I found some resistance and pressure sensitivity in the right subcostal region, associated with Liver vacuity (Matsumoto & Birch 1988, Shudo 1990) and/or the *yin wei-chong mai* (Manaka et al 1995). I also found resistance and pressure sensitivity to the sides of the navel, especially at right ST26 *wailing* and, to a lesser degree, at right ST25 *tianshu* and ST27 *daju*. This is associated with Lung vacuity (Matsumoto & Birch 1988, Shudo 1990) and the arm *yang* channels (Manaka et al 1995, Matsumoto & Birch 1988).

Palpation of the neck, especially in the supraclavicular fossa region, showed a general tightness, in particular around ST11 *qishi* and ST12 *quepen*, indicating the *yin wei-chong mai* and *yin qiao-ren mai* (Manaka et al 1995, Matsumoto & Birch 1988). With her knees raised and feet flat on the table, I palpated the six 'polar channel' reflex areas on her calves as described by Manaka et al (1995) and found the left Liver-Small Intestine reflex area to be very sensitive and tight.

At this stage I had largely confirmed my original suspicion regarding the Liver vacuity pattern and presence of Blood stasis. For further confirmation I had Margaret turn onto her abdomen while I looked for additional signs such as pigmentation and moles. As suspected, I found extensive pigmentation in the interscapular region with occasional moles dotted over the back, typical of moderately-advanced to advanced stages of Blood stasis (Manaka et al 1995). I also found that the whole right paraspinal region from BL17 *geshu* to BL23 *shenshu* to be tight and swollen and quite sensitive to pressure, typical of Liver-related problems (Manaka et al 1995).

Primary clinical manifestations

- Left arm tremor.
- Drags left foot.
- Lop-sided gait and balance problems.
- Rigidity of neck and head, weakness of the left side of the body.
- Symptoms remain constant unless under stress or upset when they worsen.
- Pulse: weak and deep middle pulse; left deep pulse weaker than the right, especially the Liver and Kidney pulses.

- Palpation: abdomen soft and empty, especially at the left anterior superior iliac spine; deeper tightness in the right subcostal regions and to the left and especially the right side of the navel; tight in the supraclavicular fossa region; reaction on the medial lower portion of the left calf. Tight and swollen in the right paraspinal region.
- Skin colour: darkened complexion; relatively dark skin pigmentation in the interscapular region; moles.

At this first appointment I was already quite sure of the following: that Margaret had a primary pattern associated with a deep problem of Liver vacuity, accompanied by a relatively advanced stage of Blood stasis. What I also found, and what I had not expected, was a significant weakness of the lower and middle burners manifesting as a strong general *qi* and Blood vacuity state. Margaret didn't seem sufficiently run down to have such a soft and weak abdomen, which is usually found in someone in the first months postpartum, when very old, or with severe emotional instability or counterflow *qi*. Nor did Margaret have the chronic weak digestion, the severe lower back problems and the menstrual or urogenital problems that often accompany a state of *qi* and Blood vacuity. At this stage I was not sure what role lifestyle factors such as diet and exercise had played, but I began to strongly suspect that Margaret's pregnancies and caesarean sections were important factors in precipitating her presenting condition. My interpretation of the aetiology of Margaret's condition is given in the diagram shown in Figure 11.1.

Diagnostic and treatment patterns[5]

PRIMARY PATTERNS

Liver vacuity

In the *keiraku chiryo* system Margaret clearly had a Liver vacuity pattern (Fukushima 1991, Shudo 1990):

- Right subcostal tightness.
- Left anterior superior iliac spine puffiness and softness.
- Pigmentation and moles (Blood stasis).

- Tightness from right BL17 *geshu* to BL23 *shenshu*.
- Neurological symptoms.
- Muscle rigidity.
- Pulses: Liver and Kidney pulses weak.

Yin qiao-ren mai[6]

- Overall weakness of the abdominal muscles.
- Tight ST12 *quepen* and BL23 *shenshu*.
- Possibly low blood pressure.
- Lower and middle burner weakness.
- General vacuity.

Liver-Small Intestine polar channel pair[7]

- Right subcostal and right ST26 *wailing* reactions.
- Left calf reaction.
- The plethora of Liver and Blood stasis-related signs and symptoms (see the Liver vacuity pattern above).

Mixed *yin*

A combination of the *yin qiao-ren mai* and *yin wei-chong mai* that I call the 'mixed *yin*' pattern. This is confirmed by finding a particular configuration of *yin qiao-ren mai* and *yin wei-chong mai* signs:[8]

- Overall abdominal softness which indicates *yin qiao-ren*.
- Right subcostal and right ST25 *tianshu* to right ST27 *daju* reactions.
- ST11 *qishi* and ST12 *quepen* reactions.
- Signs of overall vacuity.

Cross syndrome

With all the Blood stasis signs, the underlying Liver-related pattern and the right subcostal, lower left abdominal quadrant reactions, I could also identify a 'cross syndrome' pattern. This is a common pattern of Manaka's *yin-yang* channel balancing system. It combines the treatment of the *yang wei-dai mai* on the left with the *yin wei-chong mai* on the right.[9] At an early stage this was not a strong treatment option, however, as Margaret's general vacuity improved, this pattern would probably emerge more clearly.

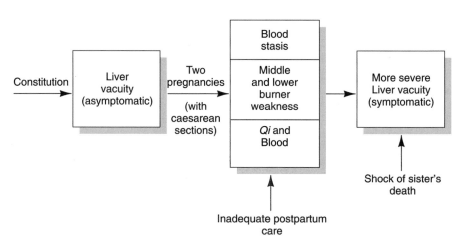

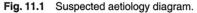

Fig. 11.1 Suspected aetiology diagram.

Assessing treatment priorities

The 'Liver vacuity' root treatment would involve using lightly inserted (1 mm) or non-inserted supplementation techniques with very thin needles (0.14–0.18 mm) on relevant points on the Liver and Kidney channels. This would typically be followed by treating secondary *yin* channel and *yang* channel manifestations with lightly inserted or non-inserted needle techniques as the whole picture unfolds in response to treating the first points. This treatment flow is typical of the blind *toyo hari* practitioners described in Fukushima (1991).

The '*yin qiao-ren mai*', 'Liver-Small Intestine', 'mixed *yin*' and 'cross syndrome' root treatment patterns would all involve using thin (0.18–0.20 mm), lightly inserted needles (2 mm) with ion-pumping cords attached at relevant points for step one. This would be followed at step two by *kyutoshin* moxa on the handle of the needles at relevant back *shu* points[10] and/or *chishin,* leaving the needles in at reactive *yang* channel points (light needling). This technique typically involves tapping in 0.16–0.20 mm gauge needles and advancing them to a maximum depth of 5 mm, usually around 2–3 mm, as detailed by Birch & Ida (1996). Step three would possibly involve structural adjustment exercises. Manaka et al (1995) discuss details of the various treatment options at each of the steps of treatment in this system.

The patient had a significant underlying vacuity with considerable Blood stasis present and I knew that I would have to first address these issues before putting emphasis on the Liver vacuity problem. The presence of the Blood stasis also required me to use bloodletting with or without cupping techniques[11] as part of the symptom control and root treatment. However, because of the underlying vacuity pattern and my perception of Margaret as a patient of high sensitivity, I delayed the bloodletting technique. I would first have to improve her underlying vacuity and assess her response to treatment and also the level of stimulation I could apply without overdosing, which is a common problem in sensitive or very vacuous patients (Manaka et al 1995).

The underlying vacuity and Blood stasis predicted a long course of therapy with gradual improvement: strong vacuity patterns take time to improve and Blood stasis is by its very nature stubborn (Manaka et al 1995).

The first treatment

At the first visit I did not have sufficient time to undertake a complete treatment (usually three to five steps). Since I planned to concentrate on treating the *yin qiao-ren mai* and mixed *yin* over the next few weeks, I decided to start the treatment by taking advantage of Manaka's *yin-yang* channel balancing model, related to his octahedral structure-function model of the channels and extraordinary vessels.[12] I did this by treating the Liver-Small Intestine polar channel pair on the first visit. My thought process at this time was a blur of intuitive insight and rational logic. If she had a Liver pattern, how would she respond if I focused on that first? How would she respond if I took advantage of the left-right (*yin-yang*) polarity of the octahedron by treating the right (healthier) side of the body to affect the left (symptomatic) side of the body?'[13] In the past I have had significant success when treating clear cases of one-sided symptoms using the polar channel pair treatment approach. Would Margaret also respond well to this treatment?

Before beginning treatment I briefly discussed my findings with Margaret. I told her that the primary problem lay in the channel which starts at the big toes, runs up the legs, up through the Liver and Gallbladder and ascends to the head to end at the crown. I discussed how this primary problem was compounded by more general problems of weakness and stagnation, possibly resulting from the pregnancies and caesarean deliveries. I also explained how this assessment could account for her neurological and muscular symptoms.

I then explained that the needles I use are disposable and many times thinner than the needles she used as a nurse, and that they would be applied in stages. First shallowly in the hands and feet, and then on the back, neck and shoulders, each addressing the primary problems. Finally I would apply various techniques in various locations to address the specific symptoms. Once this explanation was complete I proceeded with the treatment.

I located the points by palpation[14] and cleaned each with alcohol. The needles were inserted to right SI3 *houxi*, SI8 *xiaohai*, LIV2 *xingjian* and LIV8 *ququan* with ion-pumping (IP) cords attached for 10 minutes. I then had Margaret sit up while I inserted *hinaishin* (intradermal needles) to right BL18 *ganshu* and bilateral GB21 *jianjing* (see box). I gave her instructions on how to care for these retained needles, making my usual joke about these 'needles-to-go' being comparable to 'take-away-food'. This was all I had time to do at this first visit.

First treatment procedures

STEP ONE

I used 40 mm long, 0.20 mm gauge needles inserted to a depth of 2 mm in the direction of the flow of the channel and retained for 10 minutes in the following points:

- LIV2 *xingjian*, right, black clip IP cord attached.

- LIV8 *ququan,* right, red clip IP cord attached.
- SI3 *houxi*, right, red clip IP cord attached.
- SI8 *xiaohai*, right, black clip IP cord attached.

The red clip has a diode in it so the current flows from black to red.

STEP TWO

I used 6 mm intradermal needles, retained for a week, in the following points:

- GB21 *jianjing*, bilateral, 2 mm insertion angled towards the shoulders.
- BL18 *ganshu,* right, 2–3 mm insertion angled towards the spine.

The ion-pumping (IP) cord) is a simple wire containing a diode which allows small (bio)electrical currents to flow from one needle to another.

Needling technique: In none of the above techniques is the modern Chinese stimulation technique of *de qi* used, as this is viewed as both counterproductive in this treatment approach and unnecessary.[15] Manaka et al (1995) specify that for correct use of the IP cords, the insertion depth should be no deeper than 2 mm, using 0.18 mm or 0.20 mm gauge needles, and that (the modern Chinese) *de qi* is never obtained. Ideally, needle techniques produce no sensation for the patient.[16]

The *hinaishin* (intradermal needles) are inserted obliquely into the skin, at strong pressure pain points, to a length of 1–3 mm, at an actual depth of 1 mm or less, and then taped and retained for up to 1 week (Akabane 1986a, Birch & Ida 1996).

At the end of the first treatment, Margaret was clearly relieved that the treatment had been painless (although she hadn't expressed concern prior to treatment). She was also in a state of great relaxation. I discussed with her the need to schedule treatments once weekly for 10 weeks and then to reassess the situation. Her condition was not like a simple pain condition where four to six treatments would usually be sufficient to allow re-assessment. I expected Margaret's treatment to be long-term and told her so and also that, if after 10 weeks there was no improvement, she should discontinue with the treatment. However, if we did see some improvement we would then have to monitor her condition closely in order to determine future treatment plans.

Reassessment treatment by treatment

Margaret returned for weekly treatment for the next 7 months, and then came for treatment every 10–28 days. In the last 14 months she has had a total of 34 treatments. After the seventh treatment I referred her for massage, since which she has had a total of five massage treatments. Based upon a treatment by treatment reassessment of symptoms I used the primary treatment patterns outlined below.

Primary treatment patterns

ROOT TREATMENT

- KID6 *zhaohai* right (black) and LU7 *lieque* left (red) with P6 *neiguan* right (black) and SP4 *gongsun* left (red) for 12 sessions.
- KID6 *zhaohai* right (black) and LU7 *lieque* left (red) for three sessions.
- P6 *neiguan* bilateral (black) and SP4 *gongsun* bilateral (red) for 10 sessions.
- P6 *neiguan* right (black) and SP4 *gongsun* right (red) with SJ5 *waiguan* left (black) and GB41 *linqi* left (red) for two sessions.
- Either LIV1 *dadun*, LIV3 *taichong* or LIV8 *ququan* were supplemented, while the IP cords were on, in 18 sessions and SP6 *sanyinjiao* was supplemented, while the cords were on, in nine sessions. LIV1 *dadun* was supplemented when Margaret complained primarily about her balance problems. To supplement, a painless insertion was made with a 0.12–0.14 mm needle (this takes a lot of practice).

Needles and heat (moxa or lamp) were used at step two on the back in all treatments after the first session.

SYMPTOM CONTROL

- Bloodletting and cupping around DU14 *dazhui* were added by the eighth session. The bloodletting and cupping were used in relatively low doses. Following the addition of this technique we started to see an improvement in Margaret's balance and stumbling problems.
- Intradermal needles were used at ear and body points in 31 sessions.
- *Enpishin* 'press-tack needles' were used in six sessions.[17] Press-tack needles (*enpishin*) are like tiny thumb tacks with a needle length of 2–3 mm.[17]
- Press-tack needles with magnets taped over them were used on body points starting from the eleventh session onwards for 20 sessions. When used with magnets, 800 gauss north facing magnets (i.e. repels the point of the compass) are taped over the press-tack needle to create a stronger effect. This technique was used in the eleventh treatment on the knot around BL15 *xinshu* with a strong effect on all symptoms.

Progress of treatment

Although Margaret had shown little change after the first abbreviated treatment, by the third treatment her neck and back became looser, more flexible and less rigid. By the sixth treatment her tremor had started to improve. By the tenth treatment her stumbling and balance problems began to improve. After the eleventh treatment there was further marked improvement in all symptoms with a continued gradual improvement through to the 24th treatment, at which point her progress began to plateau. With the exception of a very stressful period, when her tremor and balance problems flared up, she has been able to maintain her improvements, and reports being very satisfied with the progress of treatment.

Recently she went on vacation to do a lot of hiking. She had gone to the same place just before coming for her first acupuncture treatment, and had been able to do only limited hiking. This time, however, she was able to do considerably more hiking because she felt 'steadier on her feet'.

Her primary patterns have all improved. The general vacuity is better, her abdominal tone is much better, and she generally shows more of the primary Liver pattern as predicted. The Blood stasis problem has slowly improved and I have used a lot of relatively low dosage bloodletting on her. Had she not been so sensitive, with such a strong vacuity of *qi* and Blood, I would have used heavier doses of bloodletting to bring about a more rapid change. The root treatment patterns have varied, but have tended to revolve around the primary IP cord patterns that I initially identified, coupled with general supplementation of the Liver vacuity pattern.

With hindsight

For a while I was a little concerned that I was unclear about the aetiology of Margaret's condition; it seemed too simplistic to think that her problems were largely a result of postpartum complications. However, with hindsight, I'm quite convinced that this is a good explanation of her condition. I believe that if some of the principles of East Asian medicine were adopted when working with all women postpartum, women's health care would be revolutionised in the West, thereby helping to reduce the incidence of complications many years later.

NOTES

1 For English-language texts describing this system see for example Shudo (1990) and especially Fukushima (1991).

2 See also Matsumoto & Birch (1988) for a broader discussion of abdominal palpation.

3 This system was first described in the *Nan Jing* (see *Nan Jing* 18 in Unschuld 1986). Pulses: left–HT/SI, LIV/GB, KID/BL; right–LU/LI, SP/ST, PC/TB. While currently out of favour in China, it is the most widely used system in Japan and elsewhere, and was widely used historically (Birch 1992).

4 See Fukushima (1991), Matsumoto & Birch (1988) and Shudo (1990) for descriptions of these palpation methods.

5 With the utilisation of multiple competing yet complementary methods of practice comes the recognition that the so-called 'diagnosis' is actually an assessment step that primarily functions to select treatment sites and techniques, it does not seem to refer to an objective entity. It is only the assumptions that come with the utilisation and structure of our spoken and written language that imparts any further reality to it. In the absence of studies that objectively verify the 'diagnosis', I believe it better to pragmatically adopt such an approach, which is why here diagnosis and treatment are identified together.

6 See Manaka et al (1995) and Matsumoto & Birch (1988) for details.

7 For details of this patterning approach see Manaka et al (1995).

8 For the singular extraordinary vessel patterns see Manaka et al (1995).

9 Manaka found the cross syndrome pattern to be the most commonly occurring pattern, which I have also found in my experience. For details of this see Manaka et al (1995) and Matsumoto & Birch (1988).

10 Described in Akabane (1986) and Birch & Ida (1996).

11 Discussed in Birch & Ida (1996), and Manaka et al (1995). The specialist bloodletting literature of Kudo and Maruyama also has extensive discussions of the use of bloodletting methods (see Kudo 1983, Maruyama & Kudo 1982).

12 Discussed extensively in Manaka et al (1995). For a summary description of the model see Birch (1994).

13 A principle clearly articulated by Manaka (Manaka et al 1995) and also described in the *Su Wen* (Chapter 27). This principle forms the basis of the Akabane school in Japan, for discussions, see Akabane (1985) and Akabane (1986). The specific idea of treating the healthy side to affect the diseased side is also discussed in the *toyo hari* school, see Fukushima (1991).

14 Location by palpation is archetypal of the practice of acupuncture in Japan. In this instance I used light touch to locate SI3, SI8, LIV2 and pressure to locate LIV8. The first three points would show an indentation, puffiness, roughness, lack of lustre or a sense of resistance, LIV8 pressure pain and tightness.

15 Many acupuncturists in Japan consider the modern Chinese interpretation of *de qi* to be simply *shigeki ryoho*, 'stimulation therapy', thought to be nerve stimulation, a form of 'counter-irritation' (Manaka et al 1995). While popular in some schools in Japan, this technique is regarded as unnecessary and painful by many other schools, in particular the *keiraku chiryo* schools, which prefer to follow the dictum from the *Nan Jing* which specifies that it is the practitioner who should feel the *qi* in his/her left hand, not the patient (see *Nan Jing* 78 in Unschuld 1986).

16 Shudo discusses this (Shudo 1990) as do my wife and I (Birch & Ida 1996). For an interesting discussion of the differences and similarities between the Chinese and Japanese approaches to the practice of acupuncture see Manaka (1994).

17 See Birch & Ida (1996) for details of the techniques and uses of *enpishin*.

REFERENCES

Akabane K 1986a Hinaishin Ho (Intradermal needle method), 12th edn. Yokosuka, Ido no Nippon Company

Berkow R 1982 Merck Manual, 14th edn. Rahway, Merck Sharp & Dohme Research Laboratories

Birch S 1994 Dr Yoshio Manaka's *yin-yang* balancing treatment. North American Journal of Oriental Medicine 1(1): 4–8

Birch S, Ida J 1996 The clinical handbook of Japanese acupuncture. Paradigm, Brookline

Fukushima K 1991 Meridian therapy. Toyo Hari Medical Association, Tokyo

Kudo K 1983 Zusetu Shiraku Chiryo (Illustrated guide to bloodletting therapy). Shizensha, Tokyo

Manaka Y 1994 Japanese and Chinese acupuncture similarities and differences. North American Journal of Oriental Medicine 1(2): 5–9

Matsumoto K, Birch S 1988 Hara diagnosis: reflections on the sea. Paradigm, Brookline

Shudo D 1990 Japanese classical acupuncture; introduction to meridian therapy. Eastland Press, Seattle

Unschuld P U 1986 Medicine in China: *Nan Jing*: The classic of difficulties. University of California Press, Berkeley

FURTHER READING

Akabane K 1985 Chinetsukando Niyoru Shinkyu Chiryoho (Acupuncture and moxibustion therapy by heat sensitivity method), 8th edn. Yokosuka, Ido no Nippon Company

Akabane K 1986b Kyutoshin Ho (The moxa on the handle of the needle method), 6th edn. Yokosuka, Ido no Nippon Sha

Birch S 1992 Naming the unnameable: a historical study of radial pulse six position diagnosis. Traditional Acupuncture Society Journal 12: 2–13

Manaka Y, Itaya K, Birch S 1995 Chasing the dragon's tail. Paradigm Publications, Brookline

Maruyama M, Kudo K 1982 Shinpan Shiraku Ryoho (Bloodletting therapy). Seki Bundo Pub Co, Tokyo

■ Stephen Birch

Stephen has been practising acupuncture for over 13 years. He graduated from the New England School of Acupuncture after studying with Tin Yau So and Ted Kaptchuk. He spent three summers studying in Japan with Yoshio Manaka and various 'meridian therapy' practitioners, especially those of the Toyohari Association. He specialises in the practice of Japanese styles of acupuncture, and has coauthored four published texts: Five Elements and Ten Stems; Extraordinary Vessels; Hara diagnosis: reflections on the sea; and Chasing the dragon's tail. He has two other texts in press: The clinical handbook of Japanese acupuncture; Needles and Fire: the story of acupuncture's journey westward.

He taught at the New England School of Acupuncture from 1985–93 and has taught workshops on Japanese acupuncture around the USA and in the UK and Australia. He is currently completing his doctorate through the Centre for Complementary Health Studies, University of Exeter, with the theme of acupuncture research methodology. He has conducted an acupuncture study at Harvard Medical School and is currently working with a research team at Yale University School of Medicine, focusing on substance abuse. He is cochair of the Society for Acupuncture Research and a consultant to two other large funded projects in the USA. He lives in the New Haven area where he is practising acupuncture with his wife.

Elinor in the dance

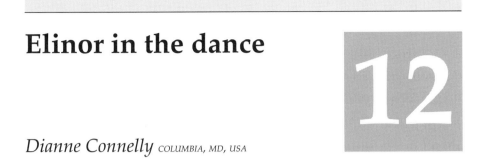

Dianne Connelly COLUMBIA, MD, USA

In writing the case you are now reading, I am keenly aware that no one is a case report. That is to say that no human being can be summarised in a few words of diagnosis, or pulse pictures, or patterns of disharmony, or Elements. Instead, I write this for you as an offering from myself, through the experiences I have had over the years of my practice. With this as my intent, I invite you to read this and cull from it what serves both you and those who come to you seeking to know who they are by being with you.

This piece is not about a patient coming to a practitioner or expert to have imbalances corrected, or even about putting in needles. I use needles according to the spirit of the points, as reminders to the patient of who they already are. For me, the traditional acupuncture examination is a loving inquiry, via the senses, into the nature of a particular person who is an incomparable constellation of life's phenomena, life's showings. The inquiry itself is part of the treatment. The person I present to you is Elinor.

A loving inquiry

Elinor is 17 years old and a student. Her parents were divorced when she was 9 years old and she now lives with her mother and younger brother. She gives painful menstrual periods as the reason she has sought treatment. She is 1.72 m tall and weighs 54.5 kg (120 lbs). Elinor appears warm and open and makes direct eye contact easily. We have some conversation about her senses, her bodily functions, and her health history. She feels herself to be in good health overall. Elinor prefers spring and summer time to the colder seasons and describes herself as 'not a morning person. I definitely prefer to stay up late and sleep late'. In childhood she had frequent sore throats and infected tonsils. It is clear from Elinor's pulses that her life force is strong and that the *wu xing (wu hsing)* are all in a fine dance with one another, with a particular calling from the Fire and its relationship to the Earth. In feeling the Three Heater, the lower *jiao (chou)* is a little cooler than the other two.

Elinor expresses concern that her menstruation is irregular and at times painful enough to cause her to miss school:

"I dread getting my period. I get the worst PMS (premenstrual syndrome). I feel horrible for days before it comes on. Normally I tend to be the kind of person who cries a lot, but before my period I get to the point where I cry at practically anything. When it comes I crave sweet and salty things that make me get really bloated. But I can't help it and I eat them anyway. The cramps are really bad. Sometimes I just have to stay in bed with a heating pad. Any position I lie in is painful."

"Have you had any other treatment for your periods?"

"Yes, I've seen my mother's gynaecologist for it. The doctor wants to put me on the pill to regulate my period. That sounds okay to me, but my mom is not wild about the idea of her daughter being on the pill at the age of 17. I mean she hasn't come right out and said that. What she says is that she thinks it would be better if we could solve this problem without my having to take medicine. But I think she's kind of freaked out by the idea of me being on birth control."

Symptoms, reminders, calls to observe life

- Painful menstrual periods, cramps, stays in bed with heating pad.
- Irregular periods.
- Premenstrual symptoms, feels 'horrible for days before'.
- Feels out of control with PMS, can feel sad and vulnerable and cranky and no fun to be around.
- Tends to cry a lot before a period and can 'cry at practically anything'.
- Warm, open, makes eye contact easily.
- Craves sweet and salty things and gets bloated.
- Prefers spring and summer.
- 'Not a morning person', likes late night hours.
- Lower *jiao* (*chou*) is cooler than the other two.
- Pulses: a strong life force in the Wood Officials but not flowing smoothly, the Fire Officials are low and the Earth Officials empty.

In being with Elinor, as with any person who asks me to be their practitioner, I am called to listen to life as it is lived through her, to listen without conclusions, even when often the patient concludes for him or herself. For example, when Elinor says she is 'the kind of person who cries a lot', I can hear that she has made a conclusion that disallows other possibilities. We, as human beings, do this all the time, I assert. In our stories, unnecessary suffering resides, both physical and emotional. What Elinor says about life will determine her peacefulness and the possibilities that are open to her. My work is to listen and assist her to reveal the distinction between phenomenon and conclusion. My offering is to be an observer, so that Elinor can open some new conversations big enough to live in, big enough for those who journey through life with her to live in.

Learning the dance

I learn the dance called Elinor by observing the following Elements showing up as present and showing up as absent:

Wood Element

She is in her youth, the springtime of her life and reflects that in how she is with me. She likes the late night hours which are the strongest time of Wood in the daily cycle. As reflected in her moods, her openness to speak, her periods and her relationships, her life is not flowing smoothly. She doesn't yet clearly see the distinctions to guide her life, the path to follow. The Officials of Wise Judgement and Planning are not yet powerfully guiding her.

Fire Element

Elinor likes summer. Heat eases her discomfort. She radiates warmth and then speaks of coldness in her body. The lower part of her abdomen is cold to touch. The pulses of the Fire Officials are low and do not reflect the strength I listen to on the Wood Officials.

Earth Element

Elinor's presenting concern, her 'ticket' to ask for assistance, relates to fertility, fecundity and the regenerative cycles of life. Earth within is calling, not as a problem, but as a calling to attend the cycles of Spring and Summer so that the harvest of her womanhood may be full. Earth is the grounding on which to stand in life. To the extent that nourishment from Fire shows up as missing, Elinor craves quick fire in the form of sweets. She does not have much energy to get moving in the morning. The pulses of the Earth Officials reflect the deficiency, the neediness of one who desires to nurture others and who does not have sufficient to give away and to ground and tend herself at the same time.

Creating a conversation

I am called to be especially rigorous as I work with Elinor, at her particular time of life, 17 cycles of seasons. Together, Elinor and I create a conversation (from the Latin *con-*, together, and *vertere*, to turn, hence we turn together). Whatever our conversation is, it must be something that she can take into life with her.

Elinor's conversation of 'PMS' is an important place to begin our inquiry. I could say that there is no such thing as 'PMS', since each person embodies life specifically and uniquely. And yet, culturally, we have created a category called 'PMS' like a thing, a 'problem' that exists that we then have to treat. Inherent in this label 'PMS' is the idea of illness, of something wrong that needs to be fixed.

With Elinor, it is essential to reveal what are the phenomena of her experience of menses, separate from the cultural conversation of 'PMS'. Without an observer present, this word 'PMS' can alienate Elinor from her own embodied living of menstruation. I ask her what 'PMS' means to her and how she experiences it. Her response is filled with unnecessary suffering — conclusions about herself and her body:

*"PMS means that I am out of control. It's what I feel right now —
like I can't get a handle on what I want to eat because I'm craving food
that's not good for me. It means I feel sad and more vulnerable than
usual. I can also get cranky and be no fun to be around. It means that I
know in a couple of days I'm going to have terrible cramps. On the
other hand I hate it when I don't get my period too. It makes me worry
about what's wrong with me. Sometimes I get scared that I might get
something like cancer and die or not be able to have children someday.
So it's kind of like I'm damned if I do and damned if I don't."*

"What is this blood for you? What is it like?"

*"Even if it weren't painful and all that, it's gross. I have to go
through all these steps to make sure people don't know I have my
period. I feel worried that at any time, some blood might show —
especially in school with other kids and boys around. I feel
embarrassed."*

"So what about boys?"

*"Well, I have a boyfriend, Mark. He's a senior. We've been together
for 10 months."*

"Who is Mark for you?"

*"I've had other boyfriends, but Mark is the first guy I've ever felt like
this about. He's very smart and funny. He's popular too, but not at all
stuck on himself. He got into a good college, so he'll be going away next
fall. He and I were talking about that last night. We both feel like we
don't want to see other people while we're apart. My mom is kind of
relieved that he's going away to school. She thinks it'll be good for me
to study more and 'get to know other people' as she says."*

"Do you and Mark make love with each other?"

*"Oh God, I knew that question was coming . . . Actually I think I was
hoping you would ask me that — I didn't quite know how to bring it
up. The first time was 7 weeks ago."*

"And what do you say about this?"

*"Well, I haven't talked a lot about it. I've spoken to my friend Sarah.
For me it was a big deal. I've had other boyfriends I was tempted to
sleep with, and some who really tried to pressure me and that kind of
thing. But it felt like the right thing to do with Mark. I was kind of
scared or nervous or whatever, but it still felt right."*

Elinor, like many young women of her age and culture is learning to
recognise herself as body, learning to know pleasure, learning to experience pain, learning to be in relationships that include her womanliness,
her loins, her sex. To serve Elinor as her practitioner-guide, the conversation I have with her about her body must be specific enough to give her
comfort as she faces new physical happenings, and as she constructs
stories about herself, so that she does not draw conclusions that are too

small to live in. The culture and subcultures she lives in run rampant with images of how a young woman 'should' be, 'should' feel, 'should' look. Even Elinor's story about the embarrassment of blood showing is a cultural narrative.

Elinor and I speak more about sex. Uncovering Elinor's world around the words 'body', 'period' and 'sex' reveals where the pain and discomfort labelled 'PMS' lives. As I listen to Elinor speak, I hear her learning to be in the world in a new way, as a woman, rather than as a child. We come back to speaking about her menses:

> *"Elinor, what might this phenomenon, this event named 'period' be calling you to? What might you learn from it?"*
> *"I'm not sure I understand what you're asking me . . ."*
> *"What if, as powerful as these pains and cravings and emotions are, your own power as a vessel for life is as strong or even stronger? What if this is a reminder of the possibility of 'woman' you are?"*
> *Elinor pauses and appears to take these words in.*
> *"I guess it's easier to think about it that way. But the pain and stuff will still be there — what about that?"*
> *"Let's see. Let's see what happens over this period that's beginning now and see whether you have a bit more freedom. If there is pain, observe it carefully and even lovingly, the way a mother would observe her baby's crying. When you come in next week we can talk about what you've observed."*

Here Elinor shows excitement and joy.

Elements and Seasons

Wood and Springtime

The rising young life force that is Elinor is learning to flow more and more smoothly into the fire which nurtures life as the partnership of mature relationships. The pulse is strong and not flowing smoothly. Elinor is learning to smooth the dance of powerful youthful Spring-like *qi (ch'i)* energy and life force.

Fire and Summertime

Coldness in the body mixed with warm openness to life signals a need for a stronger Spring *qi (ch'i)* to nourish the fires that sustain Elinor at all levels. Elinor gives off warmth to others while feeling cold within her embodied self.

Earth and Late Summer

The harvest of Late Summer depends upon the solid intensity of Spring and Summer. With Wood still learning to flow smoothly and Fire doing a dance of plenty and apparent insufficiency, the Earth squawks. There is not sufficient to produce the harvest easily, the menstrual blood is not released easily. The lower abdomen is cold. The warm rising *qi (ch'i)* is depleted before it returns downward. The labels of PMS are truly the call to paying attention. They are not the problem, they are the sign.

Callings from a birthright

I consider all of the time I spend with Elinor as 'treatment'; as attending to her, ministering through inquiring, listening, seeing, touching (holding her hand, taking pulses, feeling her body temperature, texture, moisture), savouring being with her. All I do by inserting a needle into a point, or burning moxa, is to remind Elinor of who she already is: she has had these points her whole life long, and each point is an expression, a calling from her birthright. When I am in Elinor's presence as an observer of phenomena, points arise that respond to her struggles. The presencing of each point with the needle is an answer to her call.

When I put the needle in, the point grounds her, acknowledges her strength. For example, when I needle ST40 *fenglong* (XI40) 'Abundant Splendour' on the Stomach pathway, she is reminded of her own abundance and beauty, and can dance in her life with more ease and sureness. This helps her to observe the wonder of who she is already and engage life *through* the symptoms, inquiring into them, using them, embracing the integrity of them and *then* letting them go. There is no longer a need for her to be at war with the symptoms or to perceive them as separate from herself. Healing is not opposition to symptoms — rather it is acknowledging and clearing whatever may need to be cleared, knowing that no medicine, no human being can do more than Nature will allow.

Points in the Earth and Fire serve Elinor well. Earth is associated with fertility, fecundity and the cycles of life. Being grounded and balanced, feeling centred and in harmony are gifts from Earth. Fire grants us vitality, warmth, partnership and enthusiasm. The sun is the source of Fire, with its rhythm in our lives, its presence as life-giver, its reality as part of the life cycle, its warming nourishing rays. I use the point LIV3 *taichong* (VIII 3) 'Happy Calm', an Earth point in the Wood, to remind Elinor of her smooth-flowing partnership with life, moving with life and with the flow of her periods. SI19 *tinggong* (II 19) 'Listening Palace' on the Small Intestine helps her to be a better observer of her conversations, more able to sort out the conversations that are too small for her to live in. SJ23 *sizhukong* (VI 23) 'Silk Bamboo Hollow' on the Three Heater is a powerful reminder for her: silk and bamboo are both strong and beautiful gifts of nature, like Elinor.

The acupuncture treatment

POINT PRESCRIPTION

- ST40 *fenglong* (XI40) 'Abundant Splendour' to remind her of the abundant splendour within and to dance in her life with more ease and sureness.

- LIV3 *taichong* (VIII 3) 'Happy Calm', an Earth point in the Wood, to calm the Springtime *qi (ch'i)* and for a smooth-flowing partnership with life, moving with life and with the flow of her periods.

- SI19 *tinggong* (II 19) 'Listening Palace', to be a better observer of her conversations, to be more able to sort out conversations that are too small for her to live in.
- SJ23 *sizhukong* (VI 23) 'Silk Bamboo Hollow' as a reminder of her strength and beauty, gifts of nature.

Needling technique: I use 36 gauge, 25 mm, all stainless steel needles. I use very few points in each session. Indeed, I have already treated the point by word and touch before I place the needle on the point to embody in Elinor what has already arisen in our being together. I call her attention to the point as a gift and invite her to breathe into the point as I insert the needle in her body. Sometimes the needle remains for 15 or 20 minutes to allow for movement, and other times I do needling in a flash to call forth what is already happening.

For the third and fourth points above, the needles are inserted and removed immediately. These needles stoke the fire which is further nourished by the burning of five small cones of moxa on each of the points. These points on the *yang* Officials call forth the fullness of the fire within.

A yearning for openings

In being with Elinor, I am very aware of her searching, asking for openings and movement. For instance in our conversation, Elinor's relief when I ask her about sex with her boyfriend is a yearning for an opening. Points that are windows and gates are of particular service to Elinor, to remind her of who she is, as a portal for life with freedom to move to and fro. HE7 *shenmen* (I 7) 'Spirit Gate' on the Heart meridian, SI16 *tianchuang* (II 16) and SJ16 *tianyou* (VI 16) 'Heavenly Window' on the Small Intestine and Three Heater meridians, P6 *neiguan* (V 6) 'Inner Frontier Gate' on the Pericardium (Circulation Sex) meridian and ST16 *yingchuang* (XI 16) 'Breast Window' on the Stomach meridian are all wonderful points for her.

Over time, Elinor has become easier with her periods. She misses school rarely now and will go to college in the fall. She and Mark are still together. Elinor is more contented and passionate in their sexual partnership:

> *I'm not as worried and shy about sex as I was before. I've even started talking with my mother about my relationship with Mark. She's not nearly as uptight as I thought she was!*

Elinor has become more observant and at home in her body and more comfortable with becoming a woman. Her relationships, especially with her mother, have become happier and closer.

> ### Summary of outcome
>
> - Easier with her periods, rarely missing school now.
> - More contented and passionate in her sexual relationship.
> - Less worried and shy about sex.
> - More observant.
>
> - More at home in her body.
> - More comfortable with becoming a woman.
> - Relationships have become happier and closer.

Being with Elinor

In the presence of Elinor, I as practitioner am reminded one more time that being alive is an ongoing phenomenon and not a conclusion, mine or hers. In being with Elinor, gratitude arises in me at the wonder that I am alive, and that in the great mystery of living I, like you, like all mortals dwelling on this earth must die. Still, in the presence of death, the ongoing promise of springtime lives in Elinor's presence. Elinor and I are in this 'boat' together, fellow travellers, patient and practitioner as one.

Addendum

With regard to the question about 'why' I did the case report in this way, I would respond that the whole presentation is not based on the conversation of 'Why... because'. I say that living is poetry and larger than the construct of 'why... because'. In the presence of the phenomenon Elinor, I Dianne, phenomenon, simply dance it this way — a mutual arising, a poetry of presence, life with itself. As Meister Eckhart wrote, 'The rose is without a why — it blooms because it blooms.'.

The following quote from Lieh-Tzu is a powerful reminder to me of the inherent simplicity and poetry of the practice of acupuncture:

> *My body is in accord with my mind, my mind with my energies, my energies with my spirit, my spirit with Nothing. Whenever the minutest existing thing or the faintest sound affects me, whether it is far away beyond the eight borderlands, or close at hand between my eyebrows and eyelashes, I am bound to know it. However, I do not know whether I perceived it with the seven holes in my head and my four limbs, or knew it through my heart and belly and internal organs ...*
>
> *... when I had come to the end of everything inside and outside me, my eyes became like my ears, my ears like my nose, my nose like my mouth ... My mind concentrated and my body relaxed, bones and flesh fused completely, I did not notice what my body leaned against and my*

feet trod upon, I drifted with the wind East and West, like a leaf from a tree or a dry husk, and never knew whether it was the wind that rode me or I that rode the wind. (Graham 1960)

REFERENCES

Graham A C 1960 The book of Lieh-Tzu (trans) John Murray Publishers, London

FURTHER READING

Connelly D M 1993 All sickness is homesickness. Traditional Acupuncture Institute, Columbia

Connelly D M 1994 Traditional acupuncture: the law of the Five Elements. Traditional Acupuncture Institute, Columbia

Duden B 1991 The woman beneath the skin. Harvard University Press, Cambridge, Massachusetts

Duggan R M 1995 Complementary medicine: transforming influence or footnote to history? Alternative therapies. May 1 (2)

Martin E 1987 The woman in the body: a cultural analysis of reproduction. Beacon Press, Boston

Maturana H, Varela F J 1992 The tree of knowledge. Shambhala Press, Boston and London

SOPHIA Handbook 1992 Traditional Acupuncture Institute, Columbia

Sullivan J G 1992 To come to life more fully: an east/west journey. Traditional Acupuncture Institute, Columbia

■ Dianne M Connelly

Dianne M Connelly, a practitioner of traditional acupuncture since 1971, holds a doctorate in cross-cultural medicine. She cofounded, with Robert Duggan, the Traditional Acupuncture Institute (TAI). She is author of *Traditional Acupuncture: the Law of the Five Elements* and *All Sickness is Homesickness*, Chairperson of the Board of Trustees of the TAI, and contributing columnist of *Meridians*. She is a graduate of Le Moyne College (BA), New York University (MA), Union Graduate School (PhD), and the College of Traditional Chinese Medicine in the United Kingdom (MAc), where she studied with Professor J R Worsley. Born in South Colton, New York, she lives in Columbia, Maryland and is the mother of Blaize, Jade and Caeli.

Dianne writes: "My life is about serving my patients, sharing my work with students of acupuncture, and being part of the Institute's SOPHIA programme (School of Philosophy and Healing in Action), which applies this vision in the everyday world. In SOPHIA, lay persons participate in a powerful discourse based on the ancient Chinese distinctions for life, learning concepts and skills through which they can respond to the challenges of the new millennium. Students in the Institute's acupuncture training programme also learn to embody SOPHIA's themes: 'to come to life more fully so as to serve life more wisely and more nobly' and 'all work is world work'. "I continue to practise, to write, to teach, and to present workshops and lectures on SOPHIA themes. And, Dear Readers, with you, I continue in this great dance of Life. Together we are bowing servants, caring for Life, and ever opening to the myriad possibilities of being alive."

A case of tropical acne

Shmuel Halevi ISRAEL

Esther's ship of troubles

Esther was 23 years old when she first presented herself at my clinic in Nahariya, Israel. At first glance it was almost impossible to detect any health disturbance, major or minor, from her appearance. She was a lean, good looking young woman, who expressed herself fluently although somewhat shyly. Her story, nevertheless, was rather depressing and revealed a long-term illness.

Esther's first menstruation at the age of 14½ had not been quite normal. The colour of the menses had been brown, containing many clots, there had been plenty of discharge and menstruation had lasted 7 days. Inflamed eruption of acne appeared on her face along with her first period, and after that her ship of troubles set sail. Her dermatologist first suggested antibiotics, along with regular visits to an experienced cosmetician. The antibiotics were changed many times in the course of several months, due to their failure to bring about any relief at all. Presumably because of the antibiotics, as Esther herself suspected, the eruptions wandered from her face down to her upper chest and back.

At the age of 17, for no apparent reason, the acne suddenly disappeared both from her face and trunk, and she was clear of it until she was 19 years old. At this time Esther started taking contraceptives, and discovered, a few months later, that her old problem had reappeared, in a much more serious fashion, but only upon her upper trunk. Again she was given various kinds of antibiotics, she changed her contraceptives, managed her diet and changed her dermatologist — all to no avail. The problem only seemed to worsen.

Uncovering information

When I examined her, after listening to her story, I was astonished by the extent of the phenomenon. Her entire chest and upper back were covered with large deep red papules and pustules, some of them clustered together to form areas of inflamed lesions.

Her tongue had a normal colour except for the tip and sides which were redder. The left rim was scalloped, and the tongue coating was white, thin and slippery. Palpating the pulse revealed that her left Heart *cun* position was slightly tense and somewhat hard, and so was the right Spleen *guan* position, which was also thin. Her Kidney *chi* pulse was absent on both wrists. Overall, her pulse was soft and thin with a normal rate of 72 beats.

Moving on to her trunk I was not surprised to discover that all her five *zang mu* points were very tender, especially so REN17 *tanzhong*. Also SP9 *yinlingquan* was extremely tender.

These findings naturally gave rise to a series of questions which uncovered the following information. During her early teens Esther became very fond of a certain milk product, which was very sweet and was flavoured by various fruit extracts. She used to consume this drink cold and in excess. Since her first menstruation, described above, she suffered from excessive vaginal discharges, which were white in colour, thick, and with an offensive odour. She was generally quite irritable, and inclined to inner tension. She was also fond of drinking water, had occasional bouts of excessive hunger, and disliked hot weather. Her periods were short, her menses scant, and before each menstruation she experienced lower back pain.

Summary of clinical manifestations

- Very serious acne upon the upper parts of the chest and back, deep red and inflamed pustules and comedones, filled with white pus.
- Thirst, dislike of warm weather, bouts of hunger.
- Short periods, scant menses, profuse thick white vaginal discharge with an offensive odour, low back pain before menstruation.
- Eyelids: left eyelid very red.
- Irritable, inner tension.

- *Mu* points: all major *mu* points tender, especially REN17 *tanzhong*. SP9 *yinlingquan* also tender.
- Tongue: red tip and sides; scalloped left side; white, thin and slippery coating.
- Pulse: Heart *cun* position tense and hard, Spleen *guan* position tense and thin, Kidney *chi* positions unpalpable, overall quality is soft.

Identifying the patterns of disharmony

In Chinese medicine it is usually common to define the pattern of disharmony in skin diseases by the shape and appearance of the affected lesions (Lu Shoukang 1993). Dark red and inflamed eruptions which resemble pustules and are chronic, are usually attributed to Stasis of *qi* and Blood. The dark red colour is a sign of Heat in the Blood, and the white exudate is due to pathogenic Damp. The body area on which the affected skin lesions occur is also of significance. Usually the upper parts of the body are generally considered to be mostly affected by Wind pathogen, and the lower parts of the body by Dampness (Lu Shoukang 1993). Sometimes the lesions appear in the course of body segments, such as *taiyang* or *shaoyang,* and this also may help in understanding the root of the imbalance.

Patterns of disharmony

Heat and Damp in the skin

Dark red and inflamed pustules filled with white pus.

Spleen/Stomach imbalance

(Spleen *qi xu* with Damp and Stomach Heat).

- Thirst.
- Dislike of warm weather.
- Bouts of hunger.
- Red inner left eyelid.
- Tenderness at SP9 *yinlingquan.*
- Pulse: right Spleen *guan* thin.
- Tongue: scalloped left side, both sides reddish.

***Ren/Chong* imbalance**

- Onset of condition with first menstruation — when these two vessels begin to flourish.[1]

- Second appearance after taking contraceptives.
- Location of the disease, as *chong* and *ren* disperse on the chest and back and on the face respectively.
- Tenderness at REN17 *tanzhong.*

Kidney *qi xu* and Damp-cold in the Uterus

- Scant menses.
- Profuse white vaginal discharge with offensive odour.
- Low back pain.
- Pulses: absence of the Kidney *chi* pulses, soft and thin overall pulse quality.
- Tongue: white and slippery coating.

Aetiology and pathology

In our case, as stated above, the shape and appearance of the lesions suggested a pattern of Heat and Damp stagnation. Heat in the skin is shown by the dark red papules and pustules of the skin disease, as well as by the close relationship between the Stomach organ, the *chong mai,* and the Blood. Thus, Heat penetrating the *chong mai* from the Uterus, will easily find its way both to the Stomach and the Blood. Heat generated in the Stomach due to Damp stagnation of its *zang,* the Spleen, may penetrate the Blood and the *chong mai.*

The root of this imbalance lies, of course, in the Uterus, as indicated by the time of the onset of the problem. The consumption during puberty of too many cold and milky products, may be a cause for accumulation of Damp-cold in the lower *jiao* (Shen J, personal communication, 1988). This may later give rise to disturbances in the normal functioning of the Uterus, such as dysmenorrhea and vaginal discharges. At the age of 14, when Esther begins menstruation, the *chong* and *ren* channels are energetically activated, and then Damp-cold may turn into Heat, which will travel upward along the routes of these two channels. The *ren mai* will thus carry Damp and Heat to the face, while *chong mai* might disperse this pathogen over the chest and upper back (Mei Jianghan 1993).

The imbalance between Spleen and Stomach is the result of excess Damp that weakens and clogs the Spleen, thus creating Heat within its related organ, the Stomach. Symptoms of thirst, dislike of warm weather and bouts of hunger mark this Heat, while the pulse on right *guan* position affirms it. Also the tongue, which was scalloped only on the left side and reddish on both sides, suggests a weak Spleen and the presence of Heat. A tendency of the Heat to rise to the upper parts of the body is seen mostly on the left side (due to an overriding *yang qi*). A red inner left eyelid is one sign. Another, is the red edges of the tongue.

In Western medicine too the pathogenesis of acne is understood mainly in terms of an imbalance of hormones (Merck Manual, 1982). Acne begins at puberty when the increase of androgens causes a corresponding increase in the size and activity of the pilosebaceous glands. The pilosebaceous follicle becomes blocked, leading to the formation of the comedo acnes. These are composed of sebum, keratin and bacteria. Retention of the sebaceous secretions, and dilation of the follicle, may lead to cyst formation. Rupture of the follicle, and release of the contents into the surrounding tissues, includes an inflammatory reaction which is seen as the reddening, swelling and oozing of the affected lesions.

In my experience, the administration of antibiotics in cases of inflamed skin lesions (acne, abscesses, etc.), which are the result of an internal systemic process, usually produces an aggravation of the problem, and/or diversion or precipitation to other sites of the body. This was exactly the case with Esther. The ample use of various antibiotics banished the disease from the *ren mai* domain to the *chong mai* domain.

Two years later, because of her use of contraceptives, she had a decrease of her Kidney *qi* (evidenced by low back pain, scant menses and profuse vaginal discharge), and a consequent restagnation of *chong mai*. Hormone consumption greatly affects the *chong* and *ren mai* which originate in the Uterus. As a result the acne appeared again on Esther's chest and back.

Treating the acute symptoms first

After understanding the various components of this diagnosis (Fig. 13.1), I felt it was essential to treat the presenting symptoms in the first place,

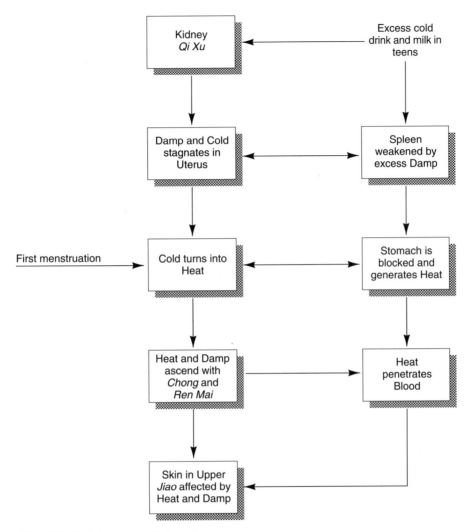

Fig. 13.1   Aetiology and pathology diagram.

putting less emphasis on the precipitating factors. Usually in chronic cases, the opposite approach would be more appropriate. However, in this case there had been too much occurring at an acute level, despite the chronic nature of the complaint.

I therefore decided to use points that cool the Blood, cool the Stomach, and resolve excess Dampness. In addition, I instructed the patient to omit heat and damp-producing foods from her diet e.g. dairy products, coffee, chocolate, alcohol, fried and greasy food. Instead she was advised to eat cooling foods such as celery, fruit, greens, etc.

Treatment procedures for the first 5 weeks

My prescription for the first set of treatments comprised two groups of points which were used alternately during the first 5 weeks, three sessions per week.

- **Group A:** P7 *daling*, P3 *quze* LI11 *quchi*, REN17 *tanzhong* , ST30 *qichong*, ST44 *neiting*, SP10 *xuehai*.
- **Group B:** SP6 *sanyinjiao*, SP9 *yinlingquan*, DU14 *dazhui*, BL16 *dushu*, BL17 *geshu*, BL40 *weizhong*.

GROUP A:

This group comprised points capable of cooling the Blood, mainly via the Stomach and Pericardium systems. P7 *daling*, P3 *quze* and REN17 *tanzhong* are situated locally to and/ or have an effect on the Pericardium (REN17 *tanzhong* is the *mu* point of the Pericardium). The Pericardium is related both to the Heart (its protector) and to the Liver (its companion in the segment of *jueyin*). Both organs, the Heart and the Liver, are closely related to the Blood. In this case, REN17 *tanzhong* served also as a local point for the affected chest region. All points were reduced by quick withdrawal manoeuvres and slow insertions. P3 *quze* was occasionally bled with a thick filiform needle (Lade 1992).

LI11 *quchi*, ST30 *qichong* and ST44 *neiting* are all situated on the *yangming* hand and leg channel. This channel is related to the Stomach and these points are renowned for their cooling ability. LI11 *quchi* is, in fact, a specialised point for skin diseases. ST30 *qichong* is the hinge, or barrier point, of the *chong mai* where the deeper *qi* of the channel ascends to the surface. This channel is generally used to balance the Stomach and, due to its location, it has a harmonising effect on the Uterus.

SP10 *xuehai* is also a specialised point for Blood disorders requiring cooling of the Blood. It makes an age-old and well-known combination with LI11 *quchi* to treat skin diseases (O'Connor & Bensky 1985). These points were also reduced as above.

GROUP B:

SP6 *sanyinjiao* and SP9 *yinlingquan* provide an excellent formula to regulate both Spleen and Kidney, water metabolism in general, and Damp accumulation in the lower *jiao* in particular (O'Connor & Bensky 1985). Thus, this pair was selected in order to resolve the vaginal discharge, promote Uterus function, and regain hormonal balance. These points were evenly manipulated.

DU14 *dazhui* and B16 *dushu* (the *shu* point of the *du* channel) have a cooling and harmonising effect on the *du* channel. The *du mai* (the collecting channel of all the *yang qi* of the body) was thus sedated, assisting in lowering the heat level in general.

B17 *geshu*, the *shu* point of the Blood, and B40 *weizhong* (Lade 1992) both have the ability to cool the Blood and to treat inflamed skin lesions

Skilful and vigorous needle technique

A characteristic of skin diseases is that they involve pathogenic changes to the tissue. This poses a challenge to the practitioner because a very skilful and vigorous needle technique is required. Chinese medicine views material changes to the tissue as both *qi* and Blood stagnation, not just *qi* stasis alone. While the bleeding of specialised points, such as P3 *quze*, has a tremendous effect on Blood stasis, I also administered different forms of manipulation in order to achieve the goal of cooling the Blood whilst moving it.

My needle techniques intended to generate strong movement of the *qi* because the *qi* moves the Blood. ST30 *qichong*, a most influential point, was manipulated to produce *qi* sensation both in the Uterus and over the chest area. After obtaining *deqi*, I intensified the local sensation by quick counter-clockwise withdrawal manipulation. I then redirected the needle tip under the skin in a proximal direction, manipulating it and massaging the skin proximally along the route of the Stomach meridian. Usually this procedure resulted in a clear *qi* sensation propagating from the lower abdomen up to the breasts or even to the throat.

Also, REN17 *tanchong* was manipulated in several directions, lifting and redirecting it each time. This gave rise to a sensation of *qi* dispersing all over the chest.

The age and general health of the patient is also of great significance when administering these needle techniques. One should adjust the extent and amplitude of the needle manipulations very carefully in order not to damage the patient's *qi* and cause undesired reactions.

Radical cleansing of the blood

During the first 5 weeks there was a reasonable reduction in both the amount of acne already existing and in newly formed lesions. The chest area had cleared quite dramatically, while the back seemed to be more stubborn.

At this stage I decided to obtain a more radical blood cleansing effect using diet therapy (Vigmour A, personal communication, 1982). I asked Esther to stop eating solid food for a whole week, and prescribed to her different juices instead. She was to drink a glass of carrot juice mixed with a small quantity of celery juice twice daily, water as much as she pleased, and a glass of almond extract once a day. All acupuncture treatments for this period were suspended. After 2 days on this fasting programme, she had a sudden rise in body temperature with perspiration, and general malaise. Even though I considered this a good sign (a release of long-term internal heat), I instructed her to stop fasting, and start eating gradually. A week later she resumed her fasting, this time without any side-effects, for one complete week. At the end of this week, and a total of 7 weeks since starting treatment, we were happy to discover that her condition had improved by 80%.

Resolving the remaining acne

Now we resumed our treatments at a rate of two sessions per week. It is worthwhile mentioning here that at this point in time Esther no longer had vaginal discharge, irritability or bouts of sudden hunger. Also her most recent periods had changed for the better. In the remaining 3 weeks of treatment, I generally used points from both groups, chosen at random, and administered two special techniques to resolve the few remaining, or newly formed, acne.

The first technique works wonders in the treatment of large boils, abscesses (whether hot or cold), and evidently, also big or tight clusters of acne pustules and comedones. The abscess or pustule is surrounded by 4–6 needles (usually gauge 30, length 40 mm), inserted shallowly beneath the bottom of the abscess, in a horizontal angle, forming a 'blossom' of needles, and pointing to the centre. This is left in situ for approximately 30 minutes. Where Cold boils, or chronic *qi xu* type boils or abscesses exist (which is not the case here), it is also recommended to administer moxa. This is done either by a moxa roll above the boil, or by warm needling of one or two of the needles in the needle-blossom.

The second technique, also applied here, involves shallow tapping of the pustules (especially those with pus), with the seven-star (plum-blossom) needle. This is done until slight bleeding and pus exudes. Immediately afterwards, a cup is laid over the wound for 20 minutes until an amount of blood is sucked out. The wound should then be cleaned and sterilised[2] (Wu Wei Ping, personal communication, 1984).

The application of these techniques gave prompt results in Esther's case, and within 2–3 days the treated wounds usually diminished and disappeared. After 10 weeks of treatment we had almost completely cured the complaint and 1 year later there had been no significant recurrence or relapse.

Outcome	
• Acne disappeared, no recurrence within a year.	• No sudden bouts of hunger.
• No vaginal discharge.	• Overall, a stronger sense of well-being and confidence.
• No irritability.	

Conclusion

Generally skin diseases respond extremely well to acupuncture. The practitioner can monitor the effect of his/her treatments objectively as the results, if any, are visible. In addition, skin diseases involving pathogenic changes of tissue are viewed in Chinese medicine as *qi* and Blood stagnation. Treatment requires the implementation of decisive needling techniques that are capable of moving the *qi* and Blood.

Another important issue is treatment frequency. Considering the goal of Blood dispersal and the severe nature of the problem, the treatments should be carried out at least three times per week. Less than this would most probably not induce the desired effect.

Experienced acupuncturists should observe the impact of their treatments during the different phases of the treatment process, and adjust their techniques accordingly. At the beginning of the treatment process, minor changes, mostly of the *qi* characteristic, should indicate whether or not the treatment is being carried out effectively. In Esther's case, the correct choice of treatment was confirmed by an immediate reduction both in the intensity of the redness and the amount of pus. In addition, decreased vaginal discharge and fewer hunger bouts also indicated a positive change. In practice, response to treatment sometimes stops and the treatment process becomes 'stuck'. A new technique or approach, often on an entirely different level, can create a dramatic response. Such was the case when I implemented a fasting technique in Esther's therapy, a decision that evidently proved itself correct.

NOTES

1   Su Wen from the Huang Di Nei Jing, Chapter 1, Discourse on the natural truth of ancient times.

2   Personal observation in Taichong, Taiwan, 1984.

REFERENCES

Lade A 1992 Acupuncture points, images and functions. Third printing. Eastland Press, Seattle
Lu Shoukang 1993 Acupuncture and moxibustion in the treatment of dermatoses. Journal of Traditional Chinese Medicine 13(1): 69–75
Mei Jianghan 1993 The extraordinary channel *chong mai* and its clinical applications. Journal of Chinese Medicine pp 27–31
Merck Manual 1982, 14th edn. Merck Sharp & Dohme Reseach Laboratories, Rahway p 2048
O'Connor J, Bensky D 1985 Acupuncture, a comprehensive text. Eastland Press, Seattle

■ Shmuel Halevi

Shmuel Halevi was born in 1951 in Israel. His interest in Chinese medicine began around 1978, after reading a book about acupuncture by Dr Felix Mann. At the time Shmuel was the owner of a small and successful printing shop in Galilee, the northern part of Israel. Since no books were available in Hebrew, nor in Israel, at that time, nor were there any Chinese schools of medicine, Shmuel studied by himself from mail-order books from abroad. In order to enhance his general medical knowledge, he took correspondence courses in biology and medicine.

Later, he enrolled at the North American College of Acupuncture and after graduating travelled to Taiwan in order to gain clinical experience. In Taiwan, Shmuel worked and studied in a number of clinics and gained experience both in acupuncture and herbal medicine. After returning to Israel, he sold his printing shop and established his own clinic in Galilee. This was one of the first acupuncture clinics in Israel, particularly in the northern, less populated, part of Israel.

During 1989 Shmuel was appointed as a senior lecturer at the School of Natural Therapies in Tel Aviv, where he lectured and demonstrated acupuncture to the first classes of this school. In 1990, after completing a course in Human Behaviour in the US, he obtained a PhD degree.

Today Shmuel runs two clinics, one in Nahariya, a tourist town on the north-west coast, and the other in Kfar Veradim, about 20 km east of Nahariya, on the hilly western region of Galilee. His patients are mostly the inhabitants of Galilee: Jews, Arabs, and Druse alike, plus occasional patients from other parts of Israel. The diversity and heterogenic nature of his patients has enriched Shmuel's clinical experience, and exposed him to other forms of natural and rural ethnic therapies, of which he takes advantage.

Shmuel is married and has three children, age 4, 17 and 21. One of his major hobbies is hiking on foot around the lovely hilly landscapes of Galilee.

Palpitations, periods and purpose

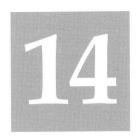

Peter Valaskatgis NEWBURY, MA, USA

An inner resolve

A female patient, Rachel, came to my office a year ago for a consultation. She had been referred to me by her meditation teacher. The patient, in practising mindfulness meditation, was very much aware of a blockage in her breathing pattern, especially during exhalation. In addition, Rachel had had a tightness in her chest for most of her life which was very much fear and anxiety related. During the consultation, Rachel decided that the anxiety and chest tightness were her main concerns, but as will become apparent, there were other issues which Rachel very much wanted to address.

Rachel was a pleasant person, 37 years of age and of medium build. What was most striking to me was her very dull-pale complexion. In talking with her, she seemed a little shy, tense, and frightened and it was my sense that the fear and tension were long-standing and not simply due to her interaction with an acupuncturist for the very first time. In talking, I also sensed in her an inner resolve and a willingness to work with strong effort on her physical concerns and emotional issues.

Palpitations and periods

Rachel also experienced daily palpitations which felt like a fluttering sensation in her chest, with her heart skipping beats. The palpitations were worse during stressful times or when very fatigued. A check-up with a medical doctor had shown no serious abnormalities.

Rachel's other concerns included her gynaecological problems. For the previous 10 years she had had abnormal Pap smears, yeast infections, Bartholin cysts[1] and uterine fibroids. The fibroids had caused heavy bleeding, leading to anaemia, and had been removed 8 years ago. After this surgery, her periods had not been so heavy, but her anaemia had continued to remain borderline. More recently, Rachel had begun spotting a few days after the last day of her period. Her periods were heavy at times and she took Anaprox to control the bleeding and cramping. Recently, she had had an ultrasound scan which had found some new small fibroids. Her gynaecologist suspected that the presence of polyps was possibly the cause of the spotting. Her periods were now regular with some pain and small clotting. Occasionally, Rachel had PMS with symptoms of breast tenderness, emotional sensitivity, and irritability.

No sense of purpose

Regarding emotional issues, Rachel felt quite fearful and anxious, trying to hide her fear by 'pushing it down'. Subsequently she became sad and depressed and this started manifesting in body tension. She also said she had difficulty in communicating feelings and thoughts. Another concern was that she had no sense of purpose and direction in her life.

With regard to my examination, her tongue was pale, slightly dry, slightly swollen, with a slightly reddish tip. There were a few very shallow cracks in the centre and very little white tongue coating. The overall quality of her pulse was thin and choppy, slightly wiry in the Liver position and weaker in the left Kidney position (i.e. in the third position). Also, she was quite pale under the inner lower eyelids.

Summary of clinical manifestations

- Chest tightness with anxiety.
- Breathing blockage on exhalation.
- Palpitations with heart skipping or fluttering, worse with fatigue or anxiety.
- Occipital headaches, monthly and stress related.
- Body tension.
- Spotting in between periods (discharge of brownish blood 3–5 days after period had stopped).
- Menstrual pain, heavy bleeding with small clots.
- Occasional PMS with breast tenderness, emotional sensitivity, irritability.
- Dull pale complexion, pale under inner lower eyelids.
- Fatigue with stress.
- Occasional dry stools.
- Sensitive to cold, and cold extremities.
- Fearful, anxious, becoming sad and depressed when hiding fear.
- No sense of purpose and direction in her life.
- Difficulty in communicating feelings and thoughts.
- Poor night vision, eye 'floaters'.
- Dry skin, at times hair falling out.
- Pulse: overall choppy and thin, slightly wiry in Liver position, weaker in Kidney position.
- Tongue: pale, slightly swollen, slightly dry, reddish tip, few very shallow cracks in centre.

Patterns of disharmony

The major pattern of disharmony was a *qi* and Blood deficiency. The weak Spleen *qi* gave rise at first to heavy bleeding and then to spotting in between periods which in turn led to a Blood deficiency. The Blood deficiency manifested in both the Liver and Heart. Over time the Heart was not only Blood deficient but also becoming *yin* deficient as evidenced by the reddish tip of the tongue.

In addition, there were signs of Liver *qi* stagnation leading to a slight stagnation of Blood as indicated by the period pain with the passing of small clots. Also, the *qi* deficiency which caused the heavy bleeding had led to a stagnation of *qi* and Blood, and this accounted for the discharge of brownish blood 3–5 days after the period had stopped.

The overall condition, in my opinion, was mainly a deficiency of *qi* and Blood with some secondary stagnation of *qi* (stagnation of Liver *qi* and stagnation of *qi* in the chest) and stagnation of Blood in the Uterus.

Evidence for patterns of disharmony

PRIMARY PATTERNS

Spleen *qi* deficiency

- Cold extremities.
- Heavy bleeding.
- Spotting in between periods.
- Tongue: pale.

General Blood deficiency

- Dry skin.
- Hair easily falling out.
- Dull pale complexion, pale under inner lower eyelids.
- Pulse: choppy and thin.
- Tongue: pale, slightly dry.

Heart Blood deficiency

- Palpitations.
- Anxiety.
- Dream-disturbed sleep.

Liver Blood deficiency

- Eye 'floaters'.
- Poor night vision.
- Fear, lack of direction (ethereal soul not rooted).

SECONDARY PATTERNS

Stagnation of *qi* the Chest

- Chest tightness.
- Restriction in the breathing pattern.

Stagnation of Liver *qi*

- Stress-related occipital headaches.
- Body tension (could also be Blood deficiency).
- PMS with breast tenderness, irritability.
- Menstrual pain.
- Pulse: wiry in Liver position.

Blood Stagnation in the Uterus

- Menstrual pain with the passing of clots.
- Uterine fibroids.
- Uterine polyps.

Heart *yin* deficiency

- Palpitations.
- Anxiety.
- Tongue: red tip, tongue cracks.

Aetiology and pathology

The emotional factors are an important cause of Rachel's patterns of disharmony. As a child she was unable to express her feelings and particularly brooded and worried, leading to the Spleen *qi* deficiency. Also, I believe there was a constitutional weakness to the Spleen *qi*. She had had too many gynaecological problems for them to have been caused by emotional factors alone.

The Heart and Liver Blood deficiency was caused by the heavy bleeding and was exacerbated by Rachel's feelings of anxiety, worry, fear and lack of direction in life. Over time, the Heart Blood deficiency led to Heart *yin* deficiency.

Rachel's unresolved and unexpressed feelings of frustration and anger, together with her inability to communicate easily, led to Liver *qi* stagnation. This, together with the chronic anxiety, contributed to stagnation of *qi* in the Chest. Long term Liver *qi* stagnation, combined with blood loss caused by the Spleen *qi* deficiency, led to stagnation of Blood in the Uterus (Fig. 14.1).

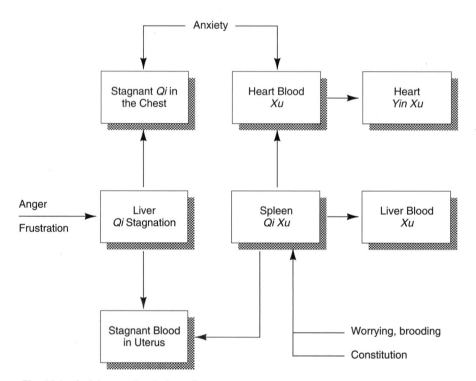

Fig. 14.1 Aetiology and pathology diagram.

Treatment issues

My treatment plan was mainly to tonify the *qi* and Blood deficiency, move the stagnation a little bit, and to try to control the excess bleeding and spotting. In treating the *qi* and Blood deficiency, I also wanted to use points to calm and strengthen the spirit. For the Heart Blood deficiency, as well as the Liver Blood deficiency and constrained Liver *qi* patterns, I thought that acupuncture and herbs could help fairly quickly (i.e. within 3–4 weeks). It was more difficult to assess how effective acupuncture would be in treating Rachel's menstrual problems but we agreed to work through two or three menstrual cycles before reassessing the situation.

I took the patient through my analysis, explaining to her that her lifestyle was relatively healthy and that 'energy medicine' would help to strengthen her both physically and emotionally and would certainly complement and enhance her experience of meditation and psychotherapy.

Although Rachel was anxious about her condition, she felt reluctant to have the D & C procedure (dilatation and curettage) recommended by her gynaecologist and was willing to postpone the operation until she had tried acupuncture. We decided on a treatment plan of two treatments per week for 4 weeks, followed by an evaluation and weekly treatments thereafter if her condition had improved. I had a very good rapport with the patient and believed that this agreed course of action was quite reasonable.

Treatment

I explained to the patient the procedure of inserting the needles and the types of response she might expect from the needle insertion and manipulation. I also explained that I used sterilised and disposable needles. The insertions went smoothly. The most significant aspect of the first treatment was that Rachel became very relaxed and her circulation improved remarkably. Her extremities became warm, she became more energised, and her facial colour changed dramatically. Her dull pale complexion changed to a brighter more 'rosy' one. This was a pleasant surprise for both of us! I sensed that at this point, Rachel realised the potential effectiveness of acupuncture and the experience certainly helped to strengthen her trust and confidence in the therapy. (I wish everyone could respond in this way the first time around!)

First treatment procedures

FIRST POINT PRESCRIPTIONS

- ST36 *zusanli* to tonify Spleen *qi* to control excess bleeding and to tonify Blood by tonifying Spleen.
- SP6 *sanyinjiao* as above and to regulate the Uterus and menstruation, to move stagnant Blood in the Uterus and to calm the mind especially when combined with HT7 *shenmen*.
- REN4 *guanyuan* to nourish Blood by strengthening Kidneys, to regulate the Uterus and to benefit the Original *yuan qi*.

- LIV3 *taichong* to promote the smooth flow of Liver *qi*, to nourish Liver Blood and to assist in calming the mind.
- HE7 *shenmen* to calm the mind and to nourish Heart Blood.
- BL15 *xinshu* to calm the mind, nourish the Heart (helping with palpitations) and to invigorate the Blood.
- BL18 *ganshu* to nourish Liver Blood and to benefit the eyes.
- BL20 *pishu* to tonify Spleen and nourish Blood.
- *Yintang* to calm the mind.
- SP1 *yinbai* with needle and moxa just prior to menstruation to regulate Blood in the Uterus and to stop excess bleeding by strengthening the Spleen's function of holding Blood.
- REN6 *qihai* which was not used in the first treatment but was used subsequently to tonify the Spleen *qi*.

This prescription was intended to tonify *qi* and Blood, calm the mind, and regulate and slightly move *qi* and Blood in the Uterus.

Needle technique: Hand insertion was used. A mild *qi* sensation was obtained for all points. Reinforcing method was used on all points except for LIV3 *taichong* where an even method was used.

Needles: For REN4 *guanyuan*, a 30 mm, 30 gauge needle was used. For all other points 25 mm, 34 gauge needles were used. Needles on the anterior body were retained for 15–20 minutes, needles on the posterior body for 10 minutes.

AUXILIARY TREATMENTS

A patent herbal remedy, Restore the Spleen Pills *gui pi wan*, was prescribed to tonify Spleen *qi* and Heart Blood, calm the mind, and control excess menstrual bleeding. In addition, craniosacral techniques based on Upledger's teachings were used (Upledger 1983). These included the 'respiratory diaphragm release' and 'thoracic inlet release', both intended to release fascial restrictions in the chest area thereby facilitating respiratory diaphragm functioning and 'freeing up breathing'. These techniques are in a sense analogous to P6 *neiguan*'s opening up of the chest but can be more powerful and immediate.

Moving through feelings

The patient experienced some interesting results once treatment began. After 3–4 weeks of treatment, the fear, anxiety, and chest tightness began to dissipate. Rachel felt much less fearful, and was more able to communicate her feelings. It was interesting that as the fear and anxiety began to lessen, she became more in touch with her anger and the way in which it manifested itself in body tension when it was not expressed. The acupuncture assisted her in moving through these feelings by continuing to strengthen *qi* and Blood and move the *qi*.

Now, after 9 months of treatment (currently at 3-weekly intervals) Rachel feels a greater sense of direction, stronger emotionally, and much more able to communicate her feelings, and 'move through them' without sticking in one place. Interestingly, there was a short period during which she found it difficult to make decisions. I added the *yuan* source point

GB40 *qiuxu* (the Gall Bladder rules decisions) and Rachel reported more ease with her decision taking.

Improvement in symptoms

As far as the physical symptoms and signs are concerned, the chest tightness no longer exists, the palpitations have improved, the tension headaches are rare, circulation has improved and facial colour and night vision are much improved.

As far as gynaecological issues are concerned, there is some improvement but work still has to be done. The PMS symptoms have improved. However, the spotting still occurs, but with a smaller amount of brownish discharge. The heavy bleeding with periods still persists. My sense is that as Rachel continues to come for treatment, I'd like to focus more on the gynaecological concerns, choosing additional points and perhaps herbal medicines that directly affect the Uterus. It's interesting to note that Rachel had always been quite anxious regarding her history of menstrual difficulties, but once her *qi* and Blood strengthened, she became more confident and less fearful. In her own words, she became 'more proactive and less victimised' by her circumstances and was able to tell her gynaecologist what medical treatments she preferred or did not prefer.

A positive experience

In closing it has been a very positive experience for me to treat this particular patient. It has been interesting observing both emotional and physical changes occurring simultaneously over time as the patient's *qi* and Blood has strengthened. I have appreciated and greatly respected her approach to her own healing process. For Rachel it has been of great benefit for her to combine, in a proactive manner, psychotherapy, the spiritual practice of meditation and self-inquiry, 'energy medicine', and Western medicine. As far as her acupuncture therapy is concerned, it will be interesting to see how much more can be done regarding her gynaecological concerns. Also, I want to add that Rachel has been very helpful in reviewing this case history for its accuracy.

Summary of outcome

Mental/emotional changes
- Much less fearful, sad and depressed.
- Able to express and communicate emotions more effectively.
- Emotions more 'free flowing'.
- Increased sense of purpose and direction.
- Decision making much easier.

Gynaecological changes

- PMS symptoms of breast tenderness, irritability, sensitivity much improved.
- Spotting still persists but smaller amount.
- Heavy bleeding still persists.
- Pain persists but varies in intensity.

Other symptom/sign changes

- Chest tightness resolved after a few treatments.

- Breathing restriction resolved.
- Complexion much improved.
- Palpitations much improved.
- Extremities warmer.
- Tension headaches less frequent.
- Night vision improved.
- Pulse: no longer choppy, now empty but stronger.
- Tongue: less pale, more normal colour, tip less red.

NOTE

1 Bartholin cysts are commonly found in chronic inflammation of the Bartholin glands which are two small glands situated beneath the vestibule, one at each side of the vaginal opening and at the base of the labia majora (Taber 1980).

REFERENCES

Kaptchuk T 1983 The web that has no weaver. Congdon & Weed, New York

Maciocia G 1989 The foundations of Chinese medicine. Churchill Livingstone, Edinburgh

Maciocia G 1994 The practice of Chinese medicine. Churchill Livingstone, Edinburgh

Taber C 1980 Taber's cyclopedic medical dictionary, 7th edn. FA Davis Philadelphia

Tierney L, McPhee S, Papaldis M 1994 Current medical diagnosis and treatment. Appleton & Lange, Norwalk Ct

Upledger J 1983 Craniosacral therapy. Eastland Press, Seattle

■ Peter Valaskatgis

I have been practising acupuncture since 1979. I studied at the New England School of Acupuncture in Watertown, Ma, USA, the International College of Oriental Medicine in Sussex, England, and the Nanjing College of Traditional Chinese Medicine in Nanjing, China. I have been a faculty member of the New England School of Acupuncture since 1981 and currently serve as chair of the Traditional Chinese Medicine department. I have also studied Chinese herbal medicine and Upledger's craniosacral therapy and I incorporate both in my clinical practice. I have been strongly influenced by my excellent training in Nanjing in 1981 where I learned to be more specific and accurate with respect to diagnosis and point selection. In recent years, I have been strongly influenced by my training in Upledger's craniosacral therapy. I have developed better palpatory skills and use these skills to find energetic restrictions in the body and, when appropriate, use a combination of craniosacral therapeutic techniques and acupuncture to remove these restrictions. These craniosacral tecniques have given me interesting insights into meridian theory and treatment.

Shouting for sympathy

Ken Shifrin OXFORD, UK

Painful episodes of endometriosis

The patient, whom I shall call Kathryn, is a long-term acupuncture patient, having first attended my clinic 10 years ago. She is a 47-year-old, professional health care worker who lives with her teenage son in Oxford. Her main complaint at the time of consultation was endometriosis. This had apparently started at the age of 14, with the onset of her menses and, after 4 years of very painful periods, she was 'officially' diagnosed at the age of 18. This condition had persisted throughout her adult life without remission, apart from during her pregnancy at the age of 30.

The attacks were random in frequency, but always occurred in the spring and again in late summer. They began with acute lumbar pain, which moved to the groin and then settled in the lower abdomen. The attacks were accompanied by exhaustion, which Kathryn believed was part of the attack and not simply the outcome of being in severe pain. Kathryn felt cold most of the time, and extremely cold during an attack.

Kathryn was taking the standard, long-term hormone treatment (danazol) prescribed for endometriosis. The help she derived from this was minimal, but the major side-effect was, to my mind, serious: at the time of consultation she had not had a period in over 7 years, due to the 'pseudo-pregnancy' effect of the medication. She would take a non-steroidal, anti-inflammatory drug during an attack, although this also had little effect. Basically, nothing had ever really helped her condition. The original consultation took place in September, in the midst of a series of painful episodes.

Summary of clinical manifestations

- Attacks of severe pain: starting with acute lumbar pain, moving to the groin and settling in the lower abdomen; accompanied by exhaustion.
- Feeling cold, extremely so during attacks.
- Swelling and pain in the knees since her 20s, susceptible to a damp environment.
- Very prone to headaches during stormy or changeable weather.
- Describes food as 'the bane of my life', always hungry, especially craves cheese, intolerant to wheat and sugar.

- Excessive urination, every 2 hours, clear and copious.
- Frequent fluid retention, especially with high salt intake; much premenstrual retention.
- Lower Burner very cold; during an attack it becomes absolutely icy.
- Long history of constipation.

- Pulse: slow and deep; Kidney pulse empty; Spleen pulse slippery; Liver pulse becomes wiry at the start of an attack.
- Tongue: pale and swollen with a frothy white coat.

Causative factor

As a Five Element practitioner, I found this a fascinating case. At the consultation, Kathryn came across as a confident, cheerful and mature woman who was very self-possessed and knowledgeable about her condition. She had a good 'front', so to speak, discussing the Western medical view of her condition and breezily commenting that 7 years without periods was a 'blessing' from her point of view, as she didn't want any more children and at least she didn't need to worry about contraception! However, it quickly became apparent that she was actually in despair about her condition; she was worried about the possible effects of long-term hormone treatment and was feeling at a low ebb. Her style was a mix of being needy and controlling: she was trying to be 'in charge' but also wanted to let go of 'coping' for a while and let someone else try to help.

In Five Element terms, Kathryn has an Earth Causative Factor.[1] Her predominant colour is yellow, the sound singing, and the odour fragrant. Most of all, she absolutely craves sympathy and understanding, and rapidly pulls the listener into her story, holding his attention while she describes the fine details. She displays the classic 'push/pull' behaviour associated with Earth, alternating between neediness and the rejection of that neediness when others attempt to respond. The way in which she tells her story, going into great detail about the awfulness of it all, and regularly circling back to repeat various crucial bits (to make sure I *really do* understand) is also emblematic of the Earth Element, and corresponds to the 'overthinking' often connected with Spleen imbalance.

Kathryn's secondary Element (known in the Five Element style as the Element 'within' the Causative Factor) is Wood. This is shown primarily by the secondary signs which accompany those given above, namely green colouring, shouting and anger. Kathryn's anger is interesting. What mostly sets her off is people not understanding her, or insufficiently or incorrectly sympathising with her. She 'shouts for sympathy' and, as soon as she gets it, the anger and shouting disappear. This confirmation that sympathy, rather than anger, is primary, strengthens the diagnosis of her Causative Factor as Earth(Wood) rather than Wood(Earth).

Zang fu disharmonies

Kathryn's symptoms point towards a complex pattern of disharmony involving the Spleen and Liver in particular. The breakdown in the transforming and transporting functions of the Spleen, the issues around food, her sensitivity to dampness and stormy weather, and the tongue and pulse all indicate Spleen *qi* deficiency with Damp. From the perspective of a Five Element practitioner, the Earth Causative Factor is considered to be the primary aetiological factor, predisposing Kathryn to Spleen dysfunction.[2] In addition, the acute abdominal pain, the wiry Liver pulse, and the accompanying anger and frustration all point to Liver *qi* stagnation and a tendency towards stasis of Liver Blood. The timing of the attacks (spring and late summer) confirms the involvement of these two organs.

The Kidneys are also in distress. Her Kidney *yang* is very weak, leading to intense coldness, low backache, exhaustion, and frequent urination. This combination of Spleen, Liver and Kidney disharmony has clearly caused great disturbance to the Uterus, which is affected by the Blood Stasis and also the Stagnation of Cold. Analysis of precisely what conditions prevail here is made more difficult by the lack of periods for many years.

Summary of diagnosis and patterns

Causative Factor: Earth

- Predominant signs: colour yellow; sound singing; and odour fragrant.
- Craves sympathy and understanding.
- Alternating neediness and rejection of neediness.

Element within Causative Factor: Wood

- Secondary signs: colour green; sound shouting; emotion anger.
- Anger and shouting disappear with sympathy.

Spleen *qi* deficiency with Damp

- Intolerance of wheat and sugar.
- Sensitivity to dampness and stormy weather.
- Attacks occur in late autumn.
- Tongue: pale.
- Pulse: slippery in the Spleen position.

Liver *qi* and Blood stagnation

- Acute and severe abdominal pain.
- Anger and frustration.
- Attacks occur in spring.
- Pulse: wiry.

Kidney *yang* deficiency

- Intense coldness.
- Low back pain.
- Exhaustion.
- Excessive urination, every 2 hours, clear and copious.
- Tongue: pale, swollen.
- Pulse: slow, deep, empty in the Kidney position.

Blood and Cold stagnation in the Uterus

- Episodes of severe pain and icy coldness in the lower abdomen.

Treatment approach

A fundamental premise of Five Element acupuncture is the notion that the elemental Causative Factor plays a major role in every individual's disease process, and that treatment is almost always directed here in the first instance. In Kathryn's case, we have a very neat match between her Causative Factor and the *zang fu* patterns of disharmony. It is noteworthy that such a match is by no means always the case, and the practitioner will often have to consider carefully the relationship between the Causative Factor and the presenting symptoms. My intention in this case was to tonify Earth, especially the Spleen, using needles and moxa. I assumed that both Wood (Liver) and Water (Kidneys) would also need attention, and there would probably be a need to warm the Lower Burner, due to the stagnation of *qi* and Blood and the presence of intense Cold.

In the Five Element style of practice, one first wants to assess:

1 Whether one's diagnosis of the Causative Factor is correct.
2 How other organs will respond when the Causative Factor is treated.

It is therefore usual to confine oneself to treating the Causative Factor alone (at least for the first few treatments), before directly intervening in other systems. Five Element acupuncture is minimalist in its approach, following the Daoist principle of *wu wei* (the 'Law of Least Action'),[3] and attempting to accomplish the greatest benefit with the least amount of intervention. Feedback from this phase informs the practitioner about how good, or poor, is the intercommunication between the organs. It also helps to guide the practitioner in his aim to treat where it is actually needed, i.e. where natural energetic cycles are unable to bring about improvement by themselves.

The Five Element protocol

Kathryn was quite apprehensive about the first treatment. She had received some acupuncture several years earlier for an unrelated, short-term problem, and had found it helpful but very painful. She needed lots of reassurance about the relatively pain-free needling style common to most Five Element practitioners![4]

The protocol of Five Element treatment includes checking, on the first visit, for the presence of 'Aggressive Energy'. Aggressive Energy is a form of pathogenic *qi* which, under the right conditions (e.g. severe acute or chronic disease or imbalance), may develop and lodge within one or more of the *zang* organs.[5] Aggressive Energy is checked by inserting needles, very superficially, in the back *shu* points of the *zang* organs. The appearance of bright or dark erythema around the needles (compared with other needles placed into non-point areas nearby) indicates the presence of Aggressive Energy. This is then drained by leaving the needles in place until the erythema clears.

Given Kathryn's medical history, I was unsurprised to find Aggressive Energy present on both the Spleen and the Liver. The needles were left in place for about 30 minutes, during which time Kathryn reported feeling progressively 'calmer', 'lighter', 'peaceful' and very relaxed. Following this, the source points of the Spleen and Stomach were tonified. (In accordance with normal Five Element procedure, the source points of the Causative Factor are the first to be needled.[6])

First treatment procedures

Draining the Aggressive Energy

- BL13 *feishu*, the back *shu* point of the Lungs.
- BL14 *jueyinshu*, the back *shu* point of the Pericardium.
- BL15 *xinshu*, the back *shu* point of the Heart.
- BL18 *ganshu*, the back *shu* point of the Liver.
- BL20 *pishu*, the back *shu* point of the Spleen.
- BL23 *shenshu*, the back *shu* point of the Kidney.

The standard technique for draining the Aggressive Energy involves placing the needles very superficially (0.1 *cun*) and, without manipulation, waiting for the erythema to appear. Where points show erythema significantly greater than the 'check' needles used nearby in non-acupoints, these needles are left in place until the erythema clears. In Kathryn's case, the erythema only appeared at BL18 *ganshu* and BL20 *pishu* and these needles were left in place for about 30 minutes.

Treating the source points

- SP3 *taibai*, the source point of the Spleen.
- ST42 *chongyang*, the source point of the Stomach.

Manipulation of the needle is minimal. For tonification, I simply rotate clockwise and remove, or for sedation I rotate anti-clockwise and retain. In this case, I used the tonification technique and did not retain the needles. I used 25 mm, 36 gauge (0.20 mm) needles.

Initial progress

Kathryn arrived a week later for her second treatment and reported feeling markedly better. She was in less pain, the abdominal swelling and discomfort were reduced and, most noticeably, her general level of energy and feeling of well-being were much improved. Although clearly still in the midst of an endometriosis 'episode', she said her ability to cope was much better; she felt stronger 'on the inside'.

Over the following few weeks, treatment focused primarily on building up Kathryn's Earth, using points such as SP4 *gongsun*, SP6 *sanyinjiao* and

SP8 *diji* ('Earth Motivator' or 'Earth Pivot', one of my personal favourites!), ST36 *zusanli*, BL20 *pishu* and BL21 *weishu*. Moxa was found to be a great help, and was used on just about everything!

After a few weeks, it was apparent that the chosen treatment strategy was proving successful, with general all-round improvement. However, the endometriosis, while much reduced in intensity, did not clear completely: some swelling and discomfort persisted. I therefore felt that I needed to use points specifically on the Lower Burner to warm the area and help to move the *qi* and Blood in the area. In the Five Element style, it is considered ideal if one can use points on the Causative Factor channels when treating a locally affected area. I chose, therefore, to use points such as ST29 *guilai*, ST30 *qichong*, SP12 *chongmen* and SP15 *daheng*, along with others such as REN4 *guanyuan*, REN6 *qihai* and REN8 *shenque*. The effect of these, combined with further treatment on command points, was extremely beneficial, and Kathryn's symptoms cleared completely.

Long-term treatment

As a practitioner of the Five Element style, I take the view that seasonal cycles are reflected in our health and well-being, and that long-term treatment can bring about powerful long-term improvements. With Kathryn, her attacks of endometriosis continued to occur, albeit with less pain and discomfort, each spring and late summer for the next few years. Treatment over this period was used primarily to support her Earth (what some might call a 'constitutional' treatment), and to deal with acute attacks as necessary. Gradually, the attacks faded away, with the last one 5 years ago, and since then Kathryn has been free of this problem.

I should also say that treatment did not focus exclusively on the physical aspects of Kathryn's imbalance. It was evident from the outset that Kathryn's mind and spirit were deeply involved in her problems. For example, she could become very rigid and 'stuck', mentally, seemingly unable to take in advice about managing her condition, and becoming negative and frustrated when another attack started. She would sometimes assume the air of a martyr, saying things like 'No one really understands what I'm going through, but it's OK, I'll just carry on and manage somehow'. There were also connections between her medical condition and her sexuality. When she began treatment, her marriage was an unrewarding, detached relationship which subsequently led to divorce. Her relationships have become much more rewarding for her over the years. She appears to have integrated the masculine and feminine sides of her nature much better, discovering that it's possible for her to be powerful, confident, and successful without having to sacrifice her soft, yielding and receptive side.

I have no doubt that this internal change has been a major part of her healing process, one which both she and I believe that acupuncture treatment helped to set in train.

Five Element acupuncture places great stock in the point names as indicators of the potential value and effect of each point, along with considerations such as the channel involved and also the area of the body where the point lies.[7] For example, to help overcome the mental rigidity and doom-laden air that would sometimes prevail, I used points such as BL46 *geguan* 'Thought Dwelling', ST24 *huaroumen* 'Lubrication Food Gate', ST25 *tianshu* 'Heavenly Pivot', SP16 *fuai* 'Abdomen Sorrow', and LIV14 *qimen* 'Gate of Hope'. When Kathryn needed a sense of perspective regarding her problems, and also help to resolve the deeper issues affecting her, I chose points such as KID25 *shengcang* 'Spirit Storehouse', SP20 *zhourong* 'Encircling Glory', ST4 *dicang* 'Earth Granary', and two 'Windows of the Sky' points, ST9 *renying* 'People Welcome' and REN22 *tiantu* 'Heaven Rushing Out'. Naturally these are only examples, and only one or two such points would be used in a single treatment.

Kathryn continues to be well, leading a productive and enjoyable life. She seems much more 'settled' somehow, more at ease within herself and has a much greater grasp on her own health and disease processes. She describes herself as being much stronger, more 'in control', and less in need of others' approval and understanding. She continues to attend for treatment, usually at the change of each season unless a specific need arises. Of course, she still has an Earth Causative Factor, so whenever any problem does crop up, she takes great pains to ensure that I *really do* understand how she feels!

The essence of Chinese medicine

Kathryn's treatment has been very rewarding for me. It has confirmed to me the power of simple, direct treatment aimed primarily at the underlying cause of a person's problems. The effectiveness of such treatment is something I find extremely gratifying. In a world where both patients and practitioners are constantly bombarded with information, and where the choice of medical interventions seems increasingly complex, the possibility that a more simple, gentle approach can relieve even seemingly intractable problems is a welcome antidote as well as a valuable lesson. J R Worsley (personal communication, 1975) would often refer to what he called the 'Su Wen treatment', the 'one needle which cured ten thousand diseases', and this ideal remains an archetype for practitioners of the Five Element style.

Another aspect of this treatment which I find inspiring, and which is reflective of Five Element practice, is the nature and quality of the interaction between myself and the patient. The central role of the rapport and connection between patient and practitioner, and the need to access the deeper levels of functioning within the patient's being (which can only happen if the practitioner can work from a deep level within him- or herself), are tenets fundamental to this tradition. From this arises the belief that effective diagnosis and treatment of patients cannot be viewed separately from the health and balance of the practitioner, and that professional and personal development must go hand in hand.

In these and other respects, I believe the Five Element style, at its root, reflects something of the profound essence of Chinese medicine, described for example in the Ling Shu Larre (1995),[8] whose authors believed that:

> *"a good practitioner's diagnosis is a connection from deep within himself to the Spirits of the patient", which would enable this "skilled artisan" to "interpret the rapport of the jing shen and go at once to the seat of the malady", acting "prudently, but without the least hesitation, controlling the manner and power of his gesture.".*

Such was the power and potential of acupuncture, that when the practitioner could truly work at this level, his or her work would become 'a masterpiece: the faultless fulfilment of infallible inspiration'. While achieving such a level may well be beyond my, or perhaps anyone's, grasp, it seems to me, nevertheless, a goal worth striving towards.

Postscript

I asked Kathryn to review her case study and when she'd read it her immediate suggestion was 'Tell them about the dream!', which I'd actually forgotten about until she reminded me. On the night after her first treatment, she dreamt that she'd walked out into her garden, to be confronted by a scene of neglect and abandonment, with all her plants smothered by twisting, writhing, nightmarish-looking vines. She picked up her tools and laboured through the night, hacking away at this 'unwelcome guest' (her words). By sunrise the task was accomplished, and she woke with 'a sense of renewal and self-confidence'.

NOTES

1 The concept of the 'Causative Factor' was originally promulgated in the West by J R Worsley in the early 1970s, and is central to the practice of Five Element acupuncture. Within each individual, one of the Five Elements is predominant, giving rise to many of our personality and behavioural traits, as well as our patterns of health and disease. Diagnosis of the Causative Factor is carried out primarily through perceiving the predominant colour, sound, odour and

emotion of the patient. Treatment of the Causative Factor forms the central core around which the treatment pattern is based. Although similar to what is sometimes referred to as 'constitutional' imbalance, the usefulness and significance of the Causative Factor in understanding human energetic function and, as the foundation of a treatment protocol in correcting disharmony, make it a truly unique and innovative addition to the theory and practice of traditional acupuncture.

Each of us has a Causative Factor 'for life', as it were. Whilst the *effects* of an individual's Causative Factor will wax and wane over time, the thing itself never disappears or changes to another Element. Put simply, whereas syndromes, pathogenic factors, etc., are reflective of *what a person has*, the Causative Factor is reflective of *who the person is*.

2 A note about aetiology may be useful here. Whilst every individual has, in Five Element terms, a Causative Factor, the origin of this in each person is a matter of speculation. Debate about this usually revolves around the 'nature versus nurture' dilemma and, as in other spheres, one rarely achieves a sense of resolution at the end! For a Five Element practitioner, the fact that someone's Causative Factor lies in Fire, Earth, Metal, etc., is the significant thing, rather than speculative notions about its origin.

Aetiological factors are therefore seen in a different context in Five Element practice, compared to the modern Traditional Chinese Medicine (TCM) style. The Causative Factor of an individual is understood to be of a different order altogether than the usual 'precipitating causes' one associates with TCM syndromes. Indeed, the Causative Factor is considered to be the predominant 'precipitating cause' in most illness, especially that of a chronic nature. The Causative Factor is likely to *predispose* the individual to disharmony and disease, primarily within the affected Element, but also, via Five Element interrelationships such as the *sheng* and *ke* cycles, in other Elements/Organs as well. Thus, although the aetiology of someone's Causative Factor may be obscure, it will nevertheless be found to be the primary aetiological factor in much human illness.

3 The principle of 'non-action' is fundamental to Daoist thought, and has always formed a central pillar of Five Element practice. It is summarised well in the following passage from Lao Tzu (Cleary 1991):

> *Small amounts are attainable,*
> *Large amounts are confusing;*
> *Subtly arrange the outcome, and nothing more.*
> *Do not use force.*

Others, apart from those schooled in the Five Element style, have also advocated this approach. Fr Claude Larre (1991), in a lecture series given at the College of Traditional Acupuncture, stated that using many points in a treatment was an attempt (usually misguided) to 'tie down' the *qi*, to force it into a pattern dictated by the practitioner, whereas a simple treatment allowed the *qi* to find its own level and realise its true potential. The notion that 'simple is best' and that the greatest gain is achieved from the smallest intervention, runs through ancient medical classics, and is a distinguishing characteristic of traditional acupuncture. For example, the Ode to the Streamer out of the Dark (Bertschinger 1991) comments 'What these doctors (who used what is known as spiritual healing) in all sincerity thought most highly of was a single needle inserted into a hole, the disease responding to the hand and it lifting.'.

4 The needle technique employed by most Five Element practitioners is more closely akin to Japanese needling styles than to modern TCM techniques, aiming to cause as little discomfort to the patient as possible.

5 There are no specific classical references to what is termed 'Aggressive Energy'. Bob Flaws (1989) speculated that Aggressive Energy is Worsley's term for *xie qi* or Evil *qi*, and pointed out that, over time, Evil *qi* will tend to accumulate in the *zang* organs as Evil heat. He went on to support the notion that such a situation could be characterised as a serious block to treatment, and that superficial needling of the back *shu* points, with the needles retained, was a classically accepted method of dispersal.

6 Extensive use of the source points has always been part of the treatment protocol of Five Element acupuncture. Worsley (personal communication, 1975) described them as providing 'safety' and 'stability' in treatment, and advised that they be used both at the initial stage of treatment and also, in combination with other points, to provide a 'grounding' or 'anchoring' effect.

   Such a description is entirely consistent with the classical relationship between the source points and the *yuan* or 'Original' *qi*. Original *qi* is described by Maciocia (1989) as 'the foundation of all the *yin* and *yang* energies of the body', and, due to its close links with the *jing*, as 'the foundation of vitality and stamina'. Nan Jing 66 (Larre 1992), which discusses the relationship between the *yuan qi*, the Triple Burner, and the source points, states: 'When the *zang* and *fu* have illnesses, one needles the source.'. Claude Larre (1992) explains that the source points provide a specific place on each of the *zangfu* where these properties may be reinforced. Bearing in mind the earlier discussion of how the Causative Factor is understood, the use of source points in Five Element practice is entirely consistent with this view.

7 The significance and uses of point names are a deep and complex subject, an investigation of which is beyond the scope of this work. The medical classics are filled with references to the point names and discussions about their importance. In 'The Thousand Gold Piece Prescriptions', written in 625 AD, the author, Sun Si Miao (Ellis et al 1989) states: 'The names of the points are not nominal; each has a profound meaning.'. Other, more modern authors (Ellis et al 1989) state that the point names, whilst often veiled or poetic in style, contain intricate details about point usage and 'are guides to the system of medicine that named them'.

8 I strongly recommend the translation and commentary of Larre (1995) on the Ling Shu.

REFERENCES

Bertschinger R (trans) 1991 The golden needle: and other odes of traditional acupuncture. Churchill Livingstone, Edinburgh

Cleary T (trans) 1991 Wen-Tzu. Understanding the mysteries: further teachings of Lao-Tzu. Shambala, Boston

Ellis A, Wiseman N, Boss K 1989 Grasping the Wind. Paradigm, Boston

Flaws B 1989 Four LA blocks to therapy and TCM. Traditional Acupuncture Society Journal 6: 5–7

Larre C 1992 Chinese medicine from the classics. Heart Master/Triple Heater. Monkey Press, Cambridge

Larre C 1995 Rooted in spirit: the heart of Chinese medicine. Station Hill Press, Barrytown
Maciocia G 1989 The foundations of Chinese medicine. Churchill Livingstone, Edinburgh

■ Ken Shifrin

I am a New Yorker by origin, but mellowed (somewhat!) by 25 years of living in Britain. My interest in Oriental philosophy and medicine began in 1970, when I first encountered macrobiotics and the writings of Georges Oshawa.

I began my acupuncture studies in 1975 at the College of Traditional Chinese Acupuncture in Leamington Spa, whose classes were actually held in a local hotel! I count myself lucky to have begun work at that time. J R Worsley proved to be an immensely inspiring teacher and practitioner and both he, and the style of practice that he taught, have remained the dominant, formative influences on my work.

Having qualified in 1977, I received great support during my first few years of practice from J R Worsley, from John Hicks, former Dean of the College, and others involved with the College at the time, notably Julia Measures, Judy Becker, Allegra Wint and Meriel Darby. I have been influenced by many teachers and writers, especially Ted Kaptchuk, Steven Birch, Mark Seem and Bob Flaws. My close colleague Peter Mole has, for many years, been a great ally in my practice, teaching and political work.

Another major strand in my work developed when I began teaching at the College in 1981. I have always found teaching to be enormously rewarding, especially clinical supervision. The satisfaction derived from seeing students become practitioners is balanced by the challenge to continually develop my own abilities.

Fritz Smith, the originator of zero-balancing, also served as a wonderful role model of how to be a practitioner and teacher. I would also mention Fr Claude Larre and Elisabeth Rochat de la Vallee, whose lectures and writings on the essence of Chinese medicine have served as a permanent source of wisdom and inspiration.

The tip of the volcano

David A. Bray TORONTO, CANADA

Despair and despondency

Helen was a 39-year-old, slightly overweight woman. Her facial expression and body language indicated that she was both nervous and tense. She later explained that she had seen numerous medical practitioners regarding her presenting physical complaint, all to no avail. Not one single practitioner had been able to help her in the diagnosis, treatment or management of her condition. Helen hoped that I would be able to help her because she knew friends and acquaintances who had been treated successfully with Traditional Chinese Medicine (TCM) modalities[1]. I sensed that her belief in the positive experiences and outcomes of her friends and acquaintances had been a major factor in her decision to try another form of assessment and treatment. Helen though seemed frustrated and anxious and, as she put it, was no further ahead by pursuing conventional forms of treatment in reaching a diagnosis, treatment or resolution of her main presenting complaint. However, she expressed a healthy curiosity in TCM and desired a similar success story to that of her friends who had sought to be treated using a TCM approach.

Chronic right nipple discharge

Helen described a long history of premenstrual syndrome (PMS) as well as her main problem of tenderness, and a continuous serous discharge from her right nipple. The problem had begun after the weaning of her second child, almost 7 years ago, which was also when her husband had left her. She was clearly agitated and anxious about the problem with her right breast and indicated that the PMS was something she had learned to live with.

Upon inquiry into the onset of the presenting complaint Helen became tearful, although very emotionally controlled. Her first child was conceived at the age of 29, followed by the birth of her second child 2 years later. Very shortly after the birth of her second child her husband decided to terminate their marriage and to separate. Clearly, Helen still bore much resentment, indicated by her tone of voice and the defensive body posture which she assumed while relating this history to me. Helen further went on to tell me that both her mother and grandmother had died of breast cancer. As she related this part of the story to me, Helen's angry, defensive tone and body language turned frail and she was truly afraid that she might also die in this way. At this time Helen was a single mother who worked full-time in a stressful, high power profession in order to support her two children.

Throughout the interview Helen would tell of her problems and concerns sighing and belching frequently and pointing or indicating that her right breast was her only problem. I noted that Helen would frequently point to her right breast while relating other problems to me, indicating that she felt this problem was related to many factors. She was also concerned about the appropriateness and applicability of TCM to help her resolve her condition. I reassured Helen that TCM might be able to help if she would let me explain and discuss TCM's interpretation and explanation of the nature and presentation of her complaint.

After the first interview I proceeded to explain to Helen some of TCM's rationale in terms of interpreting clinical signs and symptoms as well as the standard traditional techniques of pulse and tongue assessment, and the information that was gathered from these methods. Her curiosity was piqued by TCM's rationale and approach, although I could sense a very deep level of frustration and disappointment in the inability of other medical practitioners and specialists to resolve her condition.

Main clinical manifestations

Her tongue was reddish with a slightly greasy yellow coating, particularly on the centre and on the right lateral margin. There was very little coating on the left lateral margin. After the tongue assessment the patient added that at times she felt nauseous with a sense of constriction in her throat. Her pulse was slightly rapid and wiry, especially in the middle positions and particularly on the left.

Further questioning revealed that Helen quite often felt nauseous, although not to the point of vomiting, and was diagnosed as having chronic gastritis. Headaches were regular, diagnosed by her physician as tension headaches. Persistent right shoulder pain was mentioned, and was ascribed by her to her stressful position at work. Chronic pasty bowel movements were also noted. Menstruation was regular, although at times would arrive after several days of perimenstrual breast tenderness and irritability. The passage of dark red clotted blood was the norm for the first 2 or 3 days of flow, after which her menstruation seemed to end abruptly.

Inquiry into previous medical practitioners she had seen included several general practitioners and specialists who were unable to definitively diagnose or advise on management for her main complaint. Repeated physical examination, tissue biopsy, mammography, ultrasound and culturing of the discharge revealed no active disease process or infection. Helen anxiously indicated that while she had been assured that nothing had been missed or overlooked by other practitioners, she felt that something more serious was going on. Other than the occasional anodyne to relieve her headaches and a combination antacid and digestive enzyme, the patient took no prescriptive medication.

Helen openly discussed the stress in her life and further related her level of frustration, anger and disappointment in her physical condition and her life in general as a single mother caring for two children. At this point dietary intake, home life and work, and the need to have more time for relaxation were discussed. Given her hectic lifestyle, her diet comprised many fatty and difficult-to-digest foodstuffs such as dairy products (yoghurt, cheese and milk shakes), nuts and convenience foods. At this point I felt a shift in Helen's attitude as I inquired into issues that were seemingly unrelated (according to her understanding at this time) to her isolated complaint of a chronic right nipple discharge. I asked questions and inquired into areas of her life that other practitioners had not, and seemed interested in more than just the 'problem'.

Summary of clinical manifestations

- Chronic serous discharge from the right nipple.
- Tenderness at the right nipple.
- Persistent right shoulder pain.
- Belching and sighing.
- Angry, defensive tone.
- Tearful.
- Bitter pasty taste in the mouth.
- Dark clotted menstruation for the first 2–3 days of flow.
- Emotional constraint and control.
- Emotional lability.
- Emotional stress, frustration, anxiety, anger, irritability, resentment.
- Gastritis, nausea.
- Low back pain.
- Malar flush.
- Pasty bowel movements with sensation of burning on evacuation.
- Premenstrual tension, perimenstrual breast tenderness.
- Sense of constriction in the throat.
- Tension headaches.
- Thirst.
- Tiredness, low energy.
- Tongue: reddish with a slightly greasy coating noted especially on the centre and right lateral lingual margin, little coating on the left lateral margin. The tongue was devoid of coating at the root.
- Pulse: slightly rapid, wiry and rolling especially noted in the left and right middle positions, especially on the left. The pulse was hollow, especially in the left rear position.

Identifying the patterns of disharmony

The major sources for the diagnostic approach included standard TCM assessment of tongue and pulse as well as all information gathered in the initial interview, including additional commentary from the patient. There were seemingly contradictory signs and symptoms, which did not interfere with or figure in the working assessment and treatment plan. I was most concerned about eliciting patient compliance and understanding of the TCM rationale and approach. No actual disease process or pathology had been determined by Helen's conventional primary physicians, therefore I felt confident in my working assessment and treatment plan.

Patterns of disharmony

Liver *qi* stagnation, Heat invading the Stomach

- Discharge from the right nipple.
- Emotional stress, frustration, anxiety, anger, resentment.
- Emotional constraint and control.
- Emotional lability.
- Tiredness, low energy.
- Tension headaches.
- Sense of constriction in the throat.
- Premenstrual tension, perimenstrual breast tenderness, irritability.
- Dark clotted menstruation.
- Belching and sighing.
- Gastritis, nausea.
- Thirst.
- Tongue: reddish.
- Pulse: rapid, wiry.

Damp-heat in the Spleen and Stomach

- Chronic serous discharge from the right nipple, exiting along the Stomach channel.

- Belching.
- Gastritis.
- Bitter pasty taste in the mouth.
- Pasty bowel movements with sensation of burning on evacuation.
- Tiredness, low energy.
- Tongue: reddish with a slightly greasy coating noted especially on the centre and right lateral lingual margin.
- Pulse: slightly rapid and rolling bilaterally in the middle positions.

Kidney and Liver *yin* deficiency

- Emotional stress, frustration, anxiety.
- Thirst, sense of constriction in the throat.
- Tiredness, low energy.
- Low back pain.
- Malar flush.
- Tongue: reddish and devoid of coating at the root.
- Pulse: rapid and hollow especially in the left rear position.

Aetiology and pathology

Yin xu of Kidney will give rise to *yin xu* of Liver and consequently give rise to constraint and the formation of Heat (Fig. 16.1). Emotional factors coupled with dietary factors may give rise to Stagnation and Heat in the Stomach. Heat oppression in the Stomach will further oppress the

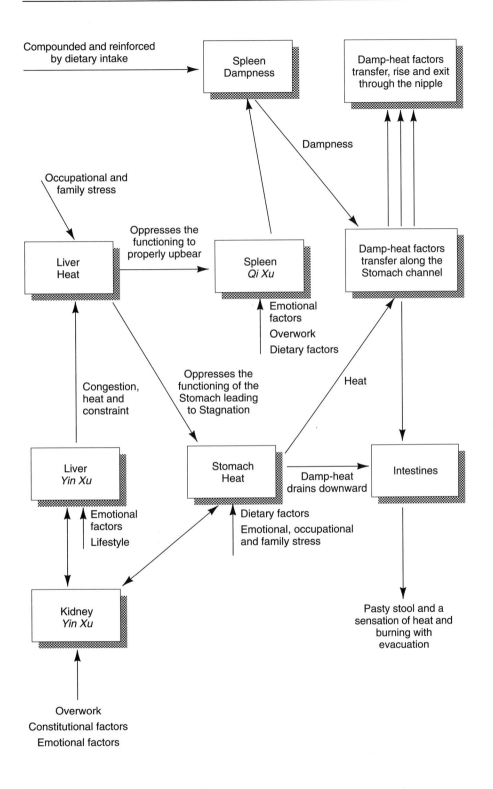

Fig. 16.1 Aetiology and pathology diagram.

functioning of its paired organ the Spleen, and the factors of Damp Spleen will then couple with Heat to form Damp-heat. Mental depression will adversely affect the patency of Liver *qi* and over consumption of fatty food will bring about Stagnation of Heat in the Stomach channel. Heat in the Stomach affects the downbearing function of the Stomach *qi* and gives rise to nausea and thirst with the factors of Heat and Dampness transferring to the Stomach channel. According to TCM theory, the nipples are located on the Stomach channel and the breasts are where the Liver meridian is distributed. Heat and Damp accumulation in the Stomach coupled with stagnation of Liver *qi* may give rise to the Dampness and Heat rising and exiting through the nipple(s), presenting as a discharge clinically.

Eliciting trust and compliance

The prime factor in order to elicit patient compliance was to explain the condition as perceived by TCM standards of assessment and to provide an appreciation of the patho-physiology as related to Helen's prime presenting complaint. The first and foremost change required was one of diet. The patient was counselled on which foodstuffs to minimise and, if possible, eliminate so that they would not further 'feed' the condition. The second factor to be addressed was a reduction in the patient's levels of stress. I encouraged her to seek help from a professional counsellor to address emotional issues. As all of this was explained to Helen there was a very definite shift in her attitude and she no longer felt helpless or victimised by her condition. She became aware of the active role she could play in her return to good health.

The patient reacted favourably to the treatment plan and was enthusiastic about ways in which her situation might be resolved. I sensed that she no longer viewed her complaint as a pathological chronic problem for which there was no answer, explanation or solution. As time progressed I sensed a growing trust and belief in a possible resolution to her compliant. Helen became more interactive, asking questions with enthusiasm, offering more information and suggesting herself how change might be possible. This shift elicited both trust and compliance as well as a commitment to the process. No prognosis was given other than an explanation that chronic conditions did sometimes take time to respond. Helen recognised that after all this time there had been no change in her condition since the initial appearance of 'the symptoms', and added that 'good things take time'. She felt empowered to participate in her recovery and to move both emotionally and physically from a pattern that had troubled her for almost 7 years.

The first treatment

Treatment commenced upon the initial visit as both the patient and I agreed that there was no time like the present. Helen's enthusiasm and hopefulness were quite high at this time. I explained to her the rationale and methodology that would be used to treat her, capitalising on the fact that everything was clearly explained in the initial consultation. Helen appeared anxious about acupuncture because it was a new experience for her and she anticipated some physical pain. I slowly and carefully explained the procedure as I began inserting the needles, and when the third needle was being inserted she inquired when I would begin! By using technique and verbal distraction she had been unaware that the procedure had even started. Helen then appeared anxious and I reassured her that we were almost finished with the insertion of the needles. After insertion I instructed her to relax, breathe deeply, and not to be overly preoccupied with all that had been discussed. At the end of the first treatment she appeared very relaxed and commented that she could not remember how long it had been since she had felt so relaxed. I urged her to try to hold on to the moment and to remember it in times of stress or when she felt at a loss or in despair.

My only hopes and expectations for the first treatment were to elicit her compliance and trust. I explained that lasting results could only be achieved with successive reinforcing treatments coupled with lifestyle and dietary changes. At the end of the first treatment I urged Helen to call me if she had any questions or wished to discuss any changes of which she was unsure. This was followed up by phone calls to detail both the positive changes and the difficulties that she was experiencing. I advised her to carry on in this way, trying to prevent the solution from becoming another problem for her.

Treatment procedures

FIRST TREATMENT

- SI1 *shaoze* disperses Heat, removes obstruction from the channel. It is traditionally used in the treatment of diminished lactation and mastitis and it is an empirical point for breast abscess. It is also the Well point of the SI channel.

- ST34 *liangqiu* clears the channels, pacifies the Stomach, removes obstructions from the channels, subdues rising Stomach *qi*, and is used for gastritis and mastitis. It is the Accumulating point of the Stomach channel.

- GB42 *diwuhai* is classically combined with ST34 *liangqiu* in the treatment of mastitis. It is an adjunct point in the treatment of low back pain.

- GB40 *qiuxu* is a Source point of the GB channel and promotes the smooth flow of Liver *qi*.

- GB21 *jianjing* adjusts *qi* circulation and removes obstruction of *qi* in the chest and hypochondriac regions.

- LIV3 *taichong* is a Source point of the Liver channel and is used for sore and congested throat, for relieving constraint, and for dysmenorrhoea.
- ST36 *zusanli* is a uniting point of the Stomach channel, it orders the Spleen and Stomach and regulates the *qi* and Blood.
- ST18 *rugen* lowers Stomach Fire in order to eliminate accumulation and stagnation of pathogenic factors.
- LIV13 *zhangmen* regulates the Liver *qi*, regulates the circulation of *qi* and Blood and assists the transformation and transportation of the Spleen.

Sources for these point actions are from O'Connor & Bensky (1984), Chen Xinnong (1987) and Maciocia (1989).

Needling methods: Points were needled on the afflicted side, or with bilateral insertion in the case of LIV3 *taichong*, GB40 *qiuxu*, GB21 *jianjing*, ST18 *rugen* and LIV13 *zhangmen*. Insertion was with a guide tube. For all points *de qi* was achieved. All points were needled with 30 mm needles, retained for 20 minutes with reducing method.

SUBSEQUENT TREATMENTS

Additional points were added and deleted as treatment progressed and the factors of Heat and Dampness diminished. Later treatment focused on ensuring patency of *qi*, safeguarding against the development and accumulation of Heat and Dampness and tonifying *yin*, for which I employed a different selection of points.

CHINESE HERBS

Chinese medicinal herbs were employed, initially using a combination of prescriptive herbs in the form of decoction as well as Chinese patent preparations based on the TCM patterns of discrimination as discussed earlier. The main patent formulae employed were *dan zhi xiao yao wan* (Augmented Rambling Powder) based on Rambling Powder *xiao yao wan* with the addition of Fructus Gardeniae *zhi zi* and Cortex Moutan Radicis *mu dan pi* , Soothe the Liver Pills *shu gan wan* and Healthy Breast Tablets *ru kang pien*.

Positive changes take hold

The initial improvement in digestion coupled with dietary modification and personal counselling changed both attitude and outlook, empowering Helen to become an active participant in her health care. As positive changes began to take hold both mentally and physically I sensed that the patient was becoming more aware of the relationship between psyche and soma. While there had been numerous distressing, emotional instances in her life (e.g. her relationship with her former husband, the death of both her mother and grandmother due to breast cancer, and her occupational stress) she was no longer so consumed with worry, anger and emotional baggage. She had a more positive attitude and was increasingly aware of her role in safeguarding and maintaining her own health by feeling empowered as a participant in control rather than a victim.

The immediate outcome for Helen was a change in her digestion. As a consequence of dietary changes and regular acupuncture treatments, the symptoms of belching and gastritis were ameliorated. Also, she experienced a change in the consistency of her bowel movements to a firmer and more complete evacuation with absence of burning. Over the course of the initial 6 weeks of treatment, the chronic serous discharge from the right nipple diminished in frequency and volume. After this, the breast and nipple tenderness were gradually eliminated. Over the course of the next 3 months the chronic serous discharge decreased progressively and was completely eliminated. Helen sought personal counselling as well as relaxation classes and took an interest in exercise and relaxation and took time to enjoy being with her children. There was a positive change in mental outlook. Over the next 3 months, menstruation became easier with the disappearance of clotted blood and PMS symptoms were of a shorter and less intense duration. Headaches became less frequent, mood became more even, back pain relieved, overall energy level increased and mental state improved.

A valuable learning experience

For me, this case was particularly challenging because I had not previously encountered such extreme symptoms. Using the sound rationale and methodology of TCM, I was able to gain insight into the patient's problem. However, I was most concerned with eliciting her cooperation and compliance with the treatment plan. I saw a similarity between this case and previous cases of premenstrual syndrome (PMS) that I had treated where the prime presenting complaint was breast distension. The puzzling part of this case was the discharge. Nevertheless, using approriate treatment principles, I was able to formulate a treatment plan specific to this patient's presentation.

Helen's case helped to deepen my appreciation of Chinese medicine not just as a physical/energetic form of therapy, but also as a way of understanding the relationship factors and influences resulting in a particular case presentation. This case also deepened my belief in treating each person as an individual and reinforced the importance of eliciting patient understanding and appreciation. Both practitioner and patient enter into a relationship which, if successful, provides a valuable learning experience for all involved.

NOTES

1   I define Traditonal Chinese Medicine (TCM) as being a cohesive system of thought, experience, theory and treatment. Health is a reflection of the balanced and harmonious functioning of the physiological, emotional and energetic factors in the body. TCM attempts to perceive and treat the whole person with regard to all these factors. Different modalities, such as traditional acupuncture,

Chinese herbology and manipulative therapy *tui na* as well as physical movement therapy, such as *qi gong* and *t'ai chi ch'uan,* all assist in restoring this balance. Each modality may be employed and adapted to treat each specific clinical complaint and individual.

REFERENCES

Cheng Xinnong 1987 Chinese acupuncture and moxibustion. Foreign Languages Press, Beijing

Maciocia M 1989 The foundations of Chinese medicine. Churchill Livingstone, Edinburgh

O'Connor J, Bensky D (trans) 1984 Acupuncture, a comprehensive text, 3rd edn. Shanghai College of TCM, Eastland Press, Seattle

FURTHER READING

Flaws B 1982 The path of pregnancy. Blue Poppy Press, Colorado

Nanjing College Of Traditional Chinese Medicine 1987 Concise traditional Chinese gynaecology. Jiangsu Science and Technology Publishing House, China pp 252–260

Wolfe H L 1989 The breast connection: a laywoman's guide to the treatment of breast disease by traditional Chinese medicine. Blue Poppy Press, Colorado

Xu Xiangcai 1989 The English-Chinese Encyclopaedia of Traditional Chinese Medicine, vol. 12. Higher Education Press, Beijing

Yang S Z, Liu D 1992 Fu Qing Zhu's gynaecology. Blue Poppy Press, Colorado pp 184–86, pp 248–51

Zhang Ting-Liang 1987 A handbook of traditional Chinese gynaecology. The Zhejiang College of Traditional Chinese Medicine, Blue Poppy Press, Colorado pp 118–121

Zhang Enqin 1990 Clinic of traditional Chinese medicine, vol. 2. Publishing House of Shanghai College of Traditional Chinese Medicine, Shanghai

■ David A. Bray

My initial interest and exposure to Chinese culture began over 20 years ago when I commenced the study of *T'ai Chi Ch'uan* and *Qi Gong*. It was at the urging and prompting of my T'ai Chi teacher that I took serious interest in the professional study of traditional Chinese medicine. He recognised my aptitude, interest and keen fascination for the topic. I have never lost the enthusiasm and allure that I initially experienced. Many aspects of Chinese culture, thought, and practice have permeated my life, and I feel profoundly honoured that I am able to bridge a cultural gap in many areas of my life, both professionally and personally.

I trained at the Guangzhou Institute of Traditional Chinese Medicine between 1978 and 1983. My clinical teachers emphasised the fact that in the light of all techniques, theories and modalities, the patient is always unique. I continue to be reminded of both our uniqueness as well as our similarities. A sound foundation in TCM theory provides the best foundation not only to understanding and explaining conditions or clinical presentations, but also to establishing treatment plans that are patient-specific and not based on any protocol.

I am active in the development of TCM as a profession, and teach seminars and classes on health-related topics that derive from Chinese health systems. I am a frequent contributor to public information sessions and professional associations. I maintain an extremely busy practice as I struggle to keep the balance between what has become both a passion and an obsession. I am also active as a consultant for professional and governmental agencies for establishing guidelines and criteria for standards of educational and professional practice.

Hysterectomy: is it necessary?

Felicity Moir LONDON, UK

Excessive bleeding

Lorca was a 32-year-old woman of 1.6 m and 77 kg (170 lbs). Her ethnic background was Afro-Caribbean and she was working part-time as a personal assistant. She had a grey hue to her face and a look of extreme tiredness and was relieved to sit down. Her voice was slow and quiet.

She presented with a 3-year history of multiple fibroids causing severe menorrhagia and metrorrhagia[1] and extreme stabbing pain in the abdomen with an intense heaviness and ache extending to the back and down the legs. The pain would start just before the period and last 4 days. At times it had been so severe that she had been hospitalised. She would bleed for 10 days, mostly a flood of dark red blood with large black clots until the last 2 days when she had a light-coloured flow. This bleeding occurred twice monthly and Lorca was unaware which bleeding was her period and which was mid-cycle bleeding.

A desire to have children

At this point I asked Lorca about her Western medical treatment and plan. She replied that she was seeing a gynaecologist who had recommended a hysterectomy. She was reluctant to accept this because she wanted to have children and hoped there might be some other way forward. There had been some talk of a possible myomectomy[2] (removal of the fibroids alone) but the gynaecologist was unhappy with this proposal. Lorca wanted to know whether I might be able to help. At this stage I said I would need more information. I continued with the consultation at a somewhat slower pace, being aware of the patient's fatigue.

Lorca suffered from PMS and became very moody before her period and, in particular, experienced severe bloating in her abdomen, breasts and ankles. She said that she liked heat but this was mainly as a comforter as it did not actually help the pain or bleeding.

Her appetite was good but she craved salty food and chocolate. She often felt bloated after a large meal and tended to be constipated but she regulated this by eating prunes. She slept well but always awoke feeling tired and often dizzy. She had occasional dull headaches across the forehead and sometimes had temple headaches which related to anger or stress. These had all occurred since the onset of heavy bleeding.

While she was sitting I examined her pulse and tongue. Her pulse was very weak and deep, thready and choppy. Her tongue was very pale, swollen and quivering with a thin white coat and raised reddish dark spots at the back. I asked her to lie down and then palpated her abdomen (Fig. 17.1). It was extremely swollen and felt hard. Her flesh was soft and lacked tone.

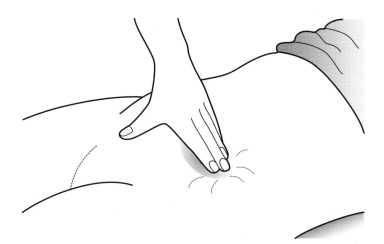

Fig. 17.1 Abdominal palpation.

Early medical history

Immediately it was apparent that I needed more information from Lorca's GP and gynaecologist and I asked Lorca if she would write a letter to say she was happy for this information to be released. (Having the consent form from the patient is necessary and speeds up the process of getting the information from the doctor or consultant. Alternatively, I give a letter to the patient to take to the doctor.)

I left Lorca lying down as it was more comfortable for her and continued to ask her about her medical history. She had had two D & Cs (dilatation and curettage[3]) 2 years and 1 year ago respectively and these had helped the bleeding and pain but only for a short time. A scan 1 year ago showed fibroids. Also 1 year ago, at a time when she was flooding heavily and in pain, she had received two blood transfusions. I was quite shocked at this point as to why she had been left with such extreme bleeding for so long without something being done as it was apparent that she was extremely anaemic. Also, why hadn't the fibroids been dealt with 2 years ago at the time of the first D & C?

Three years earlier Lorca's cycle had been 28 days with 4 days of normal bleeding and no pain. She had been on the contraceptive pill during her 20s. Just before the onset of this problem she had been very upset by a broken engagement. Her father had died at the same time as she had experienced her first pain and excessive bleeding. When asked about her current relationship she said 'OK, I suppose'. Because of her exhaustion she lived at home with her mother and only worked part-time.

Summary of clinical manifestations

- Excessive bleeding twice monthly, 10 days bleed, flooding dark red blood with large black clots, final 2 days light-coloured bleed.
- Extreme stabbing pain in the abdomen with intense heavy ache extending to back and legs.
- PMS, moody before period, severe bloating in abdomen, breasts, ankles.
- Craved salty food and chocolate.
- Bloated after a large meal, constipation.
- Awakens tired, often feels dizzy.
- Dull headaches across forehead.

- Temple headaches, related to anger or stress.
- Grey hue to face.
- Look of extreme tiredness, relieved to sit down.
- Slow and quiet voice.
- Palpation: abdomen extremely swollen, felt hard, masses; soft flesh which lacked tone.
- Pulse: very weak and deep, thready and choppy.
- Tongue: very pale, swollen, quivering, thin white coat, raised reddish dark spots at back.

The bleeding as the primary problem

While I waited for more information from the GP I needed to address Lorca's bleeding as the primary problem. This woman's body condition was very weak. From her description of the onset of the problem it would appear that the Blood *xu* was a result of haemorrhaging. Incidentally, I usually find that a choppy pulse indicates a haemorrhagic rather than a systemic cause of Blood *xu*. So the primary aim was to 'Stop Bleeding'.

Patterns of disharmony

Stagnant Blood in Uterus

- Stabbing pain, dark red blood, large black clots, masses on palpation.
- Excessive bleeding with a 10-day bleed coming twice monthly.

- Tongue: raised reddish dark spots at the back.

Qi* and Blood *xu

- Pale and grey face, tiredness, dizziness.

- Flesh lacked tone.
- Headaches across forehead.
- Bloated after a large meal.
- Menstrual flow light-coloured for the last 2 days.
- Pulse: deep, weak, thready, choppy.
- Tongue: pale, swollen, quivering.

Liver *qi* not free flowing
- PMS, moody before period.
- Temple headaches worse with stress, onset ties up with emotional trauma.

Aetiology and pathology

Excessive menstrual bleeding/haemorrhage can be caused by a number of factors which include: Heat in Blood, stasis of Blood, deficiency of *qi* and deficiency of Kidney *yin* or *yang* (Nanjing College of Traditional Chinese Medicine, 1987). In Lorca's case, given that the onset of bleeding was associated with pain, then the most likely cause was stasis of Blood which had then developed into masses in the abdomen (Fig. 17.2). The stasis disrupts the normal flow of Blood in the Blood channels and Blood breaks out of the channels. The stasis causes an accumulation of *qi* (*yang*) which manifests as pain. The *chong mai* (the Sea of Blood), which normally fills up with Blood and then discharges, no longer discharges correctly and so stasis of Blood occurs in the House of Blood (the Uterus). From a Western view, fibroids make the uterus bulky and thus enlarge the cavity so there is a greater area of endometrium to be shed at menstruation (Govan et al 1985). The haemorrhaging and the pain then causes Blood and *qi* deficiency

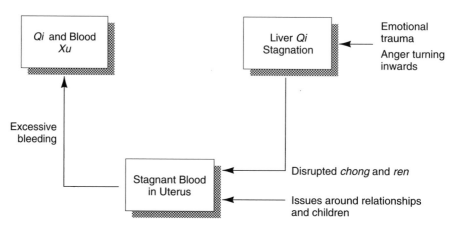

Fig. 17.2 Aetiology and pathology diagram.

and this aggravates the bleeding. In Lorca's case it could be that some of the bleeding was also from *qi xu* (the lighter flow at the end).

Lorca's history prior to the onset of symptoms was of emotional trauma from a broken engagement. This was coupled with the death of her father. Inward-turning emotions of any sort upset the function of the Liver to maintain free flowing of *qi*. This can further disrupt the smooth functioning of the *chong* and *ren* and can lead to stagnation of Blood in the Uterus. The relationship between a 'bleeding heart' and a 'bleeding womb' has long been documented and the areas where *qi* and Blood stagnate in women often relate to the specific emotional issues and life confusions being experienced (Cardinal 1984).

Treatment issues

Lorca wanted to maintain the possibility of having a baby. It might be possible to stop the bleeding and the pain but leave the masses. However it would then be unlikely for her to both conceive and maintain a pregnancy. So, with her agreement, the treatment principle was to stop the bleeding and pain so that her body condition could improve, giving her time to seek out a gynaecologist who might undertake a myomectomy if possible. Further, she needed to be stronger so as to recover well from any operation. We would continue to pursue reducing the mass as her strength recovered. Incidentally, when I did receive the report on her pelvic scan, it stated that at least five large and distinct fibroids were present, the largest two measuring 45 mm across.

Fibroids of this size, in my experience, are very difficult to resolve. They are *yin* in nature (involving stasis and immovability, and related to Blood) and therefore take a long time to treat unlike problems of *qi* or Heat. It is often the case that treatment rectifies the flow of *qi*, therefore treating the effects of the fibroids which are bleeding and painful, but does not affect the mass. If the fibroids are small it may be possible to prevent them from increasing in size. I recommend scans every 6 months to see if treatment is reducing the size of the mass. If not it is often better for patients to have an early myomectomy while the fibroid is still small, so causing less damage to the uterus. Also, because fibroids are related to oestrogen supply, once menopause is reached and the endometrium is no longer responding to oestrogen levels, it may be that the fibroid naturally starts to decrease (Merck Manual, 1977). In traditional Chinese medicine this is because the *chong mai* is no longer filling up with Blood. As a result, the stasis of Blood reduces and the regular *qi* flow resolves the mass. So, one has to weigh up the factors of age and desire to have children when analysing the effectiveness of treatment using scans.

Treatment according to stage in cycle

From end of bleeding: BL17 *geshu*, BL20 *pishu*, and BL21 *weishu* to nourish Blood and tonify post-heaven *qi*.

When pain starts: SP4 *gongsun*, P6 *neiguan*, ST29 *guilai*, and SP10

xuehai to move Blood stasis in Uterus and stop pain.

Day 5 of bleeding: SP4 *gongsun*, P6 *neiguan*, SP6 *sanyinjiao*, and moxa on SP1 *yinbai* to stop bleeding.

Treatment plan

The normal procedure when there is Blood stasis is to move the Blood but the excess bleeding had caused a more critical condition. In order to find a balance between these two states I decided to move the Blood for the first 4 days of the menstrual flow and then, on the fifth day, treat to stop the bleeding.

We agreed that Lorca would attend twice weekly. It is difficult to treat someone who is so deficient since the actual travel to and from the clinic, especially in London, is quite tiring and daily treatment is not therefore possible. As Lorca was only working part-time we agreed that she would only pay the equivalent of one consultation per week. I said that I wanted to treat her during her next three menstrual cycles by which time we should have seen some change and could then reassess the situation.

Rest was the most important issue but she was already resting. Her diet seemed adequate but I recommended Floridex and nourishing foods such as chicken soup as she was so Blood *xu*. I warned her against 'cold' foods but she did not tend to take these anyway. I noticed that each time I touched upon emotional issues she would sigh (Liver *qi* stagnation) and look more tired. I decided that she did not have the strength to deal immediately with emotional issues (if the Blood is deficient then the capacity of the Heart and Liver to resolve emotional issues is reduced). My priority was to deal with her more immediate problems.

The first treatment

It was difficult for Lorca to lie on her tummy as the fibroids caused too much pressure. I thought about treating her sitting up but she was too tired. So I had her lie on her side. This does make it difficult to apply moxa cones which is why I used a ginger slice (the moisture sticks the moxa to the slice). I explained to Lorca what I was going to do and showed her a needle and explained about moxibustion. She was not anxious or frightened. When the moxa was finished, I left the ginger slice in place until it was time to remove the needles, otherwise I feared that having opened the pores with the heat I might risk then exposing them to the relative cold.

Lorca liked the heat from the moxa very much and felt quite rejuvenated at the end of the treatment. I warned her that even though she might feel more energetic I still wanted her to rest and she should not run around doing things. I explained to her about building up her stores of energy and Blood again.

First treatment procedures

With the patient on Day 11 of her cycle, which was just after bleeding had stopped, my main aim was to nourish Blood and tonify *qi*. As the patient was so deficient I used few needles:

- BL17 *geshu* as it is the *hui* point of Blood and it nourishes Blood. I used seven moxa cones, about 12 mm tall, on a ginger slice.
- BL20 *pishu*, the back *shu* point of Spleen which nourishes post-heaven *qi*. Tonification method was used and the needles retained for 15 minutes.
- BL21 *weishu*, the back *shu* point of Stomach which, with BL20 *pishu*, nourishes post-heaven *qi*. Tonification

method was used and the needles retained for 15 minutes.

Needle technique: I used needles of 32 gauge and 1.5 *cun* in length. The needle was directed down the Bladder channel following the flow of *qi* in the channel.

Moxa for home use: The patient took home a moxa stick to use on SP1 *yinbai* from Day 5 of the bleed.

Chinese herbal patent medicine: She was also given the Chinese herbal patent medicine *yunnan bai yao* (Fratkin 1986) to take from Day 5 of the bleed until the main bleed stopped.

Controlling the bleeding

From the first cycle, the bleeding stopped occurring every 2 weeks and settled into a 26/27 day cycle with pain reduced to only 1 day, fewer large clots and reduced days of heavy bleeding followed by 5 days of spotting. She was advised to carry on the moxa on SP1 *yinbai* when spotting and this reduced the spotting. Also BL43 *gaohuangshu* with moxa on ginger was added.

At the end of 3 months her cycle was 27 days with 4 days of heavy bleeding (not flooding), followed by 4 days of spotting and small clots, and with 1 day of pain. She was feeling stronger and, as anticipated, seemed to be getting more emotional and angry about her condition. Also, she felt as if the fibroids were growing because she was more aware of them. I discussed the fact that this might be due to her increased energy as she was no longer losing so much Blood or *qi*. We decided therefore to increase treatment of the Blood stagnation by starting earlier at mid-cycle. I used:

- SP4 *gongsun* (right) with P6 *neiguan* (left) to resolve Blood stagnation in the Uterus and regulate the *chong mai*.
- The extra point *zigong* (abdomen) connected with electro (with dense at x60 cycles per second and disperse at x30 cycles per second).
- ST30 *qichong* to regulate Blood in the Uterus and regulate *chong mai*.
- SP10 *xuehai* to resolve Blood stasis and regulate menstruation.
  The needles were retained for 30 minutes.

I also prescribed Cinnamon Twig and Poria *gui zhi fu ling wan* (Nanjing College of Traditional Chinese Medicine, 1987) which moves Blood stasis in the Uterus. I chose this formula because it is gentle. (It can also be used for bleeding from Blood stasis in pregnancy.) I was concerned not to trigger off more bleeding.

Lorca proceeded well with this treatment and experienced less pain, less bleeding and, at times, even felt that the fibroids might be reducing because her abdomen didn't feel so bulky. She was always very depressed when she was bleeding and it was difficult on those days to believe that treatment was helping. Lorca's depression, I believed, had a lot to do with her fear of the excess bleeding returning. She often wanted to know if she would be able to have a baby if she had a myomectomy. Unfortunately I could not give her any clinical advice on this issue but tried to help her see that it was probably her only choice given her situation. At times, however, I myself doubted that it was the right path. Perhaps she should come to terms with a hysterectomy even though I knew that must be the last resort.

After a further 3 months of treatment she was due to have another scan to assess whether a myomectomy would be appropriate. She was apprehensive about this. Unfortunately the doctor did not turn up for the appointment and this exacerbated her anger considerably. While she waited for another appointment her frustration considerably affected her Liver *qi* and she developed a high-pitched tinnitus. It was difficult to work through this as her despondency also encompassed the acupuncture treatment. How long could the acupuncture hold the bleeding while waiting for the surgical decision? I added LIV3 *taichong* to the prescription as a means of addressing the background *qi* stagnation and the tinnitus, but otherwise maintained her treatment as before. However she was now making a lot more decisions herself and I felt it was far better for her to express, rather than suppress, her anger. We reduced the frequency of treatments to one per week because it was inconvenient for Lorca to attend more often and the pain and bleeding were very much reduced. We were now awaiting the consultation with her gynaecologist.

An operation to remove the fibroids

Lorca took a holiday as her *qi* and Blood were very much recovered, and we discussed her seeing a herbalist when she came back so that she could have a prescription more specific to her condition at that time. At this stage I temporarily stopped having direct contact with her. She started seeing a herbalist I know and I heard that the herbs were maintaining control of the bleeding. She finally had the appointment with the gynaecologist and a myomectomy was agreed. She was extremely pleased.

At this point she stopped herbs and started on Western medication for 6 months to reduce the fibroids prior to surgery. Monthly injections of Zoladex were given. This is a gonadotrophin-releasing hormone analogue which affects oestrogen supply to the fibroids and so shrinks them (British National Formulary 1992). Unfortunately she started bleeding excessively again. She was hospitalised and had a blood transfusion and a D & C, at which point one of the small fibroids came out! She was put on hormones to stop the bleeding but also returned for acupuncture treatment and together these managed to hold the bleeding long enough for her to finally have the myomectomy operation. Once she was up and moving, she had a course of eight acupuncture treatments to recover her *qi* and Blood from the operation and regulate the flow of *qi* in the Uterus. I advised that she use moxa on SP6 *sanyinjiao* and ST36 *zusanli* daily and she improved considerably. Lorca is now well but so far not pregnant.

Summary of outcome

The treatment controlled the uterine bleeding and reduced the pain so that the patient was able to pursue the operational procedure she wanted — a myomectomy. This meant that she was able to maintain the possibility of having a child, which is what she desired.

Recognising our strengths and weaknesses

In spite of the excellent results in Lorca's case I often felt perhaps I could have done more to reduce the actual masses so that she didn't need a myomectomy. In other words I doubted my original plan but rather tended to believe those stories one hears of masses that disappear 'if the practitioner has just the right touch'. Or the other ideal which we carry with us as acupuncturists, that all we need is the perfect herbal prescription to reduce the fibroids and thus eliminate the need for surgery. This idea especially came to mind when I learned that one of the fibroids had come out during the D & C. We must recognise both our strengths and weaknesses whilst understanding what it is that our patients are asking for beyond the diagnosis and needles. Rather than produce miracles we give them the power to make their own choices.

NOTES

1 Menorrhagia is an excess of menstrual blood. The norm is about 50–70 ml of blood over 3–5 days or about 12 regular tampons or pads. The heaviest bleed is on Day 1 and 2 and then it tails off. Menorrhagia is a loss of more than 80 ml for more than 5 days. Metrorrhagia refers to irregular and usually excessive bleeding at times other than menstruation.

2 Myomectomy is the removal of fibroids from the wall of the uterus thus leaving the uterus intact.

3 D & C. Dilatation refers to the expansion of the cervical canal by an instrument (a dilator) so that a curette can be inserted to scoop out the endometrial tissue in the uterus.

REFERENCES

British National Formulary (BNF) 1992 British Medical Association and Royal Pharmaceutical Society of Great Britain, London

Cardinal M 1984 The words to say it (metrorrhagia and psychoanalysis). Picador, London

Fratkin J 1986 Chinese herbal patent formulae. Institute for Traditional Medicine, Portland

Govan A D T, Hodge C, Callender R 1985 Gynaecology illustrated. Churchill Livingstone, Edinburgh

The Merck Manual 1977 Merck Sharpe & Dohme Research Laboratories, Rahway

Nanjing College of Traditional Chinese Medicine 1987 Concise traditional gynaecology. Jiangsu Science & Technology Publishing House, China

Webb A 1989 Experiences of hysterectomy. Optima, London

Zhang Ting-Liang (trans) 1987 A handbook of traditional Chinese gynaecology, Zhejiang College of Traditional Chinese Medicine, Blue Poppy Press, Colorado

■ Felicity Moir

My original training was in Western science and my first job in London was working at Guy's hospital studying genetic forms of skin cancer. Slightly disillusioned with this laboratory-based approach to disease I embarked upon a career in acupuncture doing my original training at the International College of Oriental Medicine (graduated 1980) and then at the Nanjing College of Traditional Chinese Medicine (1982). In 1983 I was involved in setting up the London School of Acupuncture and Traditional Chinese Medicine in an attempt to teach a well-defined system of medicine with historical and clinical verification based on the courses run in the People's Republic of China. I studied Chinese herbal medicine with Dr Ted Kaptchuk (1985) and have returned to Nanjing for further clinical training (1987).

One of the areas in my private practice that I have found the most rewarding to treat and the most fascinating in terms of its aetiology and pathology has been gynaecology. I also teach the subject at the London School of Acupuncture and so have put many hours into trying to understand it.

At the school we try to teach a pragmatic approach to the treatment of patients and as teachers have spent many hours discussing the difficulties we come up against as practitioners. How do we practise TCM in the West and in conjunction with scientific medicine? How do we work in recognition of our strengths and weaknesses without falling down that enormous and ultimately disappointing hole of defeat when we come up against TCM's nonomnipotence? How do we provide a holistic framework for patients when we work in isolation from mainstream medicine, and often from each other, and have no powers of direct referral? And how are we going to further our knowledge without well-organised and appropriate clinical research programmes? The answers to these questions are going to keep us busy for many more years yet!

The young woman who could only crawl

Peter Delaney BRISBANE, AUSTRALIA

Justine was the envy of her classmates and the daughter every parent hopes for. The pretty 15-year-old was popular and accomplished, a high achiever with a busy social life. It seemed there was scarcely a minute in the day that wasn't committed to some activity or other. And her loving parents were only too happy to help their middle child live life to the full.

No one suspected that Justine was to undergo an insidious change which would transform her from an energetic teenager to an invalid. Her friends would have laughed in disbelief if anyone had warned them that, within 6 months, Justine would have dropped out of classes, abandoned sports teams, and given up being chairperson of school clubs. Her family would have been aghast if they could have seen what the future held for her.

Justine's plight was brought to my notice when she was 16, after a mutual friend had called on Justine's family. As he waited on the doorstep, he heard a strange, shuffling noise behind the door. He was shocked to find Justine crawling on her hands and knees, barely able to speak. The girl who had once had the world at her feet was now too weak to walk.

Chronic fatigue with no sign of recovery

Doctors of conventional medicine had diagnosed her as suffering from chronic fatigue. The illness had started with feelings of general malaise and lethargy — symptoms which had no place in Justine's hectic life. Gradually the teenager, who relished a challenge, began to feel too tired to keep up with her daily routine which started at 5 a.m. with synchronised swimming training and ended with homework for the academic high achiever. As the weeks passed, tiredness gave way to exhaustion, and eventually to near collapse.

Her family was baffled. What was happening to the daughter who had sparkled with energy? Why wasn't she showing any signs of recovery? As she failed to respond to treatment, and as her condition deteriorated, the doctors said they could do no more to help her.

Justine's parents turned elsewhere for help. However, acupuncture, Chinese herbalism, naturopathy, homeopathy, massage and Western medicine did little to arrest her decline. The family was wary of embarking on yet another course of treatment which might result in false expectations, failure, and depression.

Yet the lives of Justine's parents and her two sisters now revolved around Justine's needs, and they refused to give up hope. Following the advice of a mutual friend, Justine's family contacted me in desperation.

Daunting prospects and a ray of hope

When I met Justine at her home, the prospects were daunting. It was shocking to see how debilitated this young woman was. She was extremely lacking in energy, and lay in her darkened bedroom day and night. She was unable to lift her head from the pillow. Her eyes were half closed and were deeply sunken into her gaunt, translucent face. She could only whisper responses. Justine had been virtually bedridden for 18 months, and was forced to crawl around the house because her legs could no longer support her. Although she had not completely lost her appetite, she had been vomiting after every meal for about 6 months.

However, an examination of her eyes revealed one ray of hope. Despite her advanced state, her *shen* was still good. As Dr J F Shen says, 'If the *shen* is intact then even the most advanced disease can be cured.' (Shen J F, personal communication, 1982).

I began the physical examination by gently touching her hands, feet and forehead to get an overall feel of Justine's energy and body temperature. The pulse and tongue were studied, the tongue being quite difficult to examine because Justine did not have the strength to poke it out. After this, I did an overall palpation of the body, examining the channels of the legs, arms, shoulders, neck, abdomen and chest. The results of these findings are detailed below.

Summary of clinical manifestations

- Total lack of energy.
- Temperature fluctuations, occasional low grade fevers.
- Vomiting after ever meal for the past 6 months, vomit lacks smell.
- Pain in neck, arms and legs; stiffness of neck, heaviness of limbs.
- Headaches: frontal, at *taiyang* and at vertex, constant dull ache.
- Muscle wasting of both legs, particularly the gastrocnemius and upper thigh muscles; lack of muscle tone.
- Extreme aversion to strong smells e.g. perfume, smoke, after-shave and

any chemical odours which left her breathless.
- Extreme difficulty in breathing, but without wheezing.
- Very pale complexion, translucent.
- Voice very weak, could only whisper.
- Distension of abdomen; has an appetite, but unable to hold food down; regurgitates after eating, but not forcefully.
- Stools tending to constipation.
- Urine dark and strong smelling.
- Itchy.
- Menstruation: little blood, irregular, 6-week cycle and lengthening, occasionally mild period pain.

- Sleep very restless with lots of dreams.
- Constant yawning.
- Very tight and painful at epigastrium.
- REN15 *jiuwei* and REN14 *juque* very tight and tender on palpation.
- Tightness and pain along the Bladder and Gall Bladder channels of the legs and neck.
- Tongue: pale, paler edges, body flaccid, very little coat, moist, unable to push tongue out.
- Pulse: right: floating, empty and a little tightness superficially; left: slippery, empty, proximal and a little slow.

Justine had had numerous medical tests, all to no avail as the results had been 'normal' time after time. These had included extensive blood tests (15 in total), a CAT scan, X-rays, ultrasounds of all abdominal organs, barium meals, an EEG and comprehensive neurological tests, all of which had been negative. In many cases similar to Justine's, a psychiatric assessment is the last avenue open to the doctors. This was not pursued in Justine's case as it was felt to be inappropriate.

Patterns of disharmony

My overall assessment of Justine was of a case of both external and internal pathology, mixed into a complex array of signs and symptoms.

Patterns of disharmony

Retained Damp pathogen
- Total lack of energy.
- Temperature fluctuations.
- Tongue: moist.
- Pulse: slippery.

Damp lodged in the channels and collaterals
- Pains in the neck, arms and legs.
- Heaviness of limbs.
- Skin moist to touch.

Spleen/Stomach *qi* deficiency
- Lack of energy, weakness.
- Dull frontal headache.
- Muscle wasting, lack of muscle tone.
- Very pale complexion, translucent.
- Regurgitation after eating, not forceful; vomit lacks smell.
- Distension of abdomen.
- Tongue: flaccid and unable to push tongue out.
- Pulse: empty.

Blood *xu*

- Reducing menstrual flow, little blood, 6-week cycle and lengthening.
- Sleep very restless, lots of dreams.
- Stools tending to constipation.
- Pale complexion.
- Tongue: pale with paler edges.

Lung *qi xu*

- Voice very weak, could only whisper.
- Breathless with perfume or smoke.
- Extreme difficulty in breathing.
- Pale and translucent complexion.
- Pulse: empty.
- Tongue: pale.

Qi stagnation in the *du* and Bladder channels

- Headaches.
- Stiff and painful neck.
- Lack of energy.
- Temperature fluctuations.
- Muscle wasting (lack of *yang qi* to nourish the limbs).
- Tightness and pain along the Bladder channels of the legs and neck.

Local stagnation in the chest and epigastrium

- Very tight and painful epigastrium.
- REN14 *juque* and REN15 *jiuwei* tight and tender on palpation.
- Regurgitation after eating.
- Difficulty breathing, but without wheezing.

Aetiology and pathology

With the benefit of hindsight, I realise now how critical that first encounter was. Justine was so weak that a softly-softly approach was crucial. It took a long time to elicit information about her physical and psychological condition. However, simultaneously, we were establishing a good rapport, which I felt would improve her chances of recovery.

Our conversation ranged from hard facts about her illness to dreams, fears, aspirations and family relationships. It transpired that Justine's family was close and loving. Her parents were supportive, but not pushy. It was Justine who set herself the punishing schedule of an all-round high achiever.

Her day had begun at 5 a.m. with synchronised swimming training, followed by more swimming training, and even more after school. She had also done cross country running and had played touch football and netball. She had become a prominent member of any school club that she joined. She had found time for all this in addition to normal schoolwork and on top of coping with the adjustments of a teenager on the brink of adulthood. There was simply no room for illness, let alone time for rest and recovery. In my experience, this is a predisposing factor in all cases of this type. Lack of recovery after illness and a busy lifestyle seem to go hand in hand. It is the main aetiological factor in this case.

Justine's condition originated from her constant overwork (reduced *qi*) and exposure to cold, damp conditions (swimming in cold water). The pathogenic factors of Cold and Damp entered her body during times of weakened *qi*. These pathogens resided in the tissue but quickly entered the interior, affecting the Stomach and Spleen. These organs lacked the available *qi* to dislodge the pathogenic factors completely. The retained Dampness disrupted the normal function of the Spleen leading to both internal and external signs of Damp.

Suddenly stoppping any form of physically demanding work will lead to a separation of *qi* and Blood. This theory has been espoused by both Dr Shen (1982) and Leon Hammer (1989). The way Dr Hammer describes it is that, because of the heavy work load, the Blood increases in volume. When work is stopped suddenly, the Blood reduces at a greater rate than the *qi*. This creates a separation of *qi* and Blood and is termed 'qi wild'. Once this happens, the body's *qi* becomes unstable and can easily lead to a variety of disturbances in the body. In this case, confinement to bed led to a *qi* stasis condition in the *ren, du* and Bladder channels due to postural constriction (*ren*) and compression (*du* and Bladder) (Fig. 18.1).

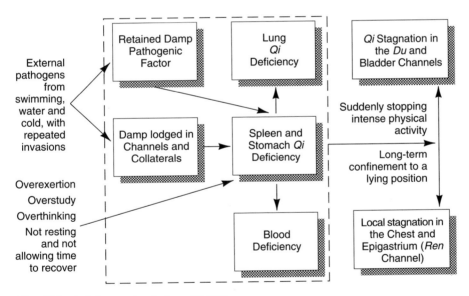

Fig. 18.1 Aetiology and pathology diagram.

Treatment issues

Justine presented interesting new problems which I had not previously encountered. All smells aggravated her condition. Perfume or smoke left her extremely breathless, and worsened her fatigue for about 1 week. So moxa, which was well indicated, could not be used. Herbs were also ruled out because her digestion was too weak and she would vomit them up. This is what had happened when she had tried to take medication in the past. Given her extreme fatigue, and past failures, it was important not to aggravate her condition. Stabilising the illness would give grounds for hope on which we could then build.

The case presented a challenge on a scale which Justine herself would have relished before her illness. I was careful to offer encouragement, without raising expectations which could prove to be false. I tried to be open and frank, because the more Justine understood her condition, the more she would feel in control of it.

I normally operate with a treatment plan, giving a specific time scale. However, I felt that this was not appropriate in Justine's case. We agreed to work together as a team, rather than as a practitioner and a patient. That meant establishing a rapport and gaining trust and cooperation.

My priorities had to be explained carefully so that Justine understood as much as possible. We had to clear the Damp, mobilise the *qi* and nourish the Stomach and Spleen's transformation and transportation functions. In particular, the vomiting had to stop.

Even though the Damp and *qi xu* were the predominant factors in this case, I believed that they were long-term issues. Therefore, I wanted to treat Justine's main presenting complaints on the first day: pain in her neck, headache with a muddled mind, vomiting and difficulty breathing. These I felt I could deal with a little more quickly, and thus gain the trust that I needed for our long journey together. By opening the *du* and Bladder channels and accessing some *yang qi* from the *du mai* I had something with which to work.

I anticipated that treatment would last at least 12 months. We would welcome improvement, but accept it as it came rather than anticipate or expect it. Only when Justine had regained some strength could we begin to think about the lifestyle changes which would be required to prevent any relapse.

First treatment procedures

POINTS PRESCRIPTION

- SI3 *houxi:* opening point of the *du mai*, relieves stiffness of the neck and headaches. Clears the Small Intestine, Bladder and the *du mai* channels. Also SI3 *houxi* clears the mind and gives clarity of thought and strength.
- BL62 *shenmai:* relaxes the sinews,

removes obstruction from the channel and clears the mind.

These two points were used in combination to strengthen the *yang* and open the channels of the back. This was important given the long-term confinement to bed which had blocked the flow of *qi* through the back. They were used in combination

as an Eight Extraordinary Vessels treatment for the *du mai*.
- DU14 *dazhui*: a meeting point of all the *yang* channels. This was tonified to regulate the nutritive *ying qi* and defensive *wei qi* and to tonify the *qi* and the *yang*. Also, it was used to clear the mind and direct clear *yang* up to the head.
- DU13 *taodao*: the meeting point of the Bladder and *du mai*. This is a good point for removing internal Heat caused by *yin* deficiency, however, its use in this case was to regulate chills and fevers.

DU14 *dazhui* and DU13 *taodao* were chosen for their clinical usefulness and also because they were *ashi* points. If the flow of *yang qi* through the *du mai* was impeded, it needed to be freed. Both points are also on the *du mai*.

Needling technique: Insertion was by hand, no guide tube was used. *Qi* was obtained at all points with mild stimulation. The needles were left in place for 5 minutes only, so as not to disperse the little *qi* present. SI3 *houxi* was inserted on the right and BI62 *shenmai* was inserted on the left: they were removed in the opposite order (Maciocia 1989, Hammer 1980). The needles used were 32 gauge, 25 mm in length.

Massage

Massage of the epigastrium was used, starting under the xiphoid process and using firm pressure, pulling downwards to REN11 *jianli*. This was done three times and seemed to have an immediate effect in removing the local stagnation, which eased Justine's breathing.

The *shen* is said to be the Emperor, and REN14 *juque* and REN15 *jiuwei* are the area of expression of the Heart *qi*, which is the store house for the *shen*. As this area was so tender, partly due to the long-term confinement to bed, I decided to use it as part of the first treatment. It was said to me in my early years as a practitioner that 'you should touch the person's pain, to let the person know that you know where they are suffering', and this seemed appropriate in Justine's case. So often we deal with what we think is important rather than what the patient wants.

Massage of this area was used so that Justine would have a physical experience of my presence, and to show that I knew where she was hurting, in her heart. Massage was used rather than needles as I wanted her to have a strong body feeling rather than a strong *qi* sensation. A *qi* sensation would possibly lead her inward, while a strong body sensation would reconnect her with her surroundings and her body as she seemed distant and detached.

Small expectations, slow improvement

Our expectations with the first acupuncture treatment were small. No response was better than an adverse one. Justine had had acupuncture in the past, and knew what to expect. However, she was vulnerable, and needed lots of time.

When I left Justine after that first meeting I was conscious that here was a complex and demanding case. I was, however, encouraged by her attitude. The determination which she had applied to her lifestyle before her illness was still present. She was now applying that same quality to her will to get better.

Over the next 10 months, we met weekly for treatment. From the beginning, Justine had an active interest in all my treatment suggestions. Later, she mentioned that I was the first practitioner to offer her a plan of treatment, and to explain the progressive stages where changes might be expected. I was willing to listen and needed to understand what she really felt. Involving her in this way seems to have been integral to her improvement, which came slowly over the ensuing months.

Touching a chord

I had taken care not to give false promises, saying I would work with her, but that she would also have to make a big effort. When I said I liked a challenge, and she was certainly that, this comment seemed to touch a chord which fitted in with her philosophy on life.

Progress was slow, and not without its setbacks. After 2 months, when the vomiting had stopped, I introduced herbs to assist in nourishing the *qi* and Blood. One of the main formulae used was Ginseng Dang Gui Ten Combination *shi quan da bu tang*. In addition, points ST36 *zusanli*, REN12 *zhongwan*, LI4 *hegu*, LIV3 *taichong* were used. Whenever an aggravation occurred I would treat it, but the frequency of incidents declined as time went on. In one of our many conversations she confided that she never lost confidence in me, and felt I was always there for her as a friend as well as a practitioner.

After 10 months, Justine had gained enough strength to start an exercise programme. This was a significant step for her. Before that, I had thought that exercise might introduce problems, and had not been prepared to take the risk. Justine had to be strong enough to cope with the physical strain of exercise, as well as the psychological frustrations she would inevitably feel as a former athlete. Treatment during this time was to clear the middle *jiao*, strengthen the function of the Stomach and Spleen, resolve Damp, and tonify Kidney and Lung *qi*.

Exercise started very gently with mild stretching of the four limbs to mobilise the *qi*. This progressed to standing for brief moments to reorient the body into a weight bearing position. Justine also started physiotherapy which included hydrotherapy and electro-muscle stimulation. This was required in order to rebuild and strengthen the wasted limbs so that Justine could walk again.

Acupuncture continued during this rebuilding process, as constant supplementation of *qi* was very important. Progress went smoothly, with only very minor setbacks. During this time, Justine had to learn that life could not be dictated by a timetable with deadlines. It was a hard lesson for her. She had been told that Chronic Fatigue lasted for 2 years, then vanished. Naturally, she was devastated when the 2 years came and went but she was still not cured.

A surprise

Once her exercise programme was established, I left Australia for 6 weeks. I hoped my absence would not create any setbacks. Whilst I was away she received a fortnightly treatment from an associate. When I returned, Justine telephoned. She was non-committal about her condition, but said she had a surprise for me. Shortly afterwards, a figure strolled up to the front door and walked in. I was speechless to see Justine not only standing, but walking. This was the first time I had seen her in an upright position. I was amazed at how tall she was, and how moved I felt.

Some months later, I was sitting outside with some friends who were over from England for their Christmas holidays. By chance, Justine called round and joined in the conversation, which covered various subjects. My friends quickly learned that Justine was studying at school, and had a holiday job working in a shop. She was tired after delivering Christmas presents but was looking forward to getting home for a swim. It would only take her a couple of minutes because she had just passed her driving test at the first attempt. There was nothing to suggest that this bright young woman had been so ill that she might not even have lived long enough to enjoy Christmas. To all intents and purposes, she was a pleasant student with nothing more to worry about than her school grades.

Justine still tires very easily, and has to pace herself. There is alarm in her family if she is just off colour, or catches a cold. However, her approach to life has changed dramatically. She has a much clearer understanding of her own health and general well-being, as well as insight into the condition of other people. Indeed, she says she now has great empathy with others who are sick, and intends to go into a healing profession.

I, too, have learned from my experience of this unusual case — particularly that we should never give up. It has also been a salutary reminder of how powerful and long-lasting an effect our words can have on our clients. Sometimes, what we say is as important as what we do!

A physician is a man working as the arbiter of human destiny.
If we are not determined there is nothing we can do.
A needle follows the principle of depth through subtlety.
We must be taught by the very best of men.
First examine the source of the disease, next apply yourself to the points.
At once you see the results — in reply to the needle, immediate effect!
Ming Dynasty Ode (Bertschinger 1991).

REFERENCES

Bertschinger R 1991 The golden needle: and other odes of traditional acupuncture. Churchill Livingstone, Edinburgh

Hammer L 1980 Eight extra meridians. American Journal of Acupuncture 8(2): 123–146

Hammer L 1989 The dragon rises, red bird flies — psychology and Chinese medicine. Station Hill Press, Barrytown

Maciocia G 1989 The Eight Extraordinary Vessels (parts 1 and 2). Journal of Chinese Medicine 29: 3–7, 30: 3–8

FURTHER READING

Bensky D, Barolet R 1990 Chinese herbal medicine: strategies and formulae. Eastland Press, Seattle

Bensky D, Gambel A, Kaptchuk T 1986 Chinese herbal medicine: materia medica. Eastland Press, Seattle

O'Connor J, Bensky D 1985 Acupuncture, a comprehensive text. Eastland Press, Seattle

Fu Di, Flaws B 1991 Aids and treatment according to traditional Chinese medicine. Blue Poppy Press, Colorado

Lee M H 1992 Overview of the diagnosis and treatment of chronic fatigue immune dysfunction syndrome according to traditional Chinese medicine. American Journal of Acupuncture 20(4): 337–347

Li Xuemei, Zhao Jingyi 1993 Acupuncture patterns and practice. Eastland Press, Seattle

Zhang Dengbu 1994 Acupuncture cases from China. Churchill Livingstone, Edinburgh

■ Peter Delaney

Peter Delaney has been in private practice in Brisbane, Australia, with his wife Mary, since 1982. Peter graduated from the Brisbane College of Traditional Acupuncture in 1981 and furthered his studies with a Diploma of Chinese Herbal Medicine in 1989. He has had training in both Traditional Chinese Medicine and Five Element acupuncture as well as shiatsu and bodywork. Even though Traditional Chinese Medicine is his main treatment style, the Five Element influence still makes its presence obvious at times. Peter has studied in China, and attended the first world congress on acupuncture and moxibustion in Beijing in 1987. From time to time Peter practises in York, England, which is Mary's home town.

Peter runs a busy practice in Brisbane which is relaxed and caring and it is not uncommon to hear laughter coming from the treatment rooms. He believes that a relaxed, light atmosphere is as important as the treatment itself.

Peter became Chairman of the Board of Directors of the Brisbane College of Traditional Acupuncture in 1985. He remained in this role for 3 years until the college amalgamated with another. Peter now runs Chinese Herbal Medicine seminars and spends time with his two sons, Aaron and Joel.

Early damage

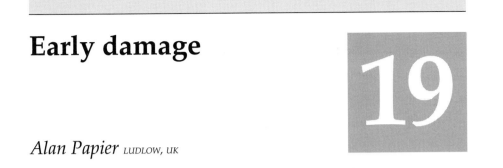

Alan Papier LUDLOW, UK

A non-practising acupuncturist

I received a phone call from Carol, a non-practising acupuncturist who had just moved to the area and wanted acupuncture treatment. She knew my name but first wanted to meet to assess whether or not she would feel comfortable receiving treatment from me. I therefore took the unusual step of inviting her for a cup of tea on my day off, whilst I was looking after my 2-year-old son.

Carol duly arrived as we had arranged. We discussed many things, and compared our respective training. Although she had originally trained as an acupuncturist, she now worked as a practising psychologist. She had received approximately 200 acupuncture treatments over the years, and had found that she was very sensitive in her response to acupuncture and hypersensitive to the insertion of needles. We then made an appointment for her first treatment.

From our very first meeting, I had made some observations. Carol was neither thin nor overweight, her physical features were all in proportion to each other, but she gave the impression of being slight of build. She was dark under the eyes, and her voice did not project well.

Permanent tiredness

Carol was 42 years old and her primary complaint was a feeling of 'depletion' — she felt tired all the time. The tiredness had been more pronounced for the last 10 years or so, but she felt that she had been tired since before puberty.

The severe tiredness began with the onset of myalgic encephalitis[1] (ME) 12 years earlier which, in turn, had started with a bad 'flu lasting 3 months and followed by an improvement in symptoms with a change of climate when the patient moved to a warmer country. The original symptoms of the 'flu were sweating, fever and weakness, followed by 'feeling weak for a few years'.

Her menstruation had been light since the onset of ME and prior to this had also been light but had included a degree of pain. Her bowels were sluggish and moved 4–5 times weekly. As a child she had suffered with fevers and sore throats and her family had a history of strokes, diabetes and heart trouble.

Nocturnal urination

The symptom which really struck me dramatically was that, since the age of 6, she had woken two to five times every night to urinate! At night, there would be a large quantity of urine and an element of urgency, while during the day her urination was normal. This was a most unusual symptom. Some children still wet the bed, even up to the age of 18, but it is very unusual for a child to wake many times every night to urinate. Between the ages of 15 and 20, she had had very bad insomnia and had woken 10–20 times each night for urination. Nocturnal urination is seen less commonly in women than in men, and it usually coincides with advancing years.

In further discussion, Carol said that she had no children and had not married. She then mentioned that she was a lesbian. It subsequently came to light that she had been sexually abused by her father and brother from the age of 4.

Suddenly, the unusual symptom of frequent nocturnal urination in a child made sense! One interpretation could be that the sexual abuse physically damaged the Kidney and Bladder organs so that their respective *qi* was not firm. Energetically, fear makes the *qi* descend (the fear being a direct result of a terrifying experience for a little girl) and the descending *qi* causes the frequency of urination. The impact must also have been profound psychologically.

Observations and interpretations

Her pulse was unusual because it had two contrasting qualities. The Heart, Liver and Stomach positions were tight and superficial. All other positions were deep and weak, especially the Kidney. The pulse rate would change every few minutes, indicating a 'nervous Heart'. According to Doctor Shen,[2] when the rate of the pulse varies significantly between the right hand and the left, then this difference in the beats per minute is indicative of a patient whose Heart is 'nervous' (Shen 1984). Moving on to the tongue, the body was red and the fur was thick and white. The tip of the tongue was redder than elsewhere and there were also red dots near the tip.

When examining the colour of the inside of her lower eye-lids, Carol removed her spectacles for the first time. I then observed that the glitter or *shen* in her eyes was greatly reduced and, in addition, there was a lack of 'feeling' in the eyes. There was also a very unusual feature on her left ear: two raised white lumps in the middle of the anti-helix. I had never seen this before. According to classical Chinese face-reading (Mar 1975), the left ear can either correspond to the first 7 years of one's life or it can represent the father's influence. In this case, both interpretations were valid. When her ear was discussed, she explained that it had been pinned back during childhood because it had stuck out too much.

Summary of clinical manifestations

- Continual feeling of tiredness.
- Sudden bouts of more severe tiredness with a need to lie down.
- Feels the cold easily.
- Light menstruation, flow lasts for 1 or 2 days.
- Bowels sluggish, 4–5 times per week.
- Copious nocturnal urination, 2–5 times per night since the age of 6.
- Reduced glitter in the eyes, lack of 'feeling' in the eyes.
- Dark area under the eyes.
- Poor sleep, restlessness, vivid dreams.
- Weak voice, voice does not project well.
- Frequent daytime urination if under stress.
- Two raised white lumps in the middle of the anti-helix of the left ear.
- History of unresolved 'flu symptoms.
- Feeling unwell with sudden or extreme changes of temperature.
- Pulses: deep and weak especially in the Kidney positions; tight in the Heart, Liver and Stomach positions.
- Tongue: red body, especially on the tip, with red dots also on the tip; thick white fur.

The patterns of disharmony

There is evidence for Kidney deficiency with many overlapping signs. A red tongue is found with Kidney *yin* deficiency. However, the thick white fur and 'feeling the cold' could easily indicate Kidney *yang* deficiency. Nocturnal urination is a symptom specific to the Kidney *qi* not being firm. However, the overall picture, especially because of the early onset of nocturnal urination, suggests a dysfunctional weakness of the Kidney organ.

According to the classics, a Kidney *yin* deficiency usually arises first causing the Heart to be unsettled and the *shen* to be disturbed (Maciocia 1989). In this case, it is a moot point to say that the Kidney pathology occurred first or is 'primary' to the disturbed Spirit. This would be similar to the chicken and egg debate. A simultaneous onset of Kidney deficiency (as manifested in the early onset of nocturnal urination) and *shen* disturbance would specifically point to the Kidneys and the Heart being in disharmony. The emotional environment within a sexually abusive family could have disturbed the *shen* even before the physical abuse occurred.

The 'pathogenic factor remaining' is the least serious pattern and the most superficial of the three. Nevertheless, it needs to be resolved before any long-term resolution of the more chronic, deeper patterns is possible.

Some of the overlapping signs could have had more than one interpretation. For example, the thick white fur could have been indicative of long-term external pathogenic Cold remaining in the body or of Kidney *yang* deficiency. The tiredness could have been due to the pathogenic factor, the Kidney deficiency, or the disturbed *shen*. Some signs in this case overlapped syndromes, but this did not dilute the essence of the diagnosis.

Patterns of disharmony

Kidney/Heart Disharmony with Heart *Shen* Disturbance

- Poor sleep, restlessness and vivid dreams.
- Reduced glitter and lack of 'feeling' in the eyes.
- Dark area under the eyes.
- Long-term copious nocturnal urination 2–5 times nightly.
- Pulse: variable, tight in Heart position, deep and weak in the Kidney positions.
- Tongue: red with redder tip.

Cold Pathogenic Factor Remaining

- Continual feeling of tiredness.
- Sudden bouts of more severe tiredness with a need to lie down in bed.
- Dislikes the cold.
- History of unresolved 'flu symptoms.
- Feeling unwell with sudden or extreme changes of temperature.
- Tongue: thick white fur.

The causes of the tiredness

Any organ's pathology can cause tiredness. In Carol's case, tiredness could have been due to her weak body condition from Kidney *yin xu*. Alternatively, it could have been due to her Heart *shen* disturbance because maintaining 'nervous energy' robs energy from other parts of the body. Together and individually these two factors can contribute to a weakened body condition (Fig. 19.1). For Carol, her weakened state meant that she could not provide her body with sufficient *qi* to protect it from external pathogenic factors. In turn, any external pathogenic factor remaining in the body would also have contributed to the tiredness.

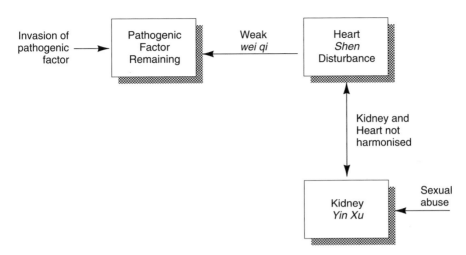

Fig. 19.1 Aetiology and pathology diagram.

Treatment

The principles of treatment were straightforward: first, resolve the external pathogenic factor remaining, then strengthen the Kidneys and calm the Heart *shen*.

Looking back, the acupuncture treatments can be divided into four phases and, within each phase, I used a different group of points. The first group of treatment points is outlined below.

First treatment procedures

POINTS PRESCRIPTION

In the first prescription, I only used four needles:

- LU7 *lieque* to release the remains of external pathogenic Cold in the body (right only).
- LI4 *hegu* to release the remains of external pathogenic Cold in the body (right only).
- P7 *daling* to calm the *shen* and reduce heat in the Heart as evidenced by red dots on a red tongue tip (left only).
- KID9 *zhubin*, the starting point of the

yinweimai. This point was used to strengthen the Kidneys and harmonise the relationship between the Kidneys and the Heart (right only).

Needling Technique: Extremely cautious needling technique was used due to the patient's sensitivity to the penetration of needles. With every treatment, the patient was able to tell me when the needle had activated the point. Minimal manual stimulation was used. In principle, all points were reduced except KID9 *zhubin* which was tonified.

Treatment variations

From the first treatment Carol felt well. Suddenly, she was having daily bowel movements and her urine was less copious during the night, although the frequency was unchanged. Her menstruation was more normal, lasting for 3 rather than 1 or 2 days. However, her stress and tiredness were unchanged.

For the second treatment, I believed it would be beneficial to strengthen the treatment by varying the first group of points. I used:

- LI4 *hegu* (left) to release the external pathogenic factor.
- HE7 *shenmen* (left) and HE5 *tongli* (right) to calm the *shen*.
- SP6 *sanyinjiao* and KID9 *zhubin* to strengthen the Kidneys.
- DU14 *dazhui* to release the external pathogenic factor and to clear the mind.

After this treatment Carol felt terrible and spent 2 days in bed crying and sleeping. Upon closer examination and with hindsight I believe the use of DU14 *dazhui* was inappropriate. In fact, her poor reaction was probably due to the fact that DU14 *dazhui's* specific function is to Clear heat, yet Carol's external pathogenic factor was from the cold! Whenever any patient has a negative reaction to a specific treatment I try, as much as possible, to trace the cause.

By the fourth treatment the thickness of the tongue fur had virtually disappeared, indicating the resolution of the external pathogenic factor. I now introduced the *second* group of treatment points:

- BL23 *shenshu* to tonify the Kidney organ directly.
- BL52 *zhishi* to reinforce the effect of BL23 *shenshu* and also to address the psychological aspect of the Kidney problem.
- Two points from KID6 *zhaohai*, KID3 *taixi* and KID7 *fuliu* to strengthen various aspects of the Kidney.
- HE7 *shenmen* to calm the Heart spirit.

The *third* group of points was introduced at the seventh treatment:

- HE7 *shenmen* to calm the *shen*.
- REN15 *jiuwei* to strongly calm the *shen*.
- REN4 *guanyuan* to tonify Kidney energy, strengthen the whole body and strengthen the Bladder.
- KID9 *zhubin* to tonify the *yinweimai* and help communication between the Heart and Kidney (Maciocia 1989, p. 430).

The *fourth* group of points was introduced at the tenth treatment and comprised BL15 *xinshu* and BL23 *shenshu* with HE3 *shaohai* and KID9 *zhubin*. Both pairs were selected to harmonise the Heart and Kidneys.

Generally speaking, the second, third and fourth groups of points all focused on strengthening the Kidney and calming the Heart *shen*. Due to Carol's sensitivity to the effects of acupuncture, she was able to verbalise the benefits of acupuncture in great detail. When she described a treatment as being 'less effective' I would vary her treatment accordingly. Chinese text books implicitly confirm this practice by providing a large selection of points for variation over an extended course of treatment. It is understood that continual use of the same points makes them less effective.[3]

Carol's case was very complicated and setbacks were inevitable. Although she had trained as an acupuncturist, she was guilty of making poor judgements concerning strategies involving her personal health. Recently, in order to 'build up her strength', she went on a walking holiday and walked for several hours in cold weather. This caused a setback where she felt considerably weaker, experiencing some symptoms similar to the original ME.

I am still treating Carol and it is interesting to note that she does not show classical symptoms of Wind-Heat or Wind-Cold in the early stages of a common cold (i.e. fever or shivering, sore throat, runny nose or sneezing). Instead, she becomes profoundly fatigued — again resembling symptoms of the original ME. Although the ME symptoms may be resolved to a certain extent, her general body condition is not yet strong enough to confront external pathogens at the superficial level of the body. In the same way, many asthmatics do not manifest symptoms of a common cold, instead their asthma worsens.

Dreaming

Recently Carol experienced dreams featuring her late father where he was 'benign' and, on a very positive note, was being 'nice to her'. She no longer feels that her 'heart is set in concrete'.

The latest stage of Carol's treatment is a group of points which, interestingly enough, is somewhat similar to her very first treatment. The points are:

- LU7 *lieque* (right only), the Master point of the *renmai*.
- KID6 *zhaohai* (first left then right), the Coupled point of the *renmai*.
- REN17 *shanzhong* and P7 *daling* (left only).

The first two needles, LU7 *lieque* on the right and KID6 *zhaohai* on the left, activate the *renmai* extra-meridian which will strengthen the Kidney and treat constitutional or very chronic problems (Maciocia 1980). The addition of KID6 *zhaohai* on the right side strengthens the effect on the

Kidney. REN17 *shanzhong* tonifies the *qi* of the entire body. Also, as a point on the *renmai*, it both reinforces and is reinforced by the Master and Coupled points and, finally, it is a meeting point of the Kidney, Lungs and Heart.

Treatment is still in progress.

Summary of outcome

- More energy.
- Less nocturnal urination, now only twice nightly.
- Feeling less stressed.

- More motivated at work.
- Dreams express some resolution to the disturbed *shen*.

Complications and challenges

This was an unusual case for me in a number of ways. Firstly, it was extremely complicated. There were three clear pathological factors, any one of which could have required a long course of treatment in an average patient. However, to have all three present in one patient made the case very challenging.

In addition, the sexual abuse with the *shen* disturbance had started almost 40 years earlier, when Carol was 4. In my opinion, pathology starting at such a young age tends to be 'embedded in the marrow' and is therefore more resistant to treatment.

In addition, it is always challenging to treat a fellow acupuncturist, regardless of whether or not they want to know about the complexities of the diagnosis and the reasons for point selection. In Carol's case, she preferred to put the treatment into my hands and sought little explanation.

Carol was also a professional psychologist and, as such, might easily have interpreted hidden meanings where none were intended. Fortunately, however, in this area my contact with Carol was relatively free of complications.

Finally, this case was particularly challenging because at the second treatment, I explained to Carol that I was considering writing up her case history for publication. Her reaction was spontaneous and concise, 'You must be confident of getting me better'.

NOTES

1   Myalgic Encephalitis (ME) is a disease entity which has only recently been named. In Western medicine there is no consensus as to its diagnosis. According to Chinese diagnosis, the main diagnostic categories are external pathogenic factor remaining or *qi, yin* or *yang* deficiency. Other names for this condition are 'postviral syndrome', 'chronic fatigue syndrome' and 'Epstein–Barr virus disease'. The disease is characterised by chronic and profound tiredness (Maciocia 1994).

2   Dr Shen is world famous for his remarkable diagnostic ability. He is able to synthesise information concerning the most subtle pulse quality, the most obscure feature of the tongue and the colour of the inner lower eyelid. Having watched Dr Shen for 20 years, I have seen how he uses Chinese face-reading. Historically, this has been used for 'fortune-telling' where a person's past and future, education and prospects are read. Dr Shen uses this in conjunction with his medical diagnosis to arrive at an accurate prognosis. In addition, face-reading is a wonderful way of assessing the personality. Not only is Dr Shen the best judge of character I have ever met, he is also the best *instant* judge of character. He is able to assess how much the individual personality affects the medical condition. His assessment includes what the patient is able or unable to understand by way of explanation regarding the cause and effects of the disease and how the individual's lifestyle may contribute towards it.

3   See the discussion on point selection in the chapter on treatment in the Essentials of Chinese Acupuncture (Beijing College of TCM 1980).

REFERENCES

Beijing College of Traditional Chinese Medicine 1980 Essentials of Chinese acupuncture. Foreign Languages Press, Beijing
Mar T 1975 Face-reading, the Chinese art of physiognomy. Signet Books New American Library, New York
Maciocia G 1989 Foundations of Chinese medicine. Churchill Livingstone, Edinburgh
Maciocia G 1994 Practice of Chinese medicine. Churchill Livingstone, Edinburgh

FURTHER READING

Shen J 1980 Chinese medicine. Educational Solutions, New York

■ Alan Papier

I first studied Chinese medicine in England, at the International College of Oriental Medicine in East Grinstead, from 1974–1977. I met Dr Shen in Boston in June 1975 when visiting an acupuncture clinic and spent the next three summers watching him work. I therefore experienced my 'crisis of integration' very early on in my professional career — seeing two completely different approaches to acupuncture, at apparent odds with each other, but each being beneficial in practice. Since 1977 I have spent a minimum of 1 week every year watching Dr Shen at work.

Dr Shen's influence permeates my professional career and I continue to see him whenever possible. As a result, I place greater emphasis on the pulse when diagnosing than do many of my colleagues (not adequately illustrated in this case history). I use face-reading when it affects the diagnosis and I try to explain the laws of cause and effect to the patient as it relates to his or her specific illness.

I attended the first Advanced Acupuncture Course in Nanjing in 1981. From 1986–1988, I attended the Chinese herbal course in London, taught by Ted Kaptchuk and Giovanni Maciocia, and I have practised Chinese herbal medicine ever since.

Currently I have a clinic attached to my home in Ludlow, Shropshire in the United Kingdom. I also work in a private clinic and at a General Practice Surgery where I see patients on the National Health Service. I am an occasional guest lecturer at colleges in the UK.

Judy, a left-handed Caucasian

Miki Shima CORTE MADERA, CA, USA

Progressive disability

Judy was a 44-year-old, single, lesbian, left-handed Caucasian school teacher. She presented 7 years ago with complaints of severe headaches, excessive fatigue, especially upon arising in the morning, pains in various joints throughout her body, depression, a general feeling of sadness, and short-term memory loss. She had a very complicated medical history including diagnosis of a mitral valve prolapse, irritable bowel syndrome 6 years ago, and possible multiple sclerosis found on an MRI scan 1 year ago. Two years prior to the diagnosis of irritable bowel syndrome the patient discontinued alcohol, tranquillisers and cigarettes, all of which she had abused for some years. With regard to her headaches, 1 year ago she was diagnosed as having aquaductal stenosis and had a shunt inserted under surgery which somewhat improved her headaches and cognition.

Judy had worked hard as a high school maths teacher for almost 20 years before becoming ill. As she became exhausted, she tried to reduce her hours by 50%, but could not even manage that. After a long battle with the state bureaucracy, she was finally assessed for complete disability allowance for 1 year. Meanwhile, she saw many physicians who all told her that she was just depressed. Despairing of traditional Western medicine, she finally decided to see a practitioner of Oriental medicine.

Tired and depressed for a long time

Prior to her first consultation with me, she had undertaken a variety of neuropsychological tests, the results indicating mild attention and concentration difficulties, some irritability, anxiety, and depression, but without any diagnosis of a mental disorder. The blood tests that I had ordered immediately after the first consultation revealed mildly elevated liver enzymes, a high level of triglycerides and a mildly depressed red blood cell count, but were otherwise unremarkable.

Judy was a lanky, pale woman with dark circles under her eyes. She was so tired and confused that she took a long time to answer any of my questions although she was very cooperative. Although there were numerous complaints, she emphasised that she had been very tired and depressed for a long time. She talked with a sad tone of voice, sitting with her back bent, and told her story very slowly. She said that she had been disabled for 2 years and might well lose her job, which made her even more anxious and nervous.

Examinations

After a quick explanation of my examination procedure, Judy changed into a gown and lay down on a table. First, I examined her pulses and found her Kidney and Spleen pulses to be extremely deficient, whereas her Heart and Liver pulses were full and wiry. The abdominal examination revealed extreme tightness of the epigastrium, upper aortic hyper-irritability, extreme weakness and tenderness of the umbilicus to deep pressure, and profound flaccidity of the lower abdomen. The tongue was damp with a thin, white coating. Meridian palpation showed tenderness in the Spleen, Kidney and Bladder muscle meridians. I did the Akabane Test (Akabane 1950) which is a Thermal Threshold Test, known as TTT, on all the *jing* points on the finger tips. I tabulated the values for both the right and left *jing* points independently. I then added them together to give a total, and subtracted them to give a deviation. These are shown in Table 20.1 as the lateral polarisations.

From these figures I calculated the extra meridian functions by adding the appropriate *jing* point values to provide new totals. By subtracting these totals for each extra meridian pair, I found the deviation. These extra meridian polarisations are shown in Table 20.2.

Table 20.1 Lateral polarisations

Meridian	R	L	Tot	Dev
FOOT				
Spleen	19	21	40	2
Liver	8	9	17	1
Stomach	9	8	17	1
Gallbladder	11	14	25	3
Kidney	32	16	48	16
Bladder	14	24	38	10
HAND				
Lung	9	12	21	3
L. Intestine	9	5	14	4
Pericardium	6	6	12	0
San jiao	5	7	12	2
Heart	8	3	11	5
S. Intestine	4	5	9	1

Table 20.2 Extra meridian polarisations

	Tot	Dev
SI3	9	29
BL62	38	29
GB41	25	13
SJ5	12	13
LU7	21	27
KID6	48	27
PC6	12	28
SP4	40	28
LU7	21	19
SP4	40	19
HT7	11	37
KID6	48	37

Finally I retabulated the *jing* point values in terms of the meridian *yin-yang* pairing to yield the deviations for the divergent meridians as shown in Table 20.3.

Table 20.3 *Yin-yang* polarisations of divergent meridian pairs

	Tot	Dev
KID	48	10
BL	38	10
LIV	17	8
GB	25	8
SP	40	23
ST	17	23
HT	11	2
SI	9	2
PC	12	0
SJ	12	0
LU	21	7
LI	14	7

Summary of clinical manifestations

- Severe headaches.
- Excessive fatigue, especially in the morning and late afternoon.
- Pains in various joints and bones.
- Depression and anxiety, palpitations.
- Short-term memory loss.
- Attention difficulties.
- Irritability.
- Paleness, dark circles under eyes.
- Tired, confused.
- Sad tone of voice.
- Burning in the eyes.
- Excessive loss of hair.
- Bleeding gums.
- Frequent sore throat.
- Stiffness in the neck and shoulders.
- Poor tolerance of heat and cold.
- Frequent day and night time sweats.
- Shortness of breath.
- Irritable bowel.
- Frequent indigestion with belching and stomach pain.

- Frequent loose bowels.
- Decreased libido.
- Occasional back pain.
- Eruptions on the forearms.
- Fibrocystic breast disease with tenderness.
- Often nervous and worried about things.
- Disturbed and interrupted sleep with intense dreaming.

- Pulse: Kidney and Spleen deficient, Heart and Liver full.
- Tongue: damp, thin white coating.
- Meridian palpation: tenderness in Spleen, Kidney and Bladder meridians.
- Abdominal examination: extreme tightness of the epigastrium with upper aortic hyper-irritability, extreme weakness and tenderness of the umbilicus to deep pressure, profound flaccidity of the lower abdomen.

Identifying the patterns of disharmony

Judy's pulses, abdomen and Akabane Test all revealed Kidney-Spleen deficiency and Liver-Heart excess.

The pulse diagnosis was uncomplicated in this case. It revealed sunken, weak pulses in the Kidneys and the Spleen, and full wiry pulses in the Heart and the Liver.

The abdominal diagnosis was the most revealing of all the diagnostic procedures. Judy had very tight epigastric spasm with hyperactivity of the aorta, denoting Heart *shen* disturbance. She also had extreme weakness in her lower abdominal muscle, signifying Kidney deficiency. Her umbilicus was also very tender to deep pressure, indicating that the Spleen was also very deficient (see Figure 20.1).

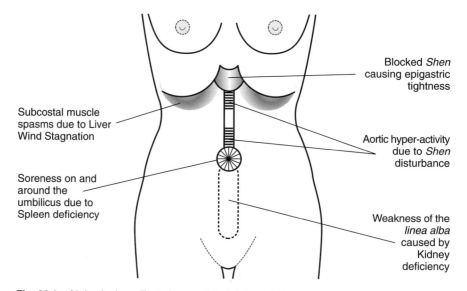

Fig. 20.1 Abdominal manifestations and their interpretation.

The Akabane Test revealed a large total count (from Table 20.1) in the Kidney meridians (n=48), and the second greatest sum was that of the Spleen meridians (n=40), signifying deficiency of *ki* (*qi*) in the meridians. At the same time, the smallest number was registered in the Small Intestine meridian (n=9), and the second smallest was in the Heart meridian (n=11), denoting *ki* (*qi*) excess.

Evidence for patterns of disharmony

Water Element (Kidney and Bladder) deficiency

- Excessive fatigue.
- Anxiety and fear.
- Excessive loss of hair.
- Poor tolerance of heat and cold.
- Frequent night sweats.
- Decreased sex drive.
- Excessive nervousness.
- Disturbed and interrupted sleep.
- Occasional back pain.
- Dark circles under eyes.
- Tenderness in Kidney and Bladder meridians.
- Profound flaccidity in the lower abdomen.
- Pulse: Kidney pulse deficient.
- Akabane result: total Kidney meridians was 48, i.e. the most deficient.

Heart *shen* disturbance

- Nervousness.
- Depression and anxiety.
- Palpitations.
- Poor heat intolerance.
- Frequent day-time sweats.
- Always worried about things.
- Disturbed sleep with intense dreaming.

- Very tight epigastrium with hyperactivity of the aorta.
- Pulse: Heart pulse excess.
- Akabane result: total Heart meridians was 11, denoting Heart excess.

Spleen *yang* deficiency

- Depressed mood all the time, tiredness.
- Concentration difficulties.
- Irritable bowel with frequent diarrhoea.
- Frequent indigestion with belching.
- Excessive phlegm congealed in the breasts resulting in cyst formation.
- Paleness.
- Tenderness in the Spleen meridian.
- Tender umbilicus to deep pressure.
- Pulse: Spleen pulse deficient.
- Akabane result: total Spleen meridians was 40, signifying Spleen deficiency.

Liver *qi* stagnation

- Severe headaches.
- Pain in various joints.
- Burning in the eyes.
- Stiffness in the neck and shoulders.
- Breast tenderness and distension.
- Irritability.
- Subcostal spasms.

Aetiology and pathology

The most chronic deficiency in Judy's meridian system is the Kidney-Bladder (Water Element) complex. Years of hard work as a maths teacher, and a long-term abuse of tobacco and alcohol has exhausted the Kidneys.

This Kidney *yin* weakness did not control the Heart *shen*, resulting in excessive anxiety and nervousness. This, in turn, weakened the Spleen, causing depression and lack of *yi* or mental capabilities, and digestive complaints. In addition the Kidney deficiency caused the Liver Blood to weaken, resulting in the Liver *hun* disturbance. Therefore, the root (*ben*) in this case was the true Kidney exhaustion, leading to Heart *shen* disturbance and Spleen deficiency. This can be illustrated in terms of the Five Elements configuration shown in Figure 20.2.

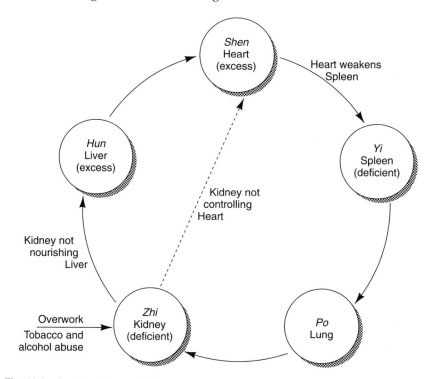

Fig. 20.2 Aetiology and pathology diagram.

Balancing the four different levels

In the Japanese system that I practise, the meridian systems have to be balanced at four different levels: the surface meridians, the muscle meridians, the extra meridians and the divergent meridians (Irie 1982). The order of acupuncture treatment is to start from the surface (*biao*) and move inwards to the organs of the *zangfu* (*li*).

First, at the level of the major surface meridians, the Japanese system places great emphasis on correcting the right-left imbalances. Either moxibustion or acupuncture is used on the back-*shu* points of the imbalanced meridians to correct the right-left imbalance. For example, if the right Kidney meridian is deficient by the Akabane Test, tonifying moxibustion or a gold needle is applied on right BL23 *shenshu* which is the Kidney *shu* point. In Judy's case I applied moxibustion to the three most deficient meridians, the Spleen, Kidney and Bladder, using BL20 *pishu* (left), BL23 *shenshu* (right) and BL28 *pangguangshu* (left) to correct the right-left imbalance of these meridians.

Second, once the major meridians are balanced, the muscle meridians are treated by releasing muscular indulation (*kori*) using special needling techniques known as *nenshin* in Japanese.

At the third level, the extra meridian system is balanced using gold and silver needles. Gold needles are used to tonify *ki* (*qi*), and silver needles are applied to sedate *ki* (*qi*). Essentially, I identified the most imbalanced extra meridian pairs (from Table 20.2) which were Heart-Kidney (37), Small Intestine-Bladder (29), Pericardium-Spleen (28) and Lung-Kidney (27). I applied a gold needle to tonify the deficient side of the pair and a silver needle to sedate the excess side e.g. a gold needle on KID6 *zhaohai* (right) and a silver needle on HE7 *shenmen* (left). Thus, I treated the four most imbalanced pairs of the extra meridians, pair by pair, using the gold-silver needling method. The needles are retained for 15–20 minutes depending on the severity of the imbalance.

Finally, at the fourth level, I attended to the imbalance of the divergent meridians. Normally, one or two of the divergent meridian pairs are selected by the Akabane test, or by *zangfu* diagnosis, for treatment by the gold-silver needling technique. The gold needle is applied at the master point of the first (K/BL), the second (GB/LIV) and the third (SP/ST) meridian pairs, and at the confluence (*he* sea) point of the fourth (HE/SI), the fifth (P/SJ) and the sixth (LU/LI) meridian pairs. The silver needle is applied at the confluence (*he* sea) point of the first, the second, and the third meridian pairs and at the master point of the fourth, the fifth and the sixth meridian pairs. See Table 20.4 for the chart.

In Judy's case the most imbalanced divergent meridian pair was the Spleen/Stomach (see Table 20.3) and the Spleen meridian was more deficient (because it has a higher number) on the left side. Therefore, the master point, ST1 *chengqi*, was needled by a gold needle on the left side and the confluence point of the Spleen, SP9 *yinlingquan*, was needled with a

Table 20.4 Master and confluence points of the divergent meridian pairs

Meridian pairs	Gold needle	Silver needle
1. Kidney/Bladder	BL1	KID10 (*yin*) BL40 (*yang*)
2. Liver/GB	GB1	LIV8 (*yin*) GB34 (*yang*)
3. Spleen/Stomach	ST1	SP9 (*yin*) ST36 (*yang*)
4. Heart/SI	HE3 (*yin*) SI8 (*yang*)	BL1
5. Pericardium/SJ	P3 (*yin*) SJ10 (*yang*)	GB12
6. Lung/LI	LU5 (*yin*) LI11 (*yang*)	ST12

silver needle also on the left. This treatment balances the *yin-yang* polarity disharmony through the *zangfu* systems. This part of balancing the divergent meridian is carried out simultaneously whilst balancing the extra meridian, and the needles are retained for 15–30 minutes, depending upon the patient's condition.

The first treatment

The whole procedure of moxibustion and acupuncture was explained to Judy before the treatment, and she was not at all apprehensive. The moxa that I used was 13–15 years old and was made into soft, soyabean-sized cones. I asked Judy to tell me when the cone got hot, and then I would remove it without cauterising the skin. Moxibustion was repeated two or three times on the same point until the skin showed faint reddening known as *hosseki* in Japan. Judy took moxibustion of the back *shu* points very well and then moved to a supine position.

I then proceeded with the extra and divergent meridian treatments with gold and silver needles. I felt expansion of *ki* (*qi*) with gold needles and constriction with silver needles in my hands. Once the needles were all in, I could feel Judy's *ki* (*qi*) moving by holding my hands about an inch over the needles. Judy lay on the table for 25 minutes very calmly without any complication. When I went back to her room to check her pulse and abdomen, she said she was very relaxed and that she could see better for some reason.

First treatment procedures

Treatment of major meridians to correct right-left imbalance:

Moxa on back *shu* points: BL20 *pishu* (left), BL23 *shenshu* (right), BL28 *pangguangshu* (left).

Treatment to balance extra meridians:

KID6 *zhaohai* (right) Gold
HE7 *shenmen* (left) Silver
BL62 *shenmai* (left) Gold
SI3 *houxi* (right) Silver
SP4 *gongsun* (left) Gold
P6 *neiguan* (left) Silver
KID6 *zhaohai* (right) Gold
LU7 *lieque* (right) Silver
Gold is for tonification and silver for sedation.

Treatment to balance divergent meridians:

ST1 *shaoze* (left) Gold
SP9 *yinlingquan* (left) Silver.

Gold is used for the master point and silver for the confluence (*he* sea) point.

Judy rested for 30 minutes with the needles in position. Her pulses and abdomen were then reexamined. The pulses were mostly balanced, but the abdomen showed deficiency of Kidney and Spleen. Therefore, traditional Chinese herbal formulae Major Six Herbs Combination *liu jun zi tang* and Rehmannia Six Combination *liu wei di huang wan* were prescribed for 2 weeks.

Improvements with treatment

From the very first treatment, Judy's pulse and Akabane Test exhibited a quick improvement. She was given two traditional Chinese herbal formulae, Major Six Herbs Combination *liu jun zi tang* and Rehmannia Six Combination *liu wei di huang wan*, which she tolerated very well. For 1 month, I saw Judy every 3 days, and her Akabane Test margins became narrower and narrower on all meridians, showing much better meridian balancing at all the four levels. During the second and the third month, I saw her once a week, and her Akabane Test results were all normal except for the left Spleen and the right Kidney meridians, indicating the chronic deficiencies at the *zangfu* level. After 3 months of treatment Judy was able to go back to teaching, and, from that time on, I saw her for 2 more years when she needed treatment.

Progress and outcome

- Headaches were very mild and infrequent within a month.
- Judy was back to part-time work within 3 months.
- Fatigue markedly better after eight treatments.
- The patient went back to her full-time job 6 months after the first treatment.
- Her joint and bone pains were greatly ameliorated
- Depression and anxiety were very much improved.

An interesting and complicated case

I have treated over 1000 cases of Chronic Fatigue Immune Dysfunction Syndrome (CFIDS), but Judy was one of the most interesting and by far the most complicated cases. Due to her extensive medical history, with many layers of emotional and physical problems, I had particularly to find out what was at the root of her problems, and to treat that instead of her superficial problems.

One of the difficulties in Judy's case was that she was left-handed and ambidextrous. I knew from my clinical experience that it was very important to correct lateral (left-right) imbalances of Judy's meridian system at all levels based on the Akabane Test in order to obtain quick clinical results.

Another interesting aspect of Judy's case was that the extra-meridian treatment was extremely effective for her emotional and psychological problems, which were the real contributing factors to her chronic exhaustion. Due to her long-term Kidney and Spleen deficiencies, Judy was losing her will to live (Kidney) and her intellect (Spleen) to function as a maths teacher. As soon as these two *zang* organs were tonified by the extra-meridian treatment and the herbs, she regained her fight to improve her physical condition and her mental concentration very quickly.

All in all, Judy was one of my most difficult CFIDS patients who had responded best to Oriental medicine. So far she is still working full time without any sign of relapse.

REFERENCES

Akabane K 1950 Method of Hinaishin (in Japanese). Ido-no-Nippon-Sha, Yokosuka
Irie D 1982 Divergent, muscle and extra-meridian treatment (in Japanese). Ido-no-Nippon-Sha, Yokosuka

FURTHER READING

Shima M 1992 Getting acupuncture back on track: what our training has been missing and how we can benefit from the Japanese empirical schools. American Journal of Acupuncture 24: 1
Shima M 1992 Shonishin: Japanese paediatric acupuncture. American Journal of Acupuncture 24: 4
Shima M 1992 The Medical I Ching: Oracle of the healer within. Blue Poppy Press, Boulder
Shima M 1992 Mysteries of the needle (Vols 1 and 2). JAAF Productions, Corte Madera

■ Miki Shima

I am a 48-year-old Japanese practitioner of acupuncture, moxibustion, herbal medicine and the medical I Ching and I live in Corte Madera, California, USA. I was trained by traditional tutorial methods in Tokyo and Osaka: in acupuncture by Dr Tadashi Irie; in herbal medicine by Dr Terutane Yamada; and in the medical I Ching by Dr Sango Kobayshi.

I came to California in 1978 after teaching traditional Chinese medical philosophy at the University of Michigan for 2 years, and passed the State Board in 1979. I was later appointed to the California Acupuncture Examining Committee for 7 years, and worked as President of the California Acupuncture Association for 2 years.

In 1987, I established the Japanese-American Acupuncture Foundation (JAAF) in California and since then I have taught over 120 clinical workshops across the United States. I have also written 'The Medical I Ching – Oracle of the Healer Within' (Blue Poppy Press) and have produced three clinical video-tapes from my past workshops on the subject of Japanese needling techniques. These are 'Mysteries of the needle', paediatric treatment 'Shonishin', and the Japanese abdominal diagnosis 'Fukushin', with two volumes for each topic (JAAF Productions).

California dreaming

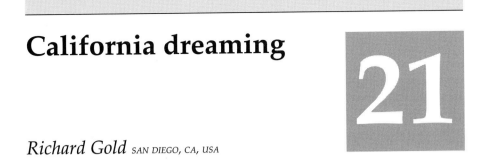

Richard Gold SAN DIEGO, CA, USA

Catherine is a 32-year-old, white female who first came to see me at my office 2 years ago. At this meeting, Catherine struck me as being extremely pale, puffy, and fatigued. Her shoulders were slumped forward and her eyes appeared tired. She had been referred to me by her study partner who was a long-time patient of mine. They were both finishing their course-work to become Licensed Psychologists, and were studying diligently for their final state licensing examinations. Catherine and I easily established a rapport, but she was extremely cautious about bestowing her trust upon another health care professional: she felt that her condition was only worsening with each additional doctor she saw.

A recurrent fever for 2 years

Catherine came to me complaining of an undiagnosed systemic infection with accompanying water retention and arthritic pain, especially in her feet and ankles. She reported that 2 years previously, when she had stopped nursing her daughter, she developed monthly fevers in the evening about 1 week prior to her menses. Prior to the onset of the recurrent fevers, she had received a 'flu vaccination. At this time, her fever reached about 101°F and was accompanied by chills. Then, 1 year later, the fevers became more frequent and persistent, reaching 103°F, with chills, vomiting and diarrhoea. At this time, she was hospitalised for 8 days. Four months later, she became acutely ill and was again hospitalised. This time there was organ involvement, with an enlarged spleen and elevated liver enzymes, in addition to the the high fever and chills. Catherine experienced extreme leg pains and a hypersensitivity (erythemanodosum) that displayed symptoms of raised red patches on her legs that became very hot and swollen and shifted locations. Recently, Catherine would awaken in the morning, still fatigued after a long night's sleep, with her eyes practically swollen shut.

At the time of our first meeting, she had been on doxycycline, an antibiotic, and spironolactone, a diuretic, for the past 7 months. In addition, because of a recently diagnosed condition of endometriosis and concern by her doctor that she should not become pregnant, she was taking the birth control pill TriPhasil.

Catherine's case was anything but a routine case for me. Catherine slowly, deliberately and directly reported her situation to me and became fatigued and morose just from the retelling. Her most recent physician had recommended that she remain on antibiotics for at least 1 year, and had told her that she might have a chronic intestinal disease known as Whipple's Disease.[1] Catherine seemed dejected and overwhelmed by her condition. As our initial interview proceeded, she seemed encouraged not only by my concern for her plight, but also by my attention to detail and my willingness to take the time to really listen to her.

After our lengthy discussion, I had Catherine put on a gown and lie down on the treatment table. At this time, I took her pulse, palpated her abdomen, and examined her tongue. The pulse was deep, deficient and thready, especially in the third position on both wrists and there was a tightness in the middle position on the left wrist. Her tongue was pale with a thin, white coat and, more notably, the tongue body was cracked and deviated to the right when presented. The abdominal palpation yielded a hardened and swollen liver and a tenderness at the left LIV13 *zhangmen* area. In addition, there was extreme tenderness in the lower right quadrant in the ileocaecal valve area at GB27 *wushu* and, on the left at ST25 *tianshu*. Overall, the abdomen was cool, swollen and lacked vitality. The aortic pulse was slightly off centre to the right.

Anything but a routine case

Additional relevant information from Catherine's history included a hospitalisation at the age of 15 for fevers and anaemia. She also reported a history of throat, tonsil and lung problems with repeated use of antibiotics. Her ears frequently felt plugged up, with an accompanying sensation of dizziness. Her blood pressure was on the low side of normal. Her eyes were often swollen and irritated. She also had a life-long problem with constipation, recurrent night sweats and intermittent periods of anaemia. She had a history of regular menses that had become increasingly painful, with a recent diagnosis of endometriosis.

Catherine's appetite was moderate, thirst was slight, and diet was marked by excessive fats, sweets, and yeasted wheat products. She had a cup of coffee daily and only occasionally drank alcohol. She exercised rarely, and then walking only, because of her fatigue and the pain in her legs and feet. She described herself as being anxious and somewhat obsessive. Catherine responded to my question about sleep and dreams by detailing a recurrent dream where she was 'totally exposed and unable to put her clothes on'. She was very happily married with one daughter, aged 4 and, because she and her husband were both back at school, they were living with her parents in order to save money. This seemed to be a good living situation with which all those involved were comfortable.

This initial interview and history took approximately 1 hour to complete. During this time, Catherine was consistently open and willing to answer all of my questions. She felt my concern for her condition and knew that I was being thorough in my approach. She could tell that I was concerned but not overwhelmed. I took detailed notes and established a chronology of events. I was interested to know what her medical doctors thought of her situation and what was their prognosis and proposed strategy. Basically, their diagnosis was inconclusive and their treatment approach was to keep Catherine on antibiotics for at least 1 year. I asked her how she felt about her situation and what she felt the future held for her. One of her primary concerns was whether she would be able to have another child and, if so, whether she would be healthy enough to carry the child. At this time, her doctors were discouraging her from even attempting to become pregnant. They had prescribed the birth control pill to prevent pregnancy and to treat the symptoms of endometriosis.

Summary of clinical manifestations

- Monthly fever, accompanied by chills, 1 week prior to menses.
- Two occurrences of persistent high fever, chills, vomiting and diarrhoea, the second time with spleen enlargement and elevated liver enzymes.
- Hypersensitivity (erythemanodosum) in the legs with painful, raised, red skin lesions surrounded by oedema and heat sensations; lesion eruptions change locations.
- Foot, ankle and leg pain, especially in the morning.
- Eyes swollen and irritated, especially in the morning.
- Eyes appear tired, shoulders are slumped and the patient is fatigued and morose at the first consultation.

- Systemic oedema.
- Pallor.
- Abdominal pain and constipation.
- Night sweats.
- Feels cold.
- Low blood pressure.
- Painful menses with endometriosis.
- Fatigue and occasional dizziness.
- Tendency to be anxious and display obsessive personality.
- Symptom picture fluctuates daily.
- Pulse: deep, deficient and thready, especially both third positions; tightness in the middle left position.
- Tongue: pale, thin white coat; tongue body cracked and deviates to the right.

Identifying the patterns of disharmony

The complexity and seriousness of this case led me to base my diagnosis on various diagnostic approaches. These approaches also helped me to encompass aspects of the case that were filled with ambiguity and uncertainty:

1 I utilised syndromes of the *zangfu* and the Eight Principles to establish the current, most pressing phenomenon.

2 The Five Elements approach allowed me to determine the oldest, most chronic and persistent imbalances.

3 Recognition of the role that Blood and *yin* deficiency had played in this case brought forth the inclusion of Fundamental Substances into the diagnostic picture.

4 Finally, because of the role played by the 'flu vaccination, recognition of toxic poison was taken into account.

The patterns of disharmony

Wind-Heat in the Blood with trapped pathogen (toxin)

- Painful, raised, red skin lesions with shifting locations.
- Lesions surrounded by heat sensations.
- Monthly fevers.
- Symptoms fluctuate daily.
- Involvement of the 'flu vaccination at the start of the pathological process.

Stagnant Liver *qi* and Blood; Internal Wind

- Eyes swollen and irritated.
- Painful menses (endometriosis).
- Dizziness.
- Abdominal pain.
- Constipation.
- Vomiting.
- Tenderness at left LIV13 *zhangmen* position.
- Elevated liver enzymes.

Spleen *qi* deficiency

- Abdominal bloating, oedema, abdomen lacks vitality.
- Fatigue.
- Obsessive personality.
- Spleen enlargement.

- Vomiting and diarrhoea with severe occurrences.
- Pulse: deficient.
- Tongue: pale.

Kidney *yang* deficiency

- Oedema of the lower extremities.
- Foot, ankle and leg pains.
- Chills.
- Anxiousness.
- Cool abdomen.
- Pulse: deep and deficient in the third positions.

Lung *qi* deficiency

- Chronic history of sore throats and lung problems.
- Propensity to recurrent sore throats and upper respiratory infections.
- Pulse: deficient.

Large Intestine *qi* deficiency

- Chronic constipation.

Blood and *yin* deficiency

- Recurrent anaemia.
- Night sweats.
- Fever associated with blood loss in menses.
- Eyes appear tired and anxious.

Aetiology and pathology

The Lung *qi* deficiency has led to deficient *wei qi*. The historic Spleen *qi* deficiency and the months of breastfeeding have led to Blood deficiency. The stagnation of the Liver Blood and *qi* has contributed to the presence of Heat in the Blood and the painful, cramping menses. The toxin from the 'flu vaccination entered a system that was already chronically Blood and *yin* deficient, adding increased Heat in the Blood. In addition, 7 months of antibiotic use had increased the Cold afflicting the Kidney *yang* and contributed to the oedema. The combined deficiencies in the Lung, Spleen, and Kidney energies have also led to the accumulation of fluids in the body. The utilisation of diuretics has further weakened the *qi* and *yang* of the Spleen and Kidneys. The deficient *qi* of the Large Intestine, together with the stagnation of the Liver energy, have contributed to the chronic constipation and irritation in the bowels (Fig. 21.1).

Catherine's pathological processes began with a Lung *qi* deficiency as manifested in recurrent throat and lung problems and begining in childhood. By the age of 15, she was hospitalised with high fevers and anaemia. This demonstrates a condition of Blood deficiency and invasion of external pathogens. According to the Five Elements, the early deficiency in Metal leads to an undernourishment of the son, Water, thus leading to a Kidney

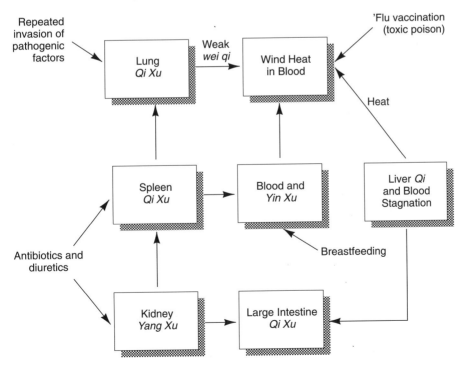

Fig. 21.1 Aetiology and pathology of *zangfu* patterns.

deficiency. This imbalance is further complicated by a tendency to Stagnation of the Liver energy. With the mother of Wood (the Kidneys) already being deficient, there is inadequate energy to move through the stagnation in the Wood (the Liver). The stagnation of Liver energy then overcontrols the Earth energy, according to the *ke* cycle, and leads to a deficient energy of the Spleen. Over time, deficient Spleen energy leads to a Blood deficient condition.

In the current situation, the *biao* (the primary manifestation) was Wind-Heat in the Blood, generated from stagnation in the Liver combined with an external toxin from the 'flu vaccination. The primary symptom was the hot, painful, raised red skin lesions that emerged suddenly and changed locations. The root disharmonies included the Lung and Spleen *qi* deficiency, the Kidney *yang* deficiency, and the stagnation of the Liver *qi* and Blood (Fig. 21.2).

Time and patience, no 'quick fix'

The primary treatment principle was to clear Wind and Heat (toxin) from the Blood in order to first affect the most pressing and external manifestations. Secondary treatment was directed at breaking Liver Blood and *qi*

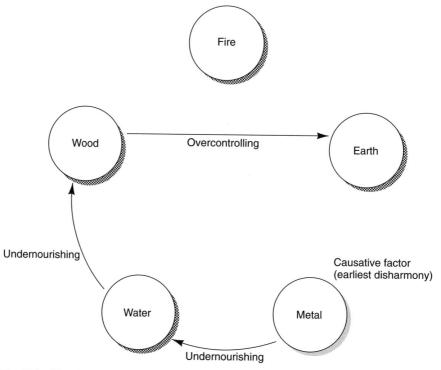

Fig. 21.2 Five Element interactions.

stagnation and resolving oedema. The third component of treatment was aimed at building the *yang* of the Spleen and Kidney, thereby nourishing and building the Blood and ridding the body of internal Cold. Fourthly, invigorating the *qi* of the Large Intestine was pursued to resolve constipation and assist in detoxifying the body. Finally, the *wei qi* was strengthened in order to ward off any opportunistic external pathogens from creating a new phase of disharmony.

I was not expecting a rapid change in the major patterns. The duration of the primary problems (2 years of recurrent fever) and the underlying chronic deficiencies, aggravated by 7 months of antibiotic use, led me to believe that treatment would require time and patience.

Joint participation in the process

Catherine recognised the seriousness and complexity of her condition. She was well aware that there was no 'quick fix'. Prior to the first treatment, I spoke with her about the fundamental principles of Chinese medicine. I did not speak in detail about diagnosis, but rather emphasised the importance of open communication and the fact that she had full access to me. Also, I made the point that we were participating in the process together. She had an active role in her treatment, and I did not want her to be simply a passive recipient of the treatment and procedures. I did not make any specific prognostic claims although I did say that I believed there would be a marked improvement over time and that, in the long-term, she could discontinue treatment by antibiotics and diuretics. Initially, I requested twice weekly treatments. I did not request that she stop her medications or come off the birth control pill. I did, however, leave open the possibility that as she improved, and with her physician's knowledge, she could be taken off her medications.

An important aspect of my approach to Catherine's treatment required dietary changes. I encouraged her to limit coffee, sweets and chocolate, all of which she used daily. She came to me on a high fat and low protein diet. This had to be reversed, with an emphasis on cooked vegetables, whole grains and a reduction in animal protein. Also, I requested that she severely limited her intake of wheat products. I invited Catherine to bring her husband along to her next treatment. At the time, he was studying to become an emergency medical technician. I knew that if he felt involved in the process, he would be able to support Catherine's dietary and lifestyle changes. When he did come along, I included him in the discussion and explained to them both my rationale and intentions. As much as possible, I explained my treatment goals in terms that were understandable from a Western medical approach.

Before beginning treatment, I spoke with Catherine about the methods I intended to use; specifically acupuncture and moxibustion. I let her know that only sterile disposable needles were used. I spoke about the importance of her being comfortable with the treatment, and let her know that at any time she could speak out if she felt uncomfortable or anxious. She was both anxious in a nervous way, and anxious to get started. I told her that an often experienced side-effect of treatment was a deep sense of calm and relaxation. I encouraged her to relax and to allow herself to be taken care of for the next period of time. My hope for the first treatment was for Catherine to be comfortable, for there to be no pain from needle insertion, for her to remain calm while receiving moxibustion, and for her to be relaxed while experiencing a small amount of *de qi* sensation from the needles. This first treatment went very well. Catherine relaxed deeply and felt cared for as a person as well as a patient. She experienced no needle discomfort.

First treatment procedures

POINTS PRESCRIPTION

- SP0 *xuehai* removes Wind and Heat from the Blood, cools and tonifies the Blood, relieves Blood stasis and regulates the menses.
- LI11 *quchi* clears Heat and cools the Blood; resolves Dampness.
- BL17 *geshu* clears Heat from the Blood, nourishes and invigorates the Blood, and tonifies *qi* and Blood.
- BL18 *ganshu* eliminates Wind, benefits the Liver, moves stagnant *qi* and benefits the eyes.
- LU7 *lieque* disperses Wind, opens the water passages, disperses Lung *qi*, circulates the *wei qi*, and is the master point of the Conception Vessel.
- ST36 *zusanli* expels Wind and Damp, resolves oedema, benefits the Spleen, tonifies *qi* and Blood, dispels Cold, brightens the eyes, regulates nutritive *qi* and *wei qi*, and regulates the intestines.
- KID7 *fuliu* resolves Damp and eliminates oedema, tonifies the Kidneys and regulates sweating.
- SP6 *sanyinjiao* strengthens the Spleen, resolves Dampness, benefits urination, promotes smooth flow of Liver *qi*, tonifies the Kidneys, nourishes Blood and *yin*, moves and

cools the Blood, and regulates the Uterus and menses.
- LIV3 *taichong* expels interior Wind and promotes the smooth flow of Liver *qi*.
- REN12 *zhongwan* tonifies the Spleen and Stomach, resolves Dampness, and is the influential point of the *fu*.

For point energetics see Maciocia (1989).

Auricular Points: Liver, Lung and Small Intestine (ileocaecal valve).

This points prescription is designed to treat the Wind and Heat in the Blood (to resolve the skin lesions), promote urination and eliminate Dampness (oedema), move Liver *qi* and Blood, and strengthen Spleen and Kidney *qi*.

Moxibustion: was applied to: SP10 *xuehai*, LI11 *quchi*, ST36 *zusanli*, KID7 *fuliu*, SP6 *sanyinjiao* and REN12 *zhongwan*. The purpose was to increase the *yang* of the Kidneys and Spleen, to resolve Damp and promote urination, and to clear the Wind from the Blood.

Needling and auxiliary techniques: Seirin #3 (20 x 40) disposable needles were used with insertion tubes. Needles were retained for 20 minutes and a slight *qi* sensation was obtained at the needles after 10 minutes. Once the needles were removed, a poultice of castor oil was applied to the lower right abdominal area and was covered with a warm hydroculator pack. The purpose of this technique was to address inflammation in the ileocaecal valve area and to promote lymphatic circulation (McGarey 1983). Whilst the poultice was in place a 10-minute foot reflexology massage was administered.

Changes to medication and diet

The initial visit took place in March, after which two treatments per week were given for a total of 15 treatments, followed by an additional 32 treatments, mostly once weekly or every two weeks. From the initiation of treatment there were positive changes, such as increased urination and reduced oedema in the legs and around the eyes, less leg and foot pain, decreased occurrence of skin lesions and pain, increased regularity of bowel movements and less fatigue. There were also significant setbacks and flare-ups.

In late March, Catherine had a flare-up of the skin lesions and leg pain. After close questioning, we discovered that she had eaten almost a quart of fresh strawberries over the weekend. I requested that she limit strawberry consumption. In early April, Catherine took herself off all medications, including the birth control pill. I supported this decision totally. The oedema was already much improved and persistent daily use of antibiotics was posing more risk than benefit. Antibiotics are considered very cold in nature. Also, their continued use made it very difficult to strengthen the *wei qi* and restore the health of the colon.

Since the beginning of our professional relationship, Catherine had spoken to me about wanting to have another child. She was concerned about being healthy enough to carry a child and was fearful of returning to poor health after giving birth. I had counselled her to concentrate on regaining her health and becoming committed to a healthy lifestyle and that, in time, the issue of pregnancy would resolve itself.

Through the spring, Catherine showed gradual improvement. Her first period after stopping the pill was light with no cramps at all. On the whole, she improved her diet significantly and began to notice that when she did not adhere to a strict diet, she suffered symptomatic flare-ups. This aware-ness encouraged her to be very disciplined with regard to her food and drink intake.

From the beginning of our treatments, I had included herbal medicine as an important part of the treatment. The primary formulae used were

Buplureum and Peony *dan zhi xiao yao san* to resolve Liver Stagnation and facilitate the menses, and Hoelen Five *wu ling san* to resolve Dampness and promote urination (Bensky & Barolet 1990). Also, three specific food supplements were used:

1 Greenmagma, a dehydrated barley grass was used daily and was prescribed to cool the Blood, provide a wide range of nutrients including protein, and to aid the bowels (Hagiwara 1985).
2 A pill composed of deodorised garlic with Coix (*Semen coicis*) was prescribed. Garlic has natural antibacterial properties whilst Coix is a natural diuretic and helps to relieve inflammation in the mucosa of the alimentary canal.
3 An acidophilus supplement was also prescribed to repopulate the colon with beneficial bacteria.

Further setbacks and flare-ups

In late June, Catherine suffered from a high fever with chills, nausea, and increased swelling of the legs. Prior to the fever, which occurred after her period, she had entertained house guests, had overextended herself, and had eaten poorly and taken some alcohol. She came for two treatments in a 4-day period, did not take antibiotics, and made a rapid recovery.

In late August, Catherine's mother-in-law became seriously ill. Whilst away to be with her, Catherine herself became ill with a sore throat, swollen glands, high fever, nausea, and vomiting. At this juncture, she took a 7-day course of the antibiotic amoxycillin, made a rapid recovery and had stabilised by the following week. Subsequent to this flare-up, she suffered from constipation, skin lesions, oedema, and leg cramps. During her menstrual period in early October, she had no fever but craved sugar and chocolate. By mid-October, there was another flare-up. This time she was at home, we were able to administer treatment and there was no antibiotic usage. The symptoms of fever and chills, yellow phlegm, and nausea and vomiting cleared up totally within 4 days. For the next 4 weeks, Catherine was in good health and had no symptoms, including no skin lesions or leg pain.

Maintaining relatively good health

Beginning mid-November, I recommended that she have treatments every other week, unless there was an acute problem. Increasingly, Catherine recognised that her symptoms worsened with dietary error and stress. This led her to become very strict with her diet and to develop stress management techniques in her daily life. As the weeks went by, Catherine maintained relatively good health. Her periods were regular, with only mild cramps or no cramps at all, and there were no fever or chills associated with the period. Occasionally, she developed painful, hot, raised red skin lesions on her lower legs. My strategy for treating these was to surround the lesion with needles, and then to directly warm the area with indirect moxibustion. This approach proved to be very effective. In addition, at each treatment, I utilised a castor oil poultice on the lower abdomen. My goal was to relieve as much as possible the persistent inflammation in the intestinal tract (Whipple's Disease).

By the following year Catherine's health had stabilised and her visits became less frequent. She had completed successfully all her state licensing examinations. When she did come for treatments, the strategy was to build her Spleen, Kidney and Lung energy, to nourish the Blood and *yin*, and to relieve any swelling or discomfort in her legs.

The dream

In July, 15 months after commencing treatment, Catherine related to me a dream. In the dream, she was pregnant. This filled her with joy. There was a strong notion of caution in the dream because her blood pressure was considered to be too low. She was informed that her blood pressure was 100/58. Upon awakening, she told her husband about the dream, and asked him to take her blood pressure, which was exactly 100/58!! After discussing this dream, and knowing how much improvement Catherine had made, I encouraged her to be open to the possibility of becoming pregnant and to feel confident of her ability to have a successful pregnancy. Also, I spoke to her about reaffirming herself as a healthy person as opposed to a sick person. I did not see Catherine again until late August. At this visit, she joyfully told me that she was 6 weeks pregnant and was feeling great and confident.

Outcome

- No raised, red, hot, swollen, painful skin lesions on the legs.
- Menses with neither painful cramps nor fevers and chills.
- Off all medications.
- Regular bowel movements.
- No abdominal pain.
- No oedema.
- Less fatigue, more energy.
- Eyes clear; no swelling and discomfort.
- No night sweats.
- Liver enzymes normal; no spleen enlargement.
- Six weeks pregnant; feeling great and confident.

Conclusion

In May, the following year, and after a short and uncomplicated labour, Catherine gave birth to a healthy 4 kg (8 lbs 14 oz) girl. She suffered no postpartum problems, either physical or mental. Her milk flourished.

Catherine's commitment to her health and healing journey led to this happy, healthy and fulfilling conclusion. Catherine had presented with very serious health problems, not fully diagnosed by Western medicine, and having taken multiple courses of prescribed drugs. Catherine's dedication to her healing and her willingness to make significant changes to her lifestyle and attitudes, were crucial to her recovery. Her patience and consistency in attending for treatments were also vital components in this process.

Having practised traditional Chinese medicine consistently since 1978, I have gained great confidence in its healing potential when applied in a rational and correct manner. Even so, with a case of this seriousness, which was complicated by prescribed drug therapies and the negative mental influences associated with an uncertain medical diagnosis, I have been reinspired by the profound effect that traditional Chinese medicine can stimulate.

Catherine's willingness to participate fully in her healing process, and my attention to including her in all decisions relating to her case, were pivotal factors in her return to health. In addition, the herbal medicines, supplementation, and external castor oil poultices played an important role in her recovery.

This case demonstrates that, even with seriously ill individuals, healing can result from a coherent and accurate diagnosis and a consistent adherence to the principles of health.

NOTE

1 Whipple's Disease is also known as Intestinal Lipodystrophy. Considered a rare disease, Whipple's is characterised by fatty stools, weight loss, a distinctive lesion of the mucosa of the jejunum and ileum, and other signs of a malabsorption syndrome. In addition, anaemia, skin pigmentation, and joint symptoms may occur. The patient commonly has abdominal pain, cough, and pleuratic pain. Treatment with intensive antibiotic therapy, followed by a maintenance therapy of tetracycline, is recommended. Untreated, the disease is considered progressive and fatal (Berkow 1992).

REFERENCES

Bensky D, Barolet R 1990 Formulae and strategies. Eastland Press, Seattle
Berkow R (ed) 1992 Merck Manual. Merck Research Laboratories, New Jersey
Hagiwara Yoshihide 1985 Green barley essence. Keats Publishing, New Canaan

Maciocia G 1989 The foundations of Chinese medicine. Churchill Livingstone, Edinburgh
McGarey W A 1983 The Edgar Cayce remedies. Bantam Books, New York

FURTHER READING

Kaptchuk T 1983 The web that has no weaver. Congdon & Weed, New York
Xinnong Cheng (ed) 1987 Chinese acupuncture and moxibustion. Foreign Language Press, Beijing

■ Richard Gold

Richard Gold is a 1972 graduate of Oberlin College with a BA degree in World Religions. In 1978, he graduated from the New England School of Acupuncture. His primary instructors, who have remained influential and inspirational in his career, were Dr Tin Yao So and Dr Ted Kaptchuk. In 1983, he earned a Doctorate in Psychology and also received his California License in Acupuncture. He has undertaken advanced clinical studies in Shanghai, China, in 1980, in Hong Kong in 1985 and in Osaka, Japan, in 1986. In 1989, Richard began his studies of the Traditional Medical Massage of Thailand (Nuad Bo-Rarn) in Chiang Mai, Thailand. Subsequently, he travelled back to Chiang Mai in 1990 and 1992 to continue these studies.

In 1982, Richard was the first President and a founding Board Member of the International Professional School of Bodywork (IPSB). In 1986, he was one of the founding Board Members of the Pacific College of Oriental Medicine in San Diego, California and in 1993 of the Pacific Institute of Oriental Medicine in New York City. Since 1989, Richard has been on the Board of Pacific Symposiums Inc. and has been a frequent lecturer at their annual conferences. Since 1990, he has been involved in the creation of instructional videos in the field of Oriental bodywork. He serves on the National Advisory Board of the American Oriental Bodywork Therapy Association (AOBTA). Richard maintains a busy clinical practice concurrently with teaching, writing, Board responsibilities, and family in San Diego, California.

Challenges that take their toll

Bernard Côté MONTREAL, CANADA

The case history presented here spans a period of 9 years. Often case presentations coming from China relate only to what I would call the first stage of treatment, i.e. the period starting from the moment when the patient first sees the practitioner and lasting anywhere from 1 week to 2 months. Usually this comprises a series of 4 to 12 treatments. Although this approach to documenting case histories is certainly relevant in acute situations, I cannot help feeling a certain sense of frustration when reading such accounts of more chronic cases. Indeed the question always remains: what happened to this patient 1 year, 2 years, or 5 years later?

My aim is not only to convey my approach to this case, but also to serve as a witness to my own evolution in the practice of Chinese medicine. Rather than trying to lull the reader with a success story, I am attempting to encourage the practitioner in his or her endeavours to develop a practice based on self-questioning and concomitant research with a rigorous analysis of results in order to reach a finer grasp of the evolutionary tendencies in the patient's energetic manifestations.

Victor and his tachychardia

Victor was 37 years old when he was seen for the first time 9 years ago. Happily married for 10 years with two daughters of 9 and 7, he worked as a college teacher and also ran a small film production company for which he was both producer and director. This work related to nature films, and he therefore regularly went into the forest by himself for many days to film wildlife, carrying heavy equipment. He also regularly went to the northern parts of Quebec to make films on wild fauna. The patient was of medium build, easy to relate to and joyful. The feeling of uneasiness he manifested during our first meeting could have been linked to the apprehension of having his state of health scrutinised or to the nature of his condition. The voice was parched and the way he delivered answers to questions was uneven in relation both to speed and strength of the voice. He smiled and laughed often when we talked about his difficulties related to health or other aspects of his life. At times, this seemed inappropriate. He was very engaging and rapport was quickly established.

Victor's chief complaint was tachycardia[1]. He presented it as a freak occurrence in his life, since apart from this problem his health had always been fine and his resistance remarkable, particularly in relation to his work. He found the limitations of tachycardia difficult to accept since his whole lifestyle revolved around physical endurance. Although he was prepared to accept the need for periods of rest, he could not really conceive of life at a slower pace. While he had consulted Western physicians, no treatment had been offered since he had never been monitored during an active episode. His father and one sister had suffered similar problems. He said his father was anxious like himself and had had heart problems although he was never able to give more precise details. In the case of his sister, tachycardia had been associated with anxiety.

His first episode happened during the night, 5 years prior to consulting me. The heart rate was of 140 beats per minute and the episode lasted for 3 minutes, after which he felt exhausted. It recurred 3 weeks later and again during the night 1 year later, after he had eaten a late meal. Episodes always happened during the night around 3.00 a.m. and a loose bowel movement alleviated the symptoms. He always felt heaviness and discomfort in the epigastric region during these episodes. He also reported experiencing some dizziness and a feeling of tingling in the shoulders and arms. He had not then suffered from an attack of tachycardia for many years, until 6 months prior to consulting me, when these episodes began to reappear at 2-monthly intervals. Since then he had felt chronically tired with a debilitating lack of enthusiasm. After each of the episodes he had great shivers and felt cold. What bothered him most at the moment of consultation was not so much the tachycardia, but rather the tremendous fatigue which he was beginning to feel on a permanent basis. He felt a constant yearning to lie down and sleep. His teaching job was perceived more and more as a burden.

Other symptoms and signs

Prior to the first onset of symptoms, Victor reported being prone to sudden and violent outbursts of anger. However, he had not experienced any such outbursts since the onset of his heart problems. Normally sleep patterns were good, with 8–9 hours of uninterrupted sleep, however he complained of still feeling tired upon waking. He also mentioned that he liked the autumn, did not like the heat and loved going by himself into the woods in the middle of winter. He reported often seeing black dots and experiencing short bouts of dizziness. Perspiration was normal. The colour of the face was uneven, pink on the cheeks, with some pale areas and a bluish tint under the eyes. He had a good appetite, liked all types of foods and ate meat or fish twice daily. He had difficulty digesting fried food, and late meals seemed to sit on his stomach all night through. Bowel movements were regular, twice a day. The patient mentioned that his micturition was less frequent than others and that his urine was very yellow and occasionally burned. He was not prone to infections like colds or 'flu.

The tongue was pale, with a thin, white coating. The pulse lacked strength at a deep level and was wiry on the surface and forceless in both *cun* positions at all levels. The speed was normal. During the physical examination there was a tendency for the skin to redden easily on palpation and discomfort on palpation of REN14 *juque* was observed. Both bone structure and muscle development seemed adequate. Calf muscle masses were well above the average. Blood pressure was 140/85.

Lifestyle issues

Victor used to drink a lot of wine but had gradually reduced his consumption. He stopped smoking 2 years prior to the initial consultation but still had the occasional cigarette. He drank daily the equivalent of 1.5 litres of fluids, including three coffees, one fruit juice and six herbal teas. He liked good food and good wine but was not overweight. He seemed to have a good constitution, was happily married, dearly loving his children, and he was enthusiastic about his filming work but weary of his teaching. He seemed to fear the prospect of being unable to carry on and unable to achieve all that he wanted to in the future. His lifestyle of travelling, overexertion from long walks, numerous freelance projects and the psychological necessity of engaging in ever more challenging projects was taking its toll on his potential to achieve all of these things at once.

Clinical manifestations

- Tachycardia, episodic, with similar problems in father and sister.
- Episodes happen at night, possibly after a late meal.
- After episodes, great shivers and feels cold.
- Chronically tired, tremendous fatigue, debilitating lack of enthusiasm.
- Heaviness and discomfort in the epigastric region during episodes, also dizziness, tingling in shoulders and arms.
- Yearns to lie down.
- Inappropriate smiling and laughing.
- Episodes alleviated by loose bowel movements.
- Likes autumn, does not like the heat.
- Sees black dots, short bouts of dizziness.
- Face colour uneven, pink on the cheeks, with some pale areas and a bluish tint under eyes.
- Difficulty digesting fried food, late meals seem to sit on his stomach all night through.

- Micturition less frequent than others, very yellow, occasionally burning.
- Fear of being unable to carry on.
- Tongue: pale, coating thin and white.

- Pulse: lacked strength at a deep level, wiry on the surface, forceless in both *cun* positions at all levels.
- Palpation: skin reddened easily, discomfort at REN14 *juque.*

Therapeutic orientation

After reviewing the initial information, it became immediately apparent that three issues would influence the therapeutic orientation.

1 Should the patient be seen by a Western physician for safety's sake prior to and during the course of treatment?
2 How could I affect, in a stable way, the symptoms and the energy balance if the lifestyle of overexertion was to be maintained?
3 Would the case be understood differently if treatment was based on short- rather than long-term considerations?

At first, I did not feel totally comfortable in treating Victor because the cardiac involvement had not been assessed satisfactorily by a Western physician. I expressed my concerns to the patient, indicating to him that if his condition did not improve within four treatments, I would continue only in consultation with his physician. The patient seemed happy with this arrangement.

I did not at that time (nor do I now), believe that the effects of any treatment would be durable if some aspects of Victor's lifestyle did not change. Nevertheless, I have never been one to overemphasise my point of view regarding a person's life path, except by changes achieved through the treatment. When treatment begins I attempt to identify (and help the patient to identify) lifestyle aspects that exacerbate the problems, and I leave to the patient the initiative of finding out how these problems should be tackled. Experience has shown me that changes are more durable if they arise within the patient as he gets better and stronger and initiates in his own way a new path in life. My position as a practitioner is to encourage any movement which is congruent with the therapeutic orientation.

In this case, quick results were necessary in order to break the pattern which had been established. Middle range objectives had to ensure the stability of any improvement and a long-term view had to satisfy the principle of treating the whole of this person with all the subtleties of his particular internal dynamics.

Patterns of disharmony

Heart *qi* deficiency

- Tachycardia.
- Inappropriate smiling and laughing.
- Tenderness at REN14 *juque.*
- Pink colouring on the cheeks.
- Triggered by periods of over-exertion, both physical and mental.
- Tongue: pale.
- Pulse: lacks strength.

Spleen and Stomach deficiency

- Chronically tired, tremendous fatigue.
- Debilitating lack of enthusiasm.
- Yearns to lie down.
- Difficulty digesting fried food; late meals seem to sit on his stomach all night.
- Tongue: pale.
- Pulse: lacks strength at the deep level.

Kidney *jing xu* and Kidney *yin xu*

- Two family members also have tachycardia.
- Pink cheeks (malar flush).
- Tachycardia episodes occur at night.
- Fear of being unable to carry on.
- Micturition less frequent, yellow, occasionally burning.

Ascendant Liver *yang*, Liver invades Spleen

- Bouts of dizziness.
- Black spots in front of eyes.
- Bouts of anger preceded initial onset of tachycardia.
- Episodes alleviated by loose bowel movements.
- Pulse: wiry on the surface.

Pathology

Heart *qi* deficiency

It was quite clear from the beginning that the patient's Heart *qi* was deficient. Tachychardia is included within the Chinese concept of palpitations and, in this case, was triggered by periods of long-term physical or mental exertion with a sensation of oppression in the chest, clearly demonstrating that the *qi* was involved. The cause related to overexertion is categorised within the *bu nei bu wai* (neither internal nor external) causes as described in the texts. If Heart *qi* is deficient, the rapidity of the heart rate tries to make up for its lack of strength. In the associations with the Five Movements (*wu xing*) theory, the inappropriate emotion of joy and laughter and the pink colour of the cheeks point in the same direction.

Spleen and Stomach deficiency

The source of acquired (*zong*) *qi* resides in the ability of the middle burner to produce adequate *qi* and Blood for all the organs. If *qi* is inconsiderately consumed, then the accelerated heart rate becomes a response to insufficient production of *qi* and Blood by the Spleen and Stomach. 'If Spleen and Stomach *qi* become decrepit and original (*yuan*) *qi* becomes insufficient, Heart Fire becomes effulgent on its own. This Heart Fire is a *yin* fire.

It starts from the lower burner and its ligation links to the Heart. The Heart does not reign, ministerial fire is its deputy. Ministerial fire is the fire of the Pericardium developing from the lower burner. It is a foe to the original *(yuan) qi.'* (Li Dong-yuan 1993).

Kidney *jing* and *yin* deficiency

The fact that two other family members suffer from similar heart problems suggests strongly that there is a factor linked to prenatal *(yuan) qi* and this has to be integrated in the understanding of the causes of the problem. In this case, this underlying cause, related to *jing*-essence, had been compensated for until the onset of the symptoms by adequate production of grain *(gu) qi* by the Spleen and Stomach and air *(kong) qi* by the Lungs. Overexertion, while injuring the production of Blood and *qi*, exacerbates Heart Fire which originates from the ministerial fire of the Kidney. This is the fire getting out of control and is associated with the deficiency of *yin*. From this association, we can understand the malar flush, the anxiety associated with the symptoms of tachycardia and the occurrence at night (Seca di Villadorata & Côté 1989).

Kidney *jing* deficiency is usually manifested in the child by poor development of bone structure and mental retardation, or premature ageing in the adult. None of these was noticeable in Victor but I had to recognise the presence of the symptom in other members of his family. Prenatal influences *(xian tian)* imply more than a genetic influence received at birth. They continue to be an ongoing force throughout life and are manifested in environmental and behavioural responses. Prenatal energy is an energy constantly acting on us

> *like the energy of a star whose light reaches us clearly but which has long ceased to exist. This energy (jing qi) is operating from conception to death, as if the individual is all through his life in a state of perpetual conception, of perpetual birth . . . in fact the adventure of this energy goes well beyond the death of the individual. (Schatz et al 1979).*

Unschuld writes that:

> *The book of changes states that the way of the well is continuous renewal. Hence the hexagram of the well is followed by that of renewal. This principle applies to the essence of the Kidneys too. (Unschuld 1990).*

Ascending Liver *yang*, Liver *qi* horizontally attacks Spleen *qi*

Victor experienced regular bouts of violent anger prior to the onset of symptoms. This suggests that the emotion of anger could have been a precipitating cause of the illness, particularly since these outbursts have since disappeared. 'The *qi* of anger rises from below and injures the *yin*' (Larre 1986). Having previously established that there was an underlying weakness in the Kidney *jing* related to prenatal factors, it can be understood how the flaring of Liver *yang* through repeated bouts of anger can stem from Liver and Kidney *yin* deficiency. Conversely, Liver stagnation generating heat and causing ascending Liver *yang*, injures the *yin* of the Heart and Kidney. It can also be understood why the anger associated with the Liver can injure Spleen *qi* throughout the *ke* cycle according to the Five Movements theory. The models revolving around Liver stagnation and Liver *yang* rising have not been retained as causative factors since the general symptomatology and morphotype of this patient did not deeply reflect this type of disharmony.

Aetiology

In understanding the aetiology, two aspects must be emphasised. The underlying cause was related to deficiency of Kidney *jing* since the problem was present in other members of the family. It was latent until other factors associated with overwork and the general process of ageing weakened the *jing* and *yin* and triggered the onset (Fig. 22.1). The symptoms appeared in a predominant context of overexertion which is included in the *bu nei bu wai* (neither internal nor external) causes. The exhaustion of *qi* and Blood led to exhaustion of Heart *qi* which, superimposed to the underlying pattern of deficient *jing qi,* led to the symptoms described. It is of interest to mention the understanding of the *bu nei bu wai* (neither internal nor external) causes of illnesses which were unfortunately often translated from the Chinese as 'other causes'. Ted Kaptchuk's use of lifestyle to describe *bu nei bu wai* seems more evocatively appropriate (Kaptchuk 1993). The *bu nei bu wai* can be understood as causes related to the interface between the *nei*, the internal, and the *wai*, the external. It includes causes which can be as profoundly internal as a weak constitution (Maciocia 1989) or external factors as in trauma. Therefore the *bu nei bu wai* causes of diseases, far from negating internal and external as causes, suggest a profound interaction between internal and external (Flaws B, personal communication, 1994).

Prior to treatment

Guiding principles of the treatments were aimed at reinforcing Spleen and Heart *qi* and at rooting Heart *qi* by supporting Kidney *yin* and *qi*. As

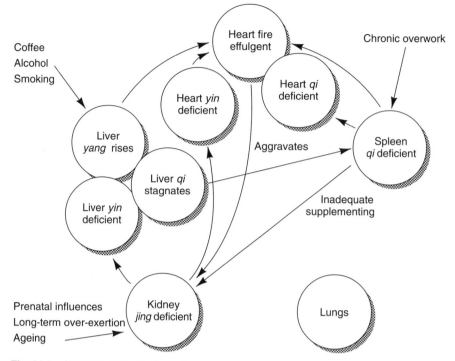

Fig. 22.1 Aetiology and pathology diagram.

Kidney *jing* is difficult to replenish, the emphasis of treatment was in supplementing the centre (*zhong qi*) to reinforce the production of postnatal *zong qi*, part of which could be directed to the Kidneys to supplement *jing* deficiency. With the *yuan qi* being supplemented, Heart source *qi* would be adequate and the Heart function would be restored. 'Spleen and Stomach are the main support for the Heart.' (Maciocia 1989).

Prior to the initial treatment, issues like chronic overexertion, excessive coffee or alcohol intake and smoking were mentioned as concerns that might hamper the successful outcome of treatment. I was convinced at first that the situation would take some time to correct and that symptoms could not rapidly be alleviated in a stable way since they seemed deeply rooted both in chronic overexertion and in the prenatal influences. While Victor accepted the fact that the course of treatment might be a prolonged one, he was greatly motivated to do what he could to help himself.

The first treatments aimed at supplementing Spleen and Stomach *qi* to complement *zong qi*, to direct this towards and reinforce the Heart, and to reinforce the Kidney.

Treatment procedures

POINTS

- ST36 *zusanli (bufa)* with moxa on needle for 10 minutes to tonify postnatal (*yuan*) *qi*.
- BL43 *gaohuangshu (bufa)* with needle and moxa, tonifies *qi* and strengthens the Essence.
- BL14 *jueyinshu (bufa)* with needle and moxa, a back *shu* point of the Pericardium, it calms the mind and nourishes the Heart.
- BL20 *pishu (bufa)* with needle and moxa roll, a back *shu* point of Spleen, it tonifies Spleen and Stomach.
- BL23 *shenshu (bufa)* with needle and moxa roll, the back *shu* point of Kidney, which tonifies Kidney and Essence, benefits the ears and nourishes Blood.
- HE5 *tongli (bufa)* with needle, a *luo* point which tonifies Heart *qi*.
- HE7 *shenmen (bufa)* a *yuan* point which nourishes Heart Blood.
- P6 *neiguan (pingbupingxie)* which regulates Heart *qi* and Blood.
- KID3 *taixi (bufa)* with needle, a Source and Earth point, tonifies *yuan qi*, original *yin* and *yang*, and tonifies the Essence.
- SP6 *sanyinjiao (bufa)* which tonifies the Spleen and the Kidneys, and nourishes Blood and *yin*.
- SP3 *taibai (bufa)* an Earth and Source point to tonify Spleen and Stomach.
- SI7 *zhizheng (bufa)* a *luo* point connecting Small Intestine with the Heart, to tonify the Heart.

- SI19 *tinggong (pingbupingxie)* with laser; it is the point of exit of the meridian and a point of experience for tinnitus.
- SJ17 *yifeng (pingbupingxie)* with laser; a point of experience for the ear.
- SJ3 *zhongzhu (pingbupingxie)* with needle, a point of experience for the ear.
- REN6 *qihai (bufa)* with needle to tonify *qi*.

Needling techniques: *Bufa* is a tonifying method, *Pingbupingxie* is an even method. In general two to three points were used bilaterally in each treatment. When strong tonification was needed, needles were not left in place and moxa was used after the needling. Dispersion was used with great care even when indicated by external invasion of pathogenic agents. Some Chinese texts mention that moxa is contraindicated in cases of Heart *yin* deficiency (Tianjin 1990, 1983). Yet, in this case, in order to tonify the *qi* adequately, moxibustion was important. Therefore all treatments included a *qi* tonifying action and most treatments included a *yin* tonifying action to temper the effect of moxa. Needles used were of 40 mm length and gauge 30 or 32.

Tuina: Tonifying techniques of *mo* (kneading), *an* (pressing), *gun* (rolling) and *yizhichantui* (one finger oscillating pressure) on the back *shu* points were integrated into the treatment.

Improvements and setbacks

Treatments were given twice weekly for 2 weeks, once weekly for 3 weeks, once monthly for 2 months and then once every 3 months. During the few days following the first treatment, the patient reported having had a bout of dizziness and tachycardia after skiing. After a rest of half an hour, he felt fine and black spots in his vision had disappeared.

It was with relief and some surprise that major improvements were witnessed soon after the initial treatments. After the first two treatments Victor had voluntarily reduced his coffee intake to one cup per day and had decided not to smoke. Improved energy levels became stable from the third treatment. Three months later he gave notice to the college where he was teaching that he had decided not to renew his contract for the following session. Another attack of tachycardia took place a month later. Three years later there was a period of frequent diarrhoea which settled after a treatment on SP6 *sanyinjiao*, KID3 *taixi*, REN6 *qihai* and ST37 *shangjuxu*.

After a 2-year gap, he returned with apologies for his absence. He complained of residual tinnitus resulting from a bad cold which had degenerated and for which he had been treated with antibiotics. The tinnitus subsided after a treatment on KID3 *taixi*, SJ3 *zhongzhu*, SI19 *tinggong* and SJ17 *yifeng*. The patient was seen 2 months later without having experienced any symptoms. His energy level seemed to be fine. His business was thriving and projects in France and Japan involved him in a lot of travelling.

For the last 2 years, Victor has been well but reports occasional tinnitus when tired, like a faint whistle. Around 6 months ago, he suffered a relapse of tiredness, but no tachycardia, following an intensive period of work in the desert of Tunisia; he then reported being constantly thirsty, and achey in the arch of both feet as he pointed to KID2 *rangu*. The pulse had changed to being thinner and more rapid. Symptoms subsided after two treatments in the same week which were oriented towards supplementing Spleen *qi* and Kidney *yin*. The patient has since been seen on a monthly basis at his request. He had one bout of tachycardia, his third since starting acupuncture treatment, which was related to overindulgence in alcohol. Now, nearly 10 years since commencing treatment, his state of health is stable.

Outcome

One bout of tachycardia in the last 6 months (three bouts in the 9 years since the onset of treatment).
Energy levels fine.

Black spots in front of eyes have disappeared.
Occasional tinnitus.
State of health stable.

The case in perspective

Victor will benefit from regular treatments, even when he is asymptomatic. He accepts this situation to the point of now insisting on receiving monthly treatments as prophylaxis. It is clear that the original *(yuan) qi* of the

Kidney is adversely affected and that it cannot be easily replenished adequately for two reasons: firstly, the replenishment of *jing* deficiency is a slow process, and secondly, he would benfit from further changes to his lifestyle. Treatments will not only facilitate *qi* production, but will also provide an opportunity to monitor changes and provide feedback on his real level of energy. Herbal medicines such as Four Gentlemen Decoction *si jun zi tang*, or Restore the Spleen Decoction *gui pi tang*, are also useful as a complement to acupuncture treatment of Spleen and Heart *qi*. They are prescribed when symptoms require such treatment. As a Kidney tonic, Six Ingredient Pills with Rehmannia *liu wei di huang wan*, is integrated into Victor's regular acupuncture treatment as a constitutional prescription.

This case puts in perspective some of the difficulties for the Western practitioner of traditional Chinese medicine in adjusting to the needs of his patients. At times, the solutions to a patient's ailments are related to aspects of his life which cannot easily be changed, or if changed suddenly, might cause some disequilibrium which would run counter to the objective of the therapy. In this case, the inevitable challenging aspects of Victor's work are both essential nutritive elements to his well being and seeds of his disharmony. Victor acknowledges this and, whilst living fully, he has to keep well within his sights the parameters affecting his health.

NOTE

1 Tachycardia is a condition in which the heart rate suddenly increases to 100 or more beats per minute. It may last for minutes or hours or even days, ending as abruptly as it began. Arterial blood pressure may fall and clinical manifestations may be similar to those of shock, or cardiac failure may develop with or without signs of shock (Holvey 1989).

REFERENCES

Holvey D (ed) 1989 The Merck Manual. Merck Research Laboratories

Kaptchuk T 1993 La toile sans tisserand. Satas, p 92

Larre C 1986 Par Cinq Institut Ricci. France, pp 41–43

Li, Dong-yuan 1993 Pi Wei Lun. Treatise on the Spleen and Stomach. Blue Poppy Press, Boulder, pp 83–84

Maciocia G 1989 The foundations of Chinese medicine. Churchill Livingstone, Edinburgh

Schatz J, Larre C, Rochat de la Vallée É 1979 Les energies du corps. Éditions So-Wen s.a.s., Milan

Seca di Villadorata M, Côté B 1989 Acupuncture en médecine clinique. Éditions Maloine-Décarie, Paris and Montreal

Tianjin No 1 Hospital of Chinese Medicine 1980 *Shi yong zhenjiu xue*. Kexue jishu chubanshe, China

Tianjin zhonyixue yuan 1983 *Zhenjiu zhiliao xue*. Renmin weisheng chubanshe, China

Unschuld P 1990 Forgotten traditions of ancient Chinese medicine. Paradigm, Boston

FURTHER READING

Bensky D, Barolet R 1992 Chinese herbal medicine formulae and strategies. Eastland Press, Seattle

Shanghai Institute of Chinese Medicine 1988 *Zhongyi Tuina Xue*. Renmin weisheng chubanshe, China

■ **Bernard Côté**

Bernard studied acupuncture with Jack Worsley in Leamington Spa and practised in London from 1978 to 1982. He honed his training with courses by Ted Kaptchuk, Claude Larre, John Shen and others. He practises in Montreal where he studied modern and classical Chinese language at McGill University. Tuina and Chinese herbology have been integrated into his acupuncture practice. He studied Tuina with Dr Yang Dapeng at the Tianjin Institute of Traditional Chinese Medicine and worked in the acupuncture department of Tianjin Hospital No.1, PRC, in 1987 under the supervision of Dr Shi Xuemin. He has directed seminars on traditional Chinese medicine in Montreal since 1983. He teaches clinical students at the department of acupuncture of the Collège de Rosemont, where training is under the auspices of the Ministry of Education of Quebec. He is coauthor with M. Sca di Villadorata of 'Acupuncture en Médecine Clinique' published in 1989 by Maloine-Décarie in Paris and Montreal.

Out of my head and into my heart

Leon Hammer INDIAN LAKE, NY, USA

Developing a liking for each other

Dr Z is a 40-year-old prematurely balding married professional and father of three children. He is 1.8 m in height, weighs 72 kg (158 lbs) and stands erect with an obviously lithe and well muscled body. His affect seemed somewhat flat and his voice lacked modulation. However, his manner was soft and friendly and we developed a liking for each other at first contact.

Physical complaints

His presenting complaint was persistent severe and debilitating upper respiratory infections along with severe and increasing fatigue. These had followed a sudden attack of meningitis one and a half years earlier when he had been caring for his wife and children who were suffering from 'flu at the time. At our first meeting he was wheezing and coughing with heaviness in the chest, achey 'flu symptoms and pain in his right flank at GB25 *jingmen*.

Since the attack of meningitis he had experienced great weakness and fatigue, repeated upper respiratory infections with headaches, weakness of his lower back, deep chills in the spine accompanied by numbness, vertigo of the 'spinning room' variety with mild nausea when overworked or lacking sufficient sleep.

In addition he had had intermittent diarrhoea one to four times a week, four or five times a day, which was loose and watery to muddy with tenesmus. There was no blood or mucus and no burning sensation. There was little pain and it was explosive only four times a year. Dr Z was most comfortable in the morning and the diarrhoea increased as the day progressed. It occurred most often with meals and especially when drinking coffee, working hard, overtired or under emotional stress. Having discovered a lactose intolerance, flatulence and burping had been reduced by eliminating milk products.

Emotional complaints

A source of extreme stress had been a vicious and financially draining divorce and a long-term and equally savage struggle for custody of a teenage son from his first marriage. His son became alienated after he had been found sexually abusing Dr Z's 6-year-old son from his second marriage. Just prior to the attack of meningitis the entire situation involving his ex-wife and son had reached fever pitch. Also, at the time of our initial contact his current wife was having an affair with another man and was seriously considering leaving the patient.

Dr Z was emotionally detached, constantly working or engaged in intellectual pursuits and striving forward with no ability to retreat. At the same time he dissipated his creative energies, giving away his ideas and assuming professional responsibilities with little recompense except momentary acceptance. I could see from the beginning that this pattern of bargaining his rich inventive mind for 'love' left him feeling unfocused, unsatisfied, unaccomplished, unappreciated and very angry.

In his work he was considered very competent, imaginative, compassionate and nurturing. He was held in high regard by his colleagues, especially for his broad scholarship, his originality and for his communication skills. In his life however, there was little room for joy, pleasure and relaxation. He was always on guard and seemed more at home with struggle and psychic agony: 'I never stop fighting. I am stubborn and will wear myself down.'.

In his personal life there was little fire, ardour and passion on a heart level so that his wife experienced him as emotionally impassive except for a strong but affectionless sexual drive. For this reason, she was having an affair and was seriously contemplating separation and divorce.

It was my initial impression that Dr Z was committed to change and that we could develop a working relationship.

Physical symptoms, signs, medical history

PHYSICAL SYMPTOMS

- Severe and increasing fatigue which came suddenly 1½ years ago after an episode of meningitis.
- Persistent severe and debilitating upper respiratory infections.
- Wheezing and coughing with heaviness in the chest with achey 'flu symptoms.
- Pain in his right flank at GB25 *jingmen*.
- Weakness of his lower back.
- Deep chills in the spine accompanied by numbness, cold extremities.
- Vertigo of the 'spinning room' variety with mild nausea.
- Intermittent diarrhoea one to four times a week, four or five times a day, which is loose and watery to muddy with tenesmus.
- Thirst unrelieved by fluid intake.
- Mucosal ulcers in the mouth.
- Sensitivity to light.
- Headaches, stiff neck.
- Aching knees especially at night.
- Easily startled, restless sleep and fear of dying.

- Profound sense of emptiness and lightness and lack of clarity in his head.

SIGNS

- Pulse: Rate 96 beats per minute, changing at rest; mild cotton; generally tense to tight; deep.

Left distal position, very feeble-flat;

Right distal position, vibration;

Left middle position, tight to wiry;

Right middle position, tense;

Left proximal position, deeper, feeble-tight, Large Intestine tense;

Right proximal position, deep and tight;

Special Lung position tense, slippery, vibration.

- Tongue: wide; moderate yellow patchy coat; centre cracks; dry centre and wet on sides; centre shows some bright red colour; tremor; teeth marks; mucous threads.
- Colour: His deeper face colour was yellow especially on the sides and red superficially.
- Physiognomy: Wood and Metal body type (Shen J, personal communication, 1980)

- Eyes: Slightly injected,[1] some confluence under eyelids and blue colour shining through.
- Structural: Long-leg syndrome with right longer than the left.
- Abdomen: Costal angle below average; skin turgidity normal; overall muscular tension normal; considerable chest distress; sub-cardiac tenderness; tenderness to the right of the umbilicus; flaccid lower abdomen; upper burner cooler than middle or lower burner.

MEDICAL HISTORY

Recurring tonsillitis and upper respiratory infections; allergy to wool, and to bee stings; multiple ongoing tooth cavities and root canals; always had difficulty keeping warm; pneumonia with frequent chest colds and bronchitis; at college had severe mononucleosis; non-familial premature baldness; two episodes of 'brutal pain' with kidney infection during emotional stress 2 years ago; vasectomy.

Patterns of disharmony

Kidney *qi* and *yang* deficiency

- Ear, nose, throat, allergy and lung problems, catches cold easily since childhood; difficulty recovering from an upper respiratory infection now.
- Multiple cavities, root canals, since childhood.
- Very early baldness.
- Diarrhoea loose and watery.
- Craves warm drinks.
- Deep cold in the spine, increasing cold extremities.
- Fingers crack in cold weather.
- Knee pain, especially at night.
- Pulse: Left proximal position deep, feeble-tight; right proximal position deep, tight.

- Tongue: wide, wet except centre.
- Abdomen: flaccid lower abdomen; sub-costal angle below average; tenderness right of umbilicus.

Nervous System Tense[2]

- Hammer (1990) and Liver *qi* stagnation; Liver *yin* deficiency
- Difficulty retreating.
- Impotent rage.
- Stress, leading to diarrhoea with tenesmus.
- Dry mouth not relieved by fluid.
- Cold extremities.
- Tight muscles and nerves.
- Constantly on guard, 'always ready for emergencies'.

- Pulse: uniformly tense-tight, left middle position wiry.
- Tongue: bright red shining through, thin yellow coating.
- Eyes: confluence under eyelids, blue colour shining through sclera.
- Sound: lack of a shouting quality in voice.

Heart and Lung *qi* deficiency and Heart 'Nervous'[3]

- Susceptibility to colds.
- Circulation: fingers crack, cold in extremities.
- Biorhythm Fire type, most wide awake at night, least perspicacious in morning.
- Insomnia, restless at night and early morning awakening.
- Sadness and coldness in intimate relations.
- Pulse: feeble-flat in both the distal positions, especially the left; vibration in right distal position; rapid rate, changing at rest.
- Abdomen: cool in upper burner; subcardiac tenderness.
- Appearance: flat affect.
- Voice: lacks modulation.

Lung Damp-cold and Damp-heat

- History of recurrent pneumonia and bronchitis.
- Wheezing and coughing with heaviness in the chest.
- Pulse: right distal position, vibration; special Lung position, tense, slippery and vibration.

- Tongue: mucous threads.
- Abdomen: cool upper burner.

Spleen *qi* and *yang* deficiency

- Increasing fatigue.
- Cold diarrhoea worse as day progresses, occurs frequently with eating.
- Lactose intolerance.
- Flatulence, burping.
- Tongue: wide; teeth marks; wet on sides.
- Face colour: deep yellow colour on sides.

Stomach Heat

- Mucosal ulcers in the mouth.
- Burping.
- Intermittent sub-cardiac pain.
- Pulse: right middle position tense.
- Tongue: cracks.

Excess Cold in Channels

- Extremities increasingly cold.
- Cracking fingers in cold winter weather.
- Examination: *gwa sa* and cups positive for Cold in muscles (Shen J, personal communication, 1975).

Note: There is also a generalised *qi* deficiency which must be mentioned because it is central to the treatment in restoring the True *qi (zhen qi)* which is the sum of all the specific organ deficiencies.

Aetiology

Constitutional

- Kidney *qi* deficiency.
- 'Nervous system tense'.

Childhood

- Stress and violence in childhood from father.
- Emotional rejection by mother and lack of warmth.

- Loss of nurturing grandmother.
- Exposure to cold without adequate protection.
- Poor eating habits.

Adulthood

- Stress: divorce and custody; older child sexually abuses younger child from second marriage; infidelity of

both first and second wives; serious financial difficulties.
- Professional frustration: no publication of book, scattering of creative energies, lack of appreciation.

- Inability to retreat.
- Denial of own need for nurture and excessive energy drain caring for others.
- Very poor eating habits.

Life issues

Water phase

Kidney *qi* deficiency involves a lack of faith (Hammer 1990). Faith was indeed missing from Dr Z's life and he constantly sought to compensate for this. This lack of faith, reinforced by life experience, evolved into a deep vulnerability to being forsaken with no faith in his ability to survive rejection. Courage in the human situation is largely based on faith. His response to terror was to cry and fall to pieces. He managed fear by avoiding joy, which would expose him to hurt, and thereby, as we shall see, he inadvertently engineered the rejection he dreaded by killing the joy in others. This Kidney *qi* deficiency and its concomitant lack of faith further deprived Liver *yin* energies, giving him no sense of safety in retreat, and requiring him to always move forward without rest.

Earth phase

The critical life deficiency was Earth energy. Dr Z's underlying need and desire was to be taken care of, just as he cared for others. This he did beyond his energy and beyond all reasonable requirement, except for his own need to feel important. However, being aware of and acceding to this need was the greatest threat to his survival since the original Earth mothering condition was so hostile and full of rejection. Without substantive Earth energies there is no secure sense that 'I am', that I have a right to be here, a birthright from mother earth. One is never at rest on the planet. Dr Z's fear of acceding to the need to be nurtured reinforced the Liver *yin* deficient condition of not being able to withdraw and retreat. This, in turn deprived Dr Z of the refuge and recovery which was also necessary for the restoration of the Earth energies. The single-minded drive to build a career dampened the immediate world of family and friends. Using the concept of chakras, his heart chakra was closed, disconnecting his head from his root chakra, so that his sexual drive was dominated by power and ego considerations rather than love.

Wood phase

A function of Liver *yin* is to allow people to retreat (Hammer 1990). These energies were suppressed to obviate surrendering to his needs for a mother. Retreating, or as he experienced it, collapsing into the dangerous world of his need for nurture, was unthinkable. The idea of not pushing forward constantly filled him with terror. With Liver *yin* and the ability to retreat neutralised, Liver *yang* was uninhibited, advancing constantly, substituting the love he wanted with control and power: 'I never stop fighting. I am stubborn and will wear myself down.' (Hammer 1990, p. 160). Other important contributors to Liver *qi* stagnation were his suppression and denial of his rage at being denied and also his denial of his need for nurture and fulfilment.

Fire phase

Approval of his Heart *yin* creative energy (Hammer 1990, p. 174) was increasingly the medium of exchange for nurture. Approval as a substitute for the basic substance provided by Earth energies was sought ceaselessly. The insecurity associated with its pursuit was endlessly enervating. Pericardium *yang* energies are 'concerned with strongly and accurately reaching the correct mark with intense, focused communication' (Hammer 1990, p. 212). He will serve himself without hurting others. Pericardium *yin* and *yang* energies did not develop to direct Dr Z's Heart and creative energies towards love and fulfilment. Instead there was a scattering of his creative Heart *yin* energies, which he bartered for the love and approval he wanted and needed (Fig. 23.1). Due to this need for acceptance, to be useful and to avoid isolation, these creative Fire energies were drained by the Earth to feed others as a medium of exchange without a central focus. His bargaining with life left him frustrated, with a smouldering impotent rage. Some of the lack of ardour and commitment exhibited by the women in his life had to be attributed to the sad truth that the heat of his internal creative process had not manifested itself in relationships as joy and passion, only as sexual drive or intellectual brilliance. His affect was flat.

Treatment issues

For the purposes of discussion, the management of the 'physical body' and the 'psychological body' will be discussed separately. This is done with the understanding that, physiologically, this separation is artificial and that the treatment process is the art of delicately intertwining the two which are in reality only one. Included in this section is only a sampling of the therapeutic strategies and interventions administered over a period of 4 years.

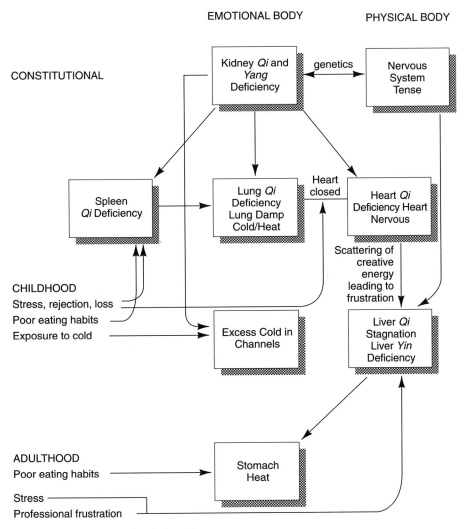

EMOTIONAL BODY   PHYSICAL BODY

CONSTITUTIONAL

Kidney *Qi* and *Yang* Deficiency — genetics → Nervous System Tense

Spleen *Qi* Deficiency

Lung *Qi* Deficiency Lung Damp Cold/Heat

Heart closed

Heart *Qi* Deficiency Heart Nervous

Scattering of creative energy leading to frustration

CHILDHOOD

Stress, rejection, loss
Poor eating habits
Exposure to cold

Excess Cold in Channels

Liver *Qi* Stagnation Liver *Yin* Deficiency

ADULTHOOD

Poor eating habits

Stress
Professional frustration

Stomach Heat

Fig. 23.1 Aetiology and pathology diagram.

It is my policy to adjust structure — the long-leg syndrome (Ewart 1972) — before I attempt other treatment unless there are more pressing immediate considerations. When structure is not corrected other interventions tend to be less effective.

However, because of Dr Z's extremely weak state, this was first postponed in favour of treating his acute external pathogenic factor and profound depletion. In the beginning more gentle magnets were often used instead of needles or moxa. The structural adjustment was made after 2 months.

Our initial thrust, achieved within 1 month, was to eliminate Damp Heat and Damp Cold from the Lungs and excess Cold from the channels, muscles, ligaments and tendons. The reason for this course of action was to eliminate the excess stagnations which were immediately involved with the acute illnesses which were draining his already deficient *qi*.

Early treatment

Gua Sha and Cups

The patient was too weak for needles or moxa at first. *Gua Sha* takes the Cold from the muscles and the cups remove it from the Blood and muscles. Used on BL12 *fengmen*, BL13 *feishu* and BL17 *geshu*, they will remove Damp Cold stagnation from the Lungs.

Acupuncture

Points used in the first few treatments included:

LU1 *zhongfu* 'Middle Palace': this is the alarm point of the Lung and overcomes stagnation in the Lungs and chest and stops the Spleen sending Damp to the Lung. It clears Heat from the upper burner. With moxa it tonifies Lung *qi*. Psychologically it welcomes the individual home, providing him with a sense of himself, making him more receptive to praise and allowing him to be pleased with himself. Its name, 'Middle Palace', implies that this point is central to the spirit, which it centres and helps a lost person find their way.

LU5 *chize* 'Cubit Marsh' expands and relaxes the chest, clears Heat, and because it is the *he* sea water point it also clears Damp in the Lungs.

LU11 *shaoshang* in combination with LI1 *shangyang* has a remarkable effect on clearing the Lung of Damp Heat. On a psychological level, LI1 *shangyang* will soften a person wearing a hard cold mask and will help them to be less obdurate and withdrawn and to communicate with others.

LI4 *hegu* 'Adjoining Valleys' alleviates exterior pathogenic conditions, especially in the Lungs, relaxes the sinews, calms and relieves tension and cleanses the body and mind of all kinds of toxicity.

REN17 *shanzhong* 'Chest Centre' regulates Lung and chest *qi*, directing rebellious *qi* downwards and is a powerful psychological point for abreactions of pent-up emotion.

Moxa on BL12 *fengmen*, BL13 *feishu*, BL17 *geshu*, BL23 *shenshu*, BL43 *gaohuangshu* is used to strengthen the protective and nourishing *qi*. Most other early to middle stage treatments centred on restoring the Kidney (and central nervous system essence), Spleen, Lung and Heart *qi* primarily with moxa.

Psychological strategies to restore *qi*

Earth and Fire strategy

We needed to help Dr Z feel safe enough to experience and gratify his infantile and adult needs for nourishment, to feel protected and to be aware of how he was selectively denying the love which others offered him. His austere quest for power created a cold ambience which was chilling the passions of others. All his Fire had gone into Liver *yang* rather than into his Heart and Pericardium *yang* and this made it more difficult for him to retreat. Restoring the Pericardium by moving his Earth energies into the Fire element, instead of having both dissipated outward, provided these protective and directive energies with the strength to make him feel safer. We were, and still are, trying to move him out of his mind and head and into his heart and gut.

Wood strategy

We wanted to support Wood with points that free and balance the Wood energies, to build the Liver *yin* so that he could retreat, and relax the Liver *yang* so that he could stop driving forward. In this way he would conserve energy for creativity and self-nourishment which he experienced when he was creative for himself.

Water strategy

The most fundamental need, at the level of the root *ben*, was to support Kidney *qi*, Essence, *yin* and *yang* for the basic fabric and foundation, and to feed the overworked Liver *yin*, as well as to give him courage to accept his infantile and adult needs for nourishment. This support also helped to restore the central nervous system which had been vulnerable due to Kidney deficiency and meningitis damage. It also helped him revitalise his mental power to focus and create.

A dragon in my heart

Dr Z was completely informed about both the diagnosis and the treatment plan and he reacted with a sense of relief that someone had listened to him and understood what he intuitively knew. Throughout our contact we established a good working relationship with a free exchange of thoughts and feelings. Dr Z tended to experience me as a 'wise elder' which I gently discouraged, taking it as a mistaken displacement of his own authority.

Lifestyle issues involved diet. More important, however, was the necessity for Dr Z to retreat from the many activities which consumed his time and energy and scattered his resources without compensation or satisfaction, except for passing gratitude. Basically he was being innocently exploited by his colleagues for whom he squandered his creative energies.

From the very beginning he began to change this pattern, to let go of dissipating responsibilities, leading to highly productive writing including a major book. 'There is a dragon in my heart waiting to be released, roaring that it wants out' and 'I am screaming to be heard'. Gradually, and clearly related to the acupuncture treatments and our discussions, his attention began also to shift to his wife and family.

Another change which he has continued faithfully is to take a long nap, for at least 1 hour, once a day. The recommendation to cut back on sexual activity has been followed less rigidly. He has consistently practised *qi gong*. He neither drinks alcohol, coffee or uses any other chemical substance. Exercise is kept in moderation.

Through acupuncture he has himself become more aware of his energy and is more able to regulate his own activity. Work load has decreased commensurate with his capacity. He has also followed the recommendation to decrease his use of sweat lodges to prevent the loss of *qi* that accompanies the excessive perspiration. His compliance with taking the herbs and treating himself at home with moxa in prescribed places, such as DU20 *baihui* and knee points, has been outstanding.

Managing middle and late stages of treatment

The emphasis shifted to restoring the True *qi (zhen qi)*. A great energy drain that needed to be controlled was the diarrhoea caused primarily by Spleen and Kidney *qi* deficiency and to a lesser degree by Liver *qi* stagnation. The diarrhoea, which was sometimes hard at first, then loose, continued to be a problem on and off during the course of treatment. Although Dr Z was willing to make many adjustments to his lifestyle, he was unable to consistently alter his diet due to the food preferences of his family. Only when his wife was convinced that she should institute these changes did this problem significantly but not completely resolve itself.

Likewise it was felt that calming the 'Heart Nervous' condition and Liver *qi* stagnation and *yin* deficient condition was essential to calm his 'Nervous System', improve his sleep, and close off these energy drains.

Some middle and late treatment strategies

Outer Associated Effect Points

These points address emotional and spiritual issues (Larre et al 1986). For example, to open his closed Heart, I first needled BL43 *gaohuangshu* and then warmed the point with moxa. To help him retreat and deal with rage and frustration, BL47 *hunmen* was needled. I used BL52 *zhishi* to restore his faith and will and to help him accept his destiny (Jarrett 1992).

Entry-Exit Points

For example, the triple burner concerns harmony especially in interpersonal relations and the Gall Bladder is the Yang aspect of Wood which is concerned with feelings, especially anger. The entry-exit combination SJ23 *sizhukong* and GB1 *tongziliao* is an 'experience' combination which opens the harmony-enhancing energies to the stuck moving energies and reduces anger and irritability (Zerinsky S, personal communication, 1983).

Windows of the Sky

These points awaken higher consciousness and the spiritual body. They help to unite the body and spirit by penetrating the ego-dominated emotional body. For example, I use SJ16 *tianyou* 'Heaven's Window' to bring warmth for those lacking in warmth, for confused vision and for anger, fear and depression (Zerinsky 1983).

Husband-Wife Imbalance

This combination was used because of his difficulty with intimate interpersonal relationships, especially in marriage. One strategy is to stimulate the Fire Horary points on the right side, SJ6 *zhigou* and P8 *laogong*, to move the Fire to the left side. Another is to use BL67 *zhiyin* and KID7 *fuliu* to move Metal to Water which was not happening for him because he was overextended in everyday activities.

Qi Gong

Kidney *qi* and *yang* are extremely difficult to nourish with acupuncture and herbs. Experience has shown that *qi gong* exercises taught by a true master are the single most effective method for enhancing Kidney *qi* and *jing*.

Herbal Remedies

Dr Z was so extraordinarily depleted that herbs were an essential aspect of his therapy since they were a daily source of nourishment. For example, I used the gentle formula Bupleurum, Cinnamon Twig and Ginger Decoction *chai hu gui zhi gan jiang tang* (Bensky & Barolet 1990) to calm the Heart, preserve *yin*, move Liver *qi*, strengthen the Spleen and build *yang*. It warms the interior and relieves thirst and dryness. A variety of herbal formulae were used throughout this period of his treatment.

Taking back control

There has been steady improvement in all areas over the past 4 years, physical and emotional. Dr Z has had fewer and fewer respiratory problems even when exposed within the family, with quick recovery, and he has had no recurrence of the central nervous system disease of meningitis.

His energy has steadily improved. He has no headaches, no weakness of his lower back, no deep chills or numbness in the spine, no vertigo, infrequent diarrhoea, no oral mucosal ulcerations, no thirst, no sensitivity to light or stiff neck, no being startled during sleep, no nightmares or dreams of abandonment, no cold extremities and no pain in his right flank.

He is no longer emotionally detached, constantly working or engaged only in intellectual pursuits, and is relieved to be able to retreat. As indicated above, he has ceased to dissipate his creative energies and is focused and productive in the areas of his personal interest. In his words, 'I am taking back control of my life and feel stronger and less like a victim', and 'I am giving up misery as a source of self-love'.

He is no longer always on guard or preoccupied with struggle. He experiences joy, pleasure and relaxation — especially in his marriage which is growing in strength, and with his children. His relationship with his wife has shifted from that of a detached father figure to one in which there is an equal give and take of nurture and support. In his words, 'I am turning my fire towards my wife and accepting nurture'.

Surrendering to his need for nurture was an important issue associated with deep primitive terror. He stated that he 'could not contain, hold or carry love', and had to give away more than he could receive. His outbursts of rage are no longer an issue. He is content being who he is and no longer feels driven, especially for recognition.

A war club in my gut

As we worked Dr Z revealed a great tension in his abdomen and pelvis. The tension in his abdomen he related to anger which 'I hold in my digestive system, like a war club in my gut'. After 3 years the tension in his abdomen suddenly relaxed. About 1 year later (i.e. recently) the tension in his pelvis, related to power issues, also relaxed dramatically. Concomitantly his preoccupation with sex changed to affection and tenderness towards his wife who in turn became more interested in sex. During this same period his ongoing panic about finances and success came to a head and then abated.

During the acupuncture treatment Dr Z experienced a great deal of meaningful imagery from which I report one episode. During a treatment he said that he felt himself 'flying, looking down on life, that everything down there is okay, that the earth is so good and beautiful, and that I am so sombre ('all work and no play') while there is so much to enjoy, so much fun in life'. He felt himself being pulled increasingly into his body and being pulled to accept love rather than be a victim.

Mental tiredness and the fear of abandonment were persistent issues for about 1 or 2 years, getting better and worse before experiencing more permanent improvement. There is still some sense of the light-headedness, rare diarrhoea and occasional restless sleep and knee pain about twice a month. As his energy has gradually improved there has always been the tendency to scatter his resources and become too involved in too many projects. Though better regulated, this aspect of his physio-psychology is still a therapeutic issue.

He panicked during the first few occasions that he developed respiratory symptoms, but he has gradually come to put these in perspective. His confidence in his physical and mental health has steadily improved. To summarise, he has gradually felt safe and strong enough to come 'out of my head and into my heart and gut'.

Summary of outcome

Steady and even dramatic improvement in all areas.

- Rare respiratory problems with quick recovery.
- No recurrence of central nervous system disease (meningitis).
- Steady improvement of energy levels.
- No headaches; no weakness and pain of lower back; no deep chills or numbness in spine; no vertigo; infrequent diarrhoea; no oral mucosal ulcerations; no thirst; no sensitivity to light or stiff neck; not startled during sleep, no nightmares or dreams of abandonment; no cold extremities, no pain in his right flank.
- No emotional detachment.
- Ability to retreat.
- Ceased to dissipate creative energies; focused and productive in areas of personal interest.
- Taking control of life; stronger, less a victim.
- 'Giving up misery as a source of self-love'.
- No longer continuously on guard or preoccupied with struggle; experiences joy, pleasure and relaxation — especially in his marriage and with his children.
- Relationship with wife shifts from detached father figure to equal give and take of nurture and support.
- No outbursts of rage; content being who he is, also less driven, especially for recognition.
- Tension in abdomen related to anger, in pelvis to power — both gone; concomitantly preoccupation with sex changes to affection and tenderness towards wife.
- Ongoing panic about finances and success peaks and abates; less sombre, more fun and pleasure.
- Mental tiredness and fear of abandonment better and worse before more permanent improvement.
- Some light-headedness, rare diarrhoea and occasional restless sleep and knee pain twice monthly.
- Safe and strong enough to come out of mind-head into heart-gut.

Limitations and changes

I found working with Dr Z to fit in with my experience of working with other relatively young people with severe chronic disease. This phenomenon has increased greatly during my years of practice.

While I feel both diagnosis and management are relatively sound in this case, the necessary slowness with which a person with severe constitutional Kidney deficiencies is able to respond, and the limits in the degree of recovery with which one is faced, does foster frustration. This emphasises the necessity for changes in lifestyle. Also, it explains the dissatisfaction one feels with even the most intelligent Westerner in understanding the need for limitations and changes.

While Dr Z did a great deal to make necessary changes and observe limitations, certain aspects of his behaviour (e.g. on vacation when all rules were suspended) made me question his real grasp of the issues. While Dr Z's ability to recover from relapses has improved considerably, it is painful to see good hard work being dissipated by a few days of indiscretion, in which the extraordinarily deficient person does not have the luxury to indulge.

NOTES

1 'Injected' is a medical term meaning many engorged red blood vessels on the sclera.

2 See Hammer (1990).

3 Shen J. Personal Communication, 1980.

REFERENCES

Bensky D, Barolet R 1990 Chinese herbal medicine, formulae and strategies. Eastland Press, Seattle
Ewart C 1972 The healing needles, the story of acupuncture and its pioneer practitioner Dr Louis Moss. Elm Tree books, London
Hammer L 1990 Dragon rises, red bird flies. Station Hill Press, Barrytown
Jarrett L S 1992 The role of human will (zhi) and the spirit of BL52. American Journal of Acupuncture 20(4): 349–359
Larre C, Schatz J, Rochat de la Vallée 1986 Survey of traditional Chinese medicine. Traditional Acupuncture Institute, Maryland

■ Leon I Hammer MD

Leon Hammer MD is a graduate of Cornell University, Cornell Medical College and the William A White Institute of Psychoanalysis and Psychiatry. Until 1971, he practised psychiatry and psychoanalysis, directed a child guidance clinic and drug abuse councils on the south-east shore of Long Island, taught at Adelphi University and was Psychiatric Consultant and Associate Professor at Southampton, New York.

After working with Fritz Perls and Alexander Lowen over a period of 8 years, he began a study of Chinese medicine in England during 1971–1974. Since then, he has followed a Chinese master, Dr John Shen, in New York City. In 1981, he spent 4 months studying Chinese medicine in Beijing, China. He has practised Chinese medicine from 1973–1989 in East Hampton and Saratoga Springs, New York. Currently, he teaches workshops in various aspects of Chinese medicine in the United States, Europe and Australia. He is author both of 'Dragon rises, red bird flies', a study of the relationship of Chinese medicine and Western psychology, and 'Contemporary Chinese pulse diagnosis'.

Like mother, like daughter

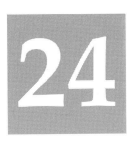

Yves Requena AIX EN PROVENCE, FRANCE

I am presenting a case study of a 49-year-old woman. I have chosen it for a specific reason: to demonstrate that acupuncture and energetic medicine can have an effect on the body, even in a genetically inherited condition. I do hope that the reader is not expecting some extraordinary exposition of traditional Chinese medicine.

Hereditary anaemia

Christine came to me suffering from palpitations and fatigue. The woman sitting in front of me was weary and exhausted, but not disheartened, and she seemed enterprising and dynamic. She was very attractive with auburn hair and green eyes. She had an aquiline face with eyebrows that arched up and a nose like a beak. This was a person who knew what she wanted but, paradoxically, she also seemed to have a shy and fearful aspect to her personality.

She had brought a concrete diagnosis with her in the form of a blood test, so my investigation was not going to be very difficult. She was suffering from chronic anaemia: when she had seen a cardiologist for her palpitations, the results of her blood tests and her fatigue had led him to suggest a blood transfusion. However, she had decided to come for acupuncture instead.

Before looking at the case from a traditional Chinese medical perspective, I would like the reader to attempt a diagnosis.[1]

Christine had an hereditary anaemia known as thalassaemia, a disease endemic to the areas bordering the Mediterranean Basin (Weatherall & Clegg 1972). It can be either homozygotic or heterozygotic. In the latter case the anaemia is moderate and it was this kind of thalassaemia that Christine had. The red blood cells vary in size or are smaller than average, leading to a defective rate of production or syntheses of the globin chain which then recurs in the composition of the haemoglobin. This decrease in production is caused by a genetic defect in the chromosomes.

Would I be able to influence this process with acupuncture?

Some contradictions

Let us return to Christine. I asked her about her fatigue. In my mind, it had to be linked to the anaemia and to the reduction of red blood cells. I was interested to find out when the Heart Blood condition that I suspected had worsened.

Christine explained:

I have to admit I tend to overexert myself. I'm doing a course in psychology. I like dancing and I go rock climbing. There's also some stress, some emotional overload. I've just started living with my partner. It's the first time in several years that I've lived with a man and I must say it's taken a lot of energy getting used to it.

In addition to her fatigue she was troubled by palpitations which would occur at various times during the day. As for other symptoms there was nothing significant except a loss of memory, which fitted in with the suspected pattern of disharmony. Also, Christine was under the care of an endocrinologist for mastitis in both breasts. Furthermore, she was slightly diabetic with a blood sugar level of 1.24 grams/litre.

The more I talked to Christine the more I became aware of the contradictions in her case: she complained of fatigue, but she was very dynamic, wilful and firm and so her exhaustion was only evident because she mentioned it.

Her complexion was pale, but only slightly. Her tongue was slightly pale with a thin coating. Her pulse was thin, but not excessively so, slightly wiry and quite rapid.

Summary of clinical manifestations

- Palpitations at various times of the day.
- Fatigued, weary, exhausted.
- Loss of memory.
- Slightly pale complexion.
- Pale, yellow, wrinkled hands.
- Mastitis in both breasts.
- Dynamic and active behaviour.
- Tendency to overexertion.
- Aquiline face.
- Sentimental behaviour.
- Shy and fearful aspect to her personality.
- Little fingers hooked.
- Hands supple and agile, small but well proportioned, gnarled and furrowed.
- Pulse: thin but not excessively so, slightly wiry and quite rapid.
- Tongue: slightly pale, thin coating

Patterns of disharmony

Heart Blood deficiency

- Palpitations.
- Fatigue, weariness, exhaustion.
- Loss of memory.
- Slightly pale complexion.
- Pale, yellow, wrinkled hands.
- Tongue: slightly pale.
- Pulse: thin but not excessively so.

Ascendant Liver *yang*

- Mastitis in both breasts.
- Dynamic and active behaviour.
- Tendency to overexertion.
- Pulse: slightly wiry.

Evaluating the terrain

I decided to make an evaluation of the terrain according to my theory of the Five Constitutions (Requena 1986a, Requena 1989).

Christine's aquiline face corresponded to Fire. I examined her hand. It was small but well proportioned, gnarled and furrowed, typical of a Wood constitution. Her little fingers were hooked however, and her hands were very supple and agile, which were to me also indications of a Fire constitution. From that moment on the terrain was obvious. As in most cases she had a double constitution: *yang* Wood and *yin* Fire.

The skin of her hands was pale, yellow and wrinkled, indicating Blood deficiency (Requena 1986b). She mentioned that these were always warning signs that she should be watching her health.

From these constitutions come the temperaments. I considered Christine to be *shao yang* and *shao yin*, that is to say Choleric and Sentimental.

A Choleric personality

To summarise the Choleric-Enthusiasts:

1 They want to be at the head of any group, because they don't like to go unnoticed. Autocratic but not coercive, they take the role of leader to get themselves noticed or simply because they are impetuous and cannot keep themselves back.
2 They are affable, ebullient, and the life and soul of the party. They can also be quick tempered.
3 They are very optimistic but also anxious. They are always in a hurry for fear of being late. They are impulsive and come to decisions quickly, which they then carry out quickly and vigorously.
4 They often take on too many things, and could be reproached for not always completing what they start.

A Sentimental personality

Fire Sentimental types can be summarised as follows:

1 They are very emotional, but internalised, introverted and hypersensitive. They do not take mishaps in their stride and dwell on them more than others; they are inclined to be pessimistic and defeatist.

2 They tend to worry about other people and themselves and are thin-skinned and susceptible to rapid mood swings.

3 They are idealists and dreamers who never renounce what they believe to be true or good. They are capable of waiting for years to get what they want. They are admirable but modest.

Evaluation of the terrain

Shao yin **Sentimental type**

- Aquiline face.
- Little fingers hooked.
- Hands supple and agile.
- Sentimental behaviour.
- Shy and fearful.

Shao yang **Choleric-Enthusiast**

- Hands small but well proportioned, gnarled and furrowed.
- Dynamic personality.
- Tendency to overexertion.

Double diagnosis, double terrain

Thus, to conclude, we have a complex picture of ascendant Liver *yang* with a primary fullness of the Gall Bladder channel, combined with a deficiency of Heart Blood. This explains the patient's dynamism and active behaviour despite the anaemia. It also explains the presence of the mastitis (fullness of the Liver/Gall Bladder).

Now that I had this double diagnosis and double terrain, I was interested to know whether, at the constitutional level, weaknesses in the Wood and Fire constitutions had manifested as early as childhood. I found it remarkable that my questioning only uncovered Fire constitution diseases e.g. viral pericarditis and throat infections, as well as diseases relating to the *shao yin* personality (deficiency of the Heart and Kidney *qi*) e.g. rheumatic fever and later, kidney stones. These are classic *shao yin* pathologies (Requena 1986a, Requena 1989).

Two months prior to attending for treatment a blood test had shown the following results:

- White blood cell count (WBC): 4.58 grams/litre (normal 4.00 to 5.70 grams/litre).
- Haemoglobin: 9.6 grams/litre (normal 12 to 16 grams/litre).

- Haematocrite: 29.5 grams/litre (normal 37 to 53 grams/litre).
- Glucose: 1.24 grams/litre (normal 0.9 to 1.0 grams/litre).

She mentioned that her fatigue had worsened since the first blood test, so it may be assumed that these indices were slightly worse at the time of her acupuncture consultation.

Acupuncture and *qi gong*

'Christine, here's what we're going to do. I want you to come for two sessions of acupuncture per week, and to come to my *qi gong* class once a week.'

For the first four sessions, the same treatment procedures were followed regularly, as described in the treatment procedure box.

Procedures for first treatments

ACUPUNCTURE

To balance the *shao yin*

The three points below belong both to the diagnosis and the strategy. They are used together to balance the *shao yin*:

- BL15 *xinshu* to strengthen Heart Blood and *yang*, used with warming needle.
- KID3 *taixi* to strengthen Kidney *qi* and benefit Essence *jing* and marrow.
- HE5 *tongli*, the *luo* connecting point of the Heart, to tonify the Blood and the *yin*, to help support the *shen* for her loss of memory, and to promote the flow of Blood back into the Heart organ and brain.

To balance the *shao yang*

The following point is used to balance the *shao yang*:

- LIV3 *taichong* to harmonise and soothe Liver *qi*, and to help with the mastitis.

Needling method: The needles are inserted and stimulated until *de qi* is obtained. On BL15 *xinshu*, I burned a 2 cm segment of moxa stick on the needle in order to tonify the Heart and Blood. The sessions lasted 20 minutes.

QI GONG

At the same time, Christine started to learn *qi gong*. I taught her the Heart sounds *ha* and *khe*, together with a sequence of movements to strengthen the Heart. In internal *qi gong*, I chose *wu dang qi gong* with 'the tiger topples the mountain', which strengthens the Heart.

Something quite strange

After four sessions of acupuncture and three sessions of *qi gong*, Christine told me that she felt less exhausted and that her energy levels were better. She began to talk more about her past and her emotional stress. When her own mother was 7 months pregnant with Christine, her partner, who was probably Christine's father, had thrown her out. Christine never knew her father. She also talked about her first husband, who had died suddenly in a car crash when she was pregnant herself.

She told me something quite strange. Her mother had developed amnesia after her partner had thrown her out. The same thing happened to Christine when she lost her husband, and she suffered from amnesia for some 2 years. She was unable to recall whole sections of her life, and sometimes she couldn't remember her own name, the date, or where she was. The amnesia was intermittent but severe.

This shows how serious the Heart Blood deficiency was becoming, to the point where the *shen* was no longer anchored, thus causing these severe lapses in memory.

For me this was the deciding factor. In the fifth session I decided that, whilst Christine was getting better, I would treat the psychological and emotional aspects of her personality by using the *shen* points of the Heart: BL44 *shentang*, HE5 *tongli* and another point which, for the time being, I will keep secret.[2] These points were used to trigger emotional release.

When I saw Christine again 2 weeks later, which was 5 weeks after she had started treatment, she was completely transformed. She was full of joy and a sense of freedom. Her hands had regained a reddish hue, and had lost their wrinkled appearance.

Here, however, is another characteristic of the *shao yang* Choleric-Enthusiasts: as soon as they get better, they disappear. Christine stopped coming for both acupuncture and *qi gong*. This was because, on my advice, she had taken a second blood test, which corroborated her improvement, even showing that her diabetes had started to improve:

- White blood cell count (WBC): 5.02 grams/litre (normal 4.00 to 5.70 grams/litre).
- Haemoglobin: 10.2 grams/litre (normal 12 to 16 grams/litre).
- Haematocrite: 32.8 grams/litre (normal 37 to 53 grams/litre).
- Glucose: 1.11 grams/litre (normal 0.9 to 1 grams/litre).

Like mother, like daughter

This encouraged me to recommend Christine to continue with regular acupuncture once fortnightly, then once monthly. I also wanted her to carry on with the *qi gong* sessions. Furthermore, I had perfected a prescription of Western herbs for her memory loss, caused by Heart Blood deficiency, which I wanted her to take. This comprised motherwort, elecampane, briarhip, chickweed, and cinchona.

Christine came to see me again 2 months later. I asked her for her permission to write this article. She was very willing and cooperative. She was in good form. Her hands were nicely coloured and she was no longer in the least bit tired.

I then asked her a question: 'Why did you come to see me for acupuncture instead of having a blood transfusion?'.

She replied thus: 'Because 4 years ago you treated my daughter for the same thing.'.

I was suprised to hear that I had treated her daughter! I had not made the connection between Christine and the young patient I remembered treating for thalassaemia 2 years previously.

Christine continued, 'She also suffered from thalassaemia, but her condition was more serious. You managed to get her better. Anyway, she couldn't handle the improvement because, psychologically, it took away her position of being the invalid.'.

'Like mother, like daughter', as we say in French.

Christine did, however, make a contract with me to come for one session of acupuncture per month.

Summary of outcome

- Lots of energy, not in the least tired.
- Full of joy with a sense of freedom.
- Hands had regained a reddish hue and lost their wrinkled appearance.
- Improvements to blood test results.

Concluding remarks

I have chosen to present this case because it is colourful and rich. Above all it illustrates the power of acupuncture, assisted by *qi gong*, to help with a genetic condition where the latitude for recovery is limited. Also, one can see the importance of psychological factors in Christine's past as well as the way in which family history repeats itself. I see this case as an example of the use of the three treatment methods: acupuncture, *qi gong* and psychotherapy. These three methods can work together for results that would otherwise seem impossible.

NOTES

1   See the box entitled Patterns of Disharmony for an answer.

2   This point I am keeping secret in order to protect the future publication of a book.

REFERENCES

Requena Y 1986a Terrains and pathology in acupuncture. Vol 1. Paradigm, Brookline
Requena Y 1986b Morphological hand diagnosis in acupuncture. Solal, Marseille
Requena Y 1989 Character and health. Paradigm, Brookline
Weatherall D J, Clegg J B 1972 The thalassaemia syndromes. Blackwell, Oxford

■ Yves Requena

Yves Requena began his studies of acupuncture with master Nguyen Van Nghi in 1971, in Marseille, during his last 3 years of medical studies. He graduated as a medical doctor and as an acupuncturist. He then spent 2 years travelling to China to improve and develop his knowledge. Since then, during subsequent years of self study, his true masters have been Soulie de Morant and the classics of Chinese medicine, the Nei Jing, the Nan Jing and the Zhen Jiu Da Cheng.

Yves is the author of the three-volumed *Terrains and Pathology in Acupuncture*, in which he develops his unique approach of using constitutions and temperaments in Chinese medicine. He is also known for his book *Character and Health* and for his studies of the energetics of Western herbs. In 1989, he created the European Institute of Qi Gong, the first professional qi gong training school in the West. For more than 15 years, he has spent half his time in his medical clinic in Aix-en-Provence and the other half travelling and teaching worldwide.

Undescended testicles

Julian Scott CAMBRIDGE, UK

I spend a lot of time treating children, perhaps more than most practitioners, so I have chosen a case history of a child. Rather than describe one of the straightforward cases, such as asthma or a digestive disturbance, I am going to write about a young boy whose testicles had not descended. Although this is a less common symptom, it nevertheless illustrates many points about the way acupuncture can help children, and in particular, the way it can affect the parent-child relationship to the benefit of both.

His beauty was striking

The child, let us call him Roy, was 5½ years old when he came to see me. The most striking thing about his appearance was his beauty, and his long, beautifully combed hair. It was not excessively long, and was not an unsuitable cut for a boy, but it attracted my attention. He was also a little pale, and rather dreamy. From his clothes he was obviously a boy, but he was a rather effeminate boy. The mother, who always came with him (I think the father had left a few years earlier), was very open, and also was a gentle person.

I found the mother and child both very likeable. There were no problems over building rapport and trust. This was partly because I already had a reputation for helping children, having successfully treated a number of children from Roy's school, which was a Steiner school. At first I did not realise that Roy attended a Steiner school, although, as I will show later, this did have a bearing on the case.

After the preliminaries were over, the mother explained to me that the doctor had recommended surgery, and that it should not be left for much longer. He was sympathetic to her request to delay surgery and to try alternative means, but he did not want to leave it much longer than another 6 months. This seemed reasonable to me. I felt, and said as much to the mother, that if nothing had happened with 6 months, then she should try something else, probably surgery.

Some surprises

The normal pattern for undescended testicles is Kidney *yang* deficiency, so I was not surprised to find that Roy's tongue was pale and wet. When I took his pulse, I was somewhat surprised to find that, although the overall quality was slightly weak, the balance of the pulse was good. That is to say that there was no noticeable weakness in the third position on either side. Nor was there any disturbance in the Lung pulse. (If the child is reasonably healthy and strong, then one would expect the pulses in the third position on both sides to be weak, and the other ones to be strong. Sometimes one sees an imbalance where the third position is only a little weak, but the Lung pulse is strong and floating.)

I was in for a further surprise upon examination for, from the boy's face, he appeared fairly plump and well-rounded. His body, concealed beneath his nice clothes, was very thin. The back in particular was without muscle from top to bottom. All the bones and ribs could be clearly felt. The main muscles along the Bladder channel felt like tight strings, rather than vibrant muscles, and the lower back was especially weak and tense. The shape of the sacrum and its spinous processes could easily be felt.

The other symptoms were not particularly special. His appetite was not all that good. In particular he had an aversion to green vegetables (a condition that is so common in children that I have come to the conclusion that perhaps green vegetables are bad for children!). His sleep was rather heavy.

Summary of clinical manifestations	
• Undescended testicles.	• Sleep rather heavy.
• Effeminate nature.	• Whole of back thin, with weak muscles.
• Flowing hair.	• Muscles on Bladder channel along the back like tight strings.
• Thin body.	
• Pale, dreamy.	• Tongue: pale and wet.
• Plump, well-rounded face.	• Pulse: overall quality weak.
• Appetite not particularly good.	

Identifying the patterns of disharmony

The very symptom of undescended testicles must be due to Kidney *qi* or Kidney *yang* deficiency, so that any information gleaned by other methods is supplementary. The tongue and pulse certainly supported this diagnosis. And so also did the feeling of the back, although here some comment needs to be made.

In an adult, if the back were thin and wasted, one would think more of Kidney *yin* deficiency. In children it is not quite the same. The strength of a child can often be determined from feeling the back. A strong child will have a firm, muscular back. If there is *yang* deficiency, the back will be weak and floppy, sometimes with excess flab, more often with thin, tight muscles. If there is *yin* deficiency, there is likely to be a hollow feeling in the back, with almost wasting of the muscles.

In a western society, children are rarely *yin* deficient. The traditional cause for *yin* deficiency in children is a long febrile disease. In the West this rarely happens because of the widespread use of antibiotics. There may be many side-effects from this treatment, and it seems likely that eventually bacteria will evolve which are resistant to all antibiotics; but for the present, this particular pattern has been wiped out. This is not to say that *yin* deficiency is unknown, but that it takes quite another form, and comes from another cause — it arises now from overstimulation from such things as TV, computer games, junk food and late nights, and presents as both *yin* and *yang* weakness, often without any trace of heat.

Pattern of disharmony

Kidney *yang* deficiency

- Undescended testicles.
- Pale.
- Back thin and wasted.
- Dreamy look.
- Tongue: pale and wet.
- Pulse: overall quality weak.

Aetiological factors

An imbalance of this kind can be due to constitutional weakness, or due to some problem that has occurred in life. From his face, it appeared that Roy's constitution was quite good. His jaw was quite large, his ears well formed, and his eyes had spirit. It therefore seemed likely that the cause was to do with something in his life. Something was preventing the Kidney energy from developing properly.

It seemed to me that there were three causes contributing to this: his mother's attitude, his father leaving home and his schooling.

I think his mother had really wanted a little girl. She was a very gentle person, and obviously related better to very gentle people. I had the feeling that she was uncomfortable with manifestations of *yang* energy in her child. This showed in little things, such as fidgeting and restlessness when the boy played with the train set, but relaxing more when the child took a book to read. While some practitioners might have communicated this to the mother, perhaps by commenting on the relationship, I tend to avoid saying anything, as I always seem to say the wrong thing, and end up upsetting everybody! Besides, as you will see, one of the wonderful effects of acupuncture is that it helps people to sort out their own relationships to their own satisfaction, which is far better than imposing my 'ideal relationship' upon the family.[1]

I think it likely also that Roy was in a mild state of shock from his father's leaving. It had had the effect of making him retire to a dream world where everything was alright, rather than engaging fully in the real world.

The school that he attended definitely encouraged these tendencies. One of the wonderful features of Steiner schools is that they encourage the development of the gentle, artistic side of children, rather than forcing them into being young adults, and developing their aggression. This produces lovely children, but for this boy, the education was a little overbalanced towards the *yin*.

Lifestyle advice

I advised the mother to give him more *yang* foods. It would have been beneficial for him to eat meat, but (not surprisingly) the mother was vegetarian, and recoiled at the idea of eating meat. In the circumstances, I advised including eggs in the diet, with more protein, especially in the form of tofu.

I was able to explain the perspective of Chinese medicine to Roy's teachers. They were fully immersed in anthroposophical philosophy, which has many similarities with Chinese philosophy. There is the idea of a soul which has to inhabit the body, and if a soul is not 'fully incarnated', then a child could become very dreamy, living partly in 'another world'. This has similarities with the Kidney being 'not firm', and so not providing proper support for the Heart. In consequence the *shen* is not housed securely, and so tends to wander off.

Roy's teachers could thoroughly agree with this picture once it had been brought to their attention. They also agreed with the dietary implications, and encouraged Roy to do more 'grounding' activities such as working with clay, rather than reading. Also they prescribed eurhythmic exercises to encourage full incarnation (these have some similarities with *qi gong* exercises.)

First treatment procedures

The principle of treatment for the first, and subsequent, treatments was to strengthen Kidney *yang*.

POINT PRESCRIPTION

- BL23 *shenshu* and BL32 *ciliao:* These two points were chosen to tonify the Kidney *yang*. They were chosen in preference to points on the front, such as REN4 *guanyuan* because of the overall weakness of the back, and because of the absence of bed-wetting.
- LIV8 *ququan:* This point was chosen because the testicles lie on the Liver channel; also because it strengthens the uro-genital system; being the Water point, it tonifies on the creative *sheng* cycle.
- KID7 *fuliu:* This point was chosen because it strengthens Kidney *yang*.

    The overall balance of the points was towards the lower part of the body, to bring the energy down to the ground.

Needling technique: All the points were needled, one after the other, using the same needle. A 12.5 mm, 34 gauge Japanese needle (with a very fine point) was used. After the arrival of *qi*, the needles were manipulated for 15 to 30 seconds, and then withdrawn. BL23 *shenshu* and BL32 *ciliao* were needled using the tonifying method i.e. small lift and thrust, with virtually no rotation. During needling, I asked the boy what he felt, and he described a warm comfortable sensation. LIV8 *ququan* and KID7 *fuliu* were needled using the moving and tonifying method. That is to say that the needle sensation travelled up the channel some way (moving), but that generally the sensation was pleasant and warm (tonifying).

After needling, moxa was used on the back points with the sparrow pecking method (tonifying).

When treating children, it can be normal for the child's pattern to change from day to day, hour to hour. However, for Roy, the above prescription was used most of the time, with only slight variations, such as adding LI4 *hegu* if he had an attack of pathogenic wind.

Progress, running and tripping out

Treatment generally went very well and Roy was quite positive about it in that he didn't raise any objection and lay down in a docile way. He seemed genuinely to enjoy coming, and certainly had no problem with the needles.

However, there was one strange time in the middle of the course of treatments, when I thought I had lost him. After about ten treatments, which were given weekly, he became much more energetic. So much so that he took up running! At first I took no special notice of this, as I regarded it as a sign of his energy returning. However, as we talked about it, it appeared that he was using his running as a way of 'tripping out'. He would choose times to run when he had had nothing to eat for several hours, for example, just before lunch when he had not had any breakfast or just before supper when he had not had any lunch. He was therefore already somewhat tired. He described to me how he would run and run (in hilly terrain) so that he got quite out of breath. He would feel more and more dreadful, until, after a few minutes, all his discomfort and tiredness disappeared. At this point, he said, he felt as light as air, and could run on and on without effort. (Work on marathon runners has shown that after about 10 miles of running, when a runner has used up all the available sugar in his body, the body then begins to break down its own muscles to provide the energy required. At this point the body also releases opium-like substances into the blood stream. They truly trip out.)

It seemed to me that this was really dangerous. On the physical level Roy was laying himself open to diabetes due to repeated hypoglycaemia, while in the short term, he was completely undoing the effects of treatment.

I explained this to him while his mother was present, making it clear to her that she was wasting her time and money. I also made it clear to Roy that he was likely to make himself very sick, and might end up having to inject himself daily with a massive needle (much larger and more painful than an acupuncture needle!). Fortunately they both heard what I had to say. (This is by no means always the case. If a child has this state of energy imbalance due to a lingering pathogenic factor, as is often the case in Kidney-deficient asthma patients, there can be a huge emotional invest-ment in the *status quo*, so that any attempt to change the way of life can meet with fierce resistance.)

After ten treatments Roy's testicles came down for most of the time. After twenty treatments his testicles were descended for all of the time. By the end of treatment (about 8 months in all, including a few maintenance treatments at 3-weekly intervals), he had gained in physical strength, and was doing better at school. His attitude had completely changed in that he was much more 'with it' and less dreamy. He was also more assertive with his mother.

Summary of outcome

- Testicles descended all the time.
- Gain in physical strength.
- Doing better at school.
- Much more 'with it', less dreamy.
- More assertive with his mother.

Diagnosis or 'gnosis'?

I have chosen this case to talk about not because the symptom is very common, but because it shows in a very simple and straightforward way some of the changes that seem to happen when a child has acupuncture. I feel that it is one of the wonders of Chinese medicine that a 'diagnosis' is really a 'gnosis' about the patient, so that in the one phrase 'Kidney *yang* deficiency' a whole pattern is described which includes favourite colour and food, a way of relating to people, and likely vices and virtues. Simply by treating Kidney *yang*, changes are effected in the whole range of the patient's experience. I would also like to say that in Roy's case conditions were favourable for a cure — his mother was in fact prepared to change, and above all, the school he attended understood the problem. This is, in fact, very rare!

NOTE

1 I suppose that what I tend to do is to just observe what goes on, and let child and mother sort things out for themselves. In the children's clinic at the time of Roy's consultation there was little time for long-winded chats. The only opportunity to talk came when applying moxa to the back *shu* points, when I talked about life in general or how Roy behaved. As you can see from this case study, however, I try to avoid giving advice, as it only seems to produce the wrong effect! Often there is just 5–10 minutes for an appointment on a busy day.

FURTHER READING

Scott J P 1991 Acupuncture in the treatment of children. Eastland Press, Seattle and Journal of Chinese Medicine (revised edition)
Scott J P 1990 Natural medicine for children. Unwin-Hyman
Scott J P, Scott S J 1991 Natural medicine for women, Gaia Books, London

■ Julian Scott

Julian Scott studied acupuncture first at the International College of Oriental Medicine (ICOM) under Dr van Buren, and then in China. Since coming back from China he has learnt enough Chinese to grope his way through the Chinese texts. He has been treating children, using acupuncture, for 18 years, and in 1984 started the Children's Clinic for Natural Therapies in Brighton, where he worked until 1989. This was a low-cost clinic, with special times for the treatment of children using acupuncture, homeopathy, herbs and cranial osteopathy. This was really a learning ground, for many patients consulted, and Julian quickly developed a feeling for what acupuncture could do for children. While at the clinic he was greatly influenced by his receptionist, Kate Diamantopolou, who was also a health visitor and was training in homeopathy at the time. He has also been influenced by the writings of Rudolph Steiner, and Buddhist teachings.

In acknowledgement, he writes: 'I would particularly like to remember my teachers, especially Dr Zhang Cai Yun, who showed me a way of needling which is almost painless. Also the many other people who have helped me in Chinese medicine, and towards an understanding of *qi*'. He treats both adults and children, but especially enjoys the humour and lightness that comes spontaneously when treating children.

A case of a gastric ulcer

Eric Marié VITRE, FRANCE

I have chosen to present this case for two main reasons. Firstly, I wanted to demonstrate that acupuncture can be effective in treating disorders which have been identified by Western medical investigations. Secondly, I wanted to show that acupuncture is not necessarily a slow and gradual therapy, and that it can produce rapid and lasting therapeutic results in serious and chronic pathologies.

Conflicts and stress

Patricia is a 33-year-old woman with a medical training, at present studying and training towards a specialisation. Most of her time and energy is therefore taken up by these studies, which limits her availability to earn a living.

At the time of her first interview she was going through a difficult period in her life, marked by worries and anxiety. She was experiencing delays in selling her apartment in Paris at a time when she needed the money to live on and to finance her studies. Conflicts in her personal life, notably a difficult relationship with another student in her group, and a bilious temperament,[1] together with overwork, some background pain from an old foot injury and various other factors, all contributed to her stress. Although Patricia's stress is well managed socially, it is nevertheless very real in its physiological effects. Patricia doesn't smoke, drinks little, and eats reasonably well without following any particular diet. She no longer exercises regularly and now lives in the country, after having lived in Paris for a long time.

Cramping stomach pains

Patricia's main complaint is cramping stomach pains, which come on suddenly and usually last for about 1 hour. The pains improve if she eats something, but then recur even more violently postprandially. On questioning her about the history of these symptoms, I learned that they first appeared 18 years ago, but in a milder form that quickly improved without treatment. Another attack 7 years later led to medical investigations and a diagnosis of a gastric ulcer. X-rays revealed the area of ulceration to be in the large flexure of the stomach. At that time, she was treated conventionally with Gastrozepin and Maalox for 1 month. The main signs and symptoms disappeared, but these would recur in a milder form from time to time, indicating a persistence of the condition.

During our first consultation, Patricia reported that she recently suffered from indigestion and vomiting after a festive meal, even though she had not overeaten. Since then she has suffered from vomiting whenever she has eaten rich sauces, especially sauces containing fresh cream. The pains have also intensified. Other signs and symptoms are presented below.

Summary of clinical manifestations

- Epigastric pains: severe, cramping, come on suddenly, last for about 1 hour, aggravated by pressure, better on eating but then recur more strongly.
- Vomiting with rich sauces and cream.
- Sleep is fretful, wakes frequently and has agitated dreams, full of confrontations, and worries about daily life.
- Appetite is fairly normal; doesn't have to eat much.
- Acid regurgitation.
- Taste not abnormal, no thirst, no dryness in the mouth.
- Slight tendency to constipation.
- Spasmodic pains in the right hypochondrium occurring with the stomach pains, or when upset during times of stress.
- Dysmenorrhoea.
- Severe PMT with distended and painful breasts.
- Slight nervous tension.
- Slight frontal headaches.
- Abdominal palpation: area around REN12 *zhongwan* very painful with pressure.
- Tongue: swollen, purplish and red at the tip, with a dry yellowish coating over the whole surface.
- Pulse: the right pulse is *xi* (thready), slightly *xian* (wiry) and slightly *hua* (slippery); the left pulse is *xi* (thready), *xian* (wiry), and *hua* (slippery).

Patterns of disharmony

Epigastric pain is classically differentiated into several syndromes: Cold invading the Stomach, Retention of Food, Stomach Fire, Stomach and Spleen *yang* deficiency, Stomach *yin* deficiency, Stasis of Blood in the Stomach and Liver *qi* invading the Stomach.

Cold invading the Stomach cannot be the diagnosis in this case since there is no improvement with heat. Furthermore, the tongue and pulse do not correspond to this syndrome.

Retention of Food cannot be considered as the main syndrome because the pains improve with eating and the condition is chronic and arises in a patient with no tendency to overeating. Furthermore, the nature of the pains and the majority of other signs and symptoms do not point towards this syndrome. However, if we consider the fact that the pains are worse after eating difficult-to-digest meals, then we could say that retention of food is an 'aggravating' or 'peripheral' syndrome in this case.

There are a few signs of Heat in the partially red tongue, the yellowish coating, the *hua* (slippery) pulse, the tendency to constipation and the acid regurgitation, but these are not conclusive as there is no thirst, no burning sensation nor any bitter taste in the mouth. There are also dreams of conflict, and some nervous tension, but no violent anger or significant irritability. I do not therefore consider Stomach Fire as the main syndrome. However, we cannot ignore the tendency to Heat production as a secondary, pathogenic factor, and we should keep this in mind.

The diagnosis of Stomach and Spleen *yang* deficiency is impossible since the pains are severe and are aggravated by pressure. Furthermore, there are no signs of Cold or *yang* deficiency (cold limbs, soft stools or water diarrhoea, fatigue, etc.). The tongue and pulse also do not support this diagnosis.

Stomach *yin* deficiency is not a possible diagnosis either since there is no thirst or dryness of the mouth, no emaciation, no dry stools, nor any general or specific constitutional signs of *yin* deficiency.

Stasis of Blood in the Stomach deserves some consideration because of the reddish purple and swollen tongue. There is often a component of Stasis of Blood in chronic, persistent and severe epigastric pain. However, the pain is neither fixed nor needle-sharp, the pulse is *hua* (slippery) and there are no other signs or symptoms relating to Blood (haemoptysis, black stools, etc.). We can therefore decide that Blood Stasis is not a primary, but a secondary syndrome.

If we take into account Patricia's disposition, with its tendency to nervous tension, irritability and susceptibility to stress (the probable cause of her pathology), together with the presenting signs and symptoms, the diagnosis of Liver *qi* invading the Stomach becomes quite clear. It should be noted that a disharmony between Liver and Stomach is often a complication of a chronic disharmony between the Liver and the Spleen. The evidence for these and the other syndromes is presented below.

Evidence for the patterns of disharmony

Liver *qi* invading the Stomach
- Epigastric pains: cramping, aggravated by pressure, initial improvement with a little food, but recur soon afterwards.
- Spasmodic pains in the right hypochondrium occuring with the stomach pains or at times of stress.
- Acid regurgitation.[2]
- Sleep disturbed by frequent waking,

with agitating and exhausting dreams of conflict concerning problems in daily life.[3]
- Nervous tension.
- Pulse: wiry.

Stasis of Blood in the Stomach

- Epigastric pain is chronic, severe and persistent.
- Tongue: reddish purple.

Stagnation of Food

- Epigastric pain worse after eating rich food and cream.
- Abdominal distension.

Stomach Fire

- Acid regurgitation.
- Tendency to constipation.
- Tongue: partially red, yellowish coating over the whole surface.
- Pulse: slippery.

Imbalance between Liver and Spleen

- Nervous tension.
- Dysmenorrhoea.
- Premenstrual syndrome with distended and painful breasts and water retention.
- Frontal headaches.
- Pulse: *xi* (thready) and *xian* (wiry).

Aetiology and pathology

The cramping pain, which is aggravated by pressure, reflects stagnation of *qi*. The Liver stores the Blood (*gan zang xue*) and stagnation of *qi* in the Liver is often the origin of Liver Blood stagnation, and from there to stagnation of Blood in the Stomach. This tendency is apparent in this case.

Finally, stagnation of food in the Stomach, from the occasional indulgence in an excess of food, increases the stagnation of Liver *qi* by compromising the *shu xie* (the free-flowing functions of the Liver) and the Spleen deficiency, by affecting the *yun hua* (the transporting and transforming functions of the Spleen). This aggravates the disharmony between the Liver and the Spleen, and eventually between the Liver and the Stomach.

To conclude, the main or central syndrome is Liver *qi* invading the Stomach and the main potential complication is Stasis of Blood in the Stomach. Stagnation of Food is a factor which can trigger an attack and Stomach Fire is an associated syndrome. The imbalance between the Liver and the Spleen is the underlying problem which needs to be addressed in the long term (Fig. 26.1).

In terms of the aetiology, there has been a long-term history of stress and conflict in Patricia's life, compounded by difficulties in her relationships. In addition, she is sensitive to her dietary intake and particularly has problems with an excess intake of rich food. It is likely that she is particularly vulnerable when these two factors occur together.

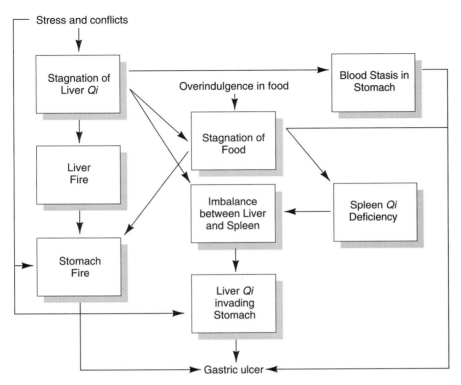

Fig. 26.1   Aetiology and pathology diagram.

Treatment issues

Treatment principles

I decide that I should begin by smoothing and dredging the Liver *qi* (*shu xie gan qi*), harmonising the Liver, Spleen and Stomach (*tiao he gan pi/wei*) and stopping the pain (*zhi tong*). If necessary, I will also allow for clearing Heat (*qing re*), and moving Blood stasis (*huo xue hua yu*).

Presenting the treatment plan

I explain to Patricia how I intend to proceed with the treatment. First address the 'branches' (*biao*), until the acute pains improve, and then harmonise and tonify the 'roots' (*ben*) in order to restore health and prevent relapses. I also explain that, for best results, the treatment sessions should be close together, and that the length of the remission from symptoms will determine the frequency of treatment.

I ask Patricia to keep a diary of her symptoms, and to record all changes in the intensity, frequency or nature of the symptoms. I suggest that she comes to see me every 2–3 days, more frequently if necessary (i.e. in case of very severe pains, or should the signs and symptoms worsen) or less frequently if she improves. I emphasise that, ideally, I would wish each subsequent treatment to take place before the benefits of the previous treatment wear off. I also explain that, in the case of an emergency, I am willing to see her at any time, without an appointment, and that I expect a similar commitment from her, for her own benefit. Patricia agrees willingly to this protocol.

Lifestyle and diet

I also ask Patricia to keep me informed of any changes in her lifestyle which may have a beneficial or detrimental effect on the outcome of the treatment.

I ask her whether she foresees any likely deviation from her usual diet as a result of socialising. She tells me that she has no forthcoming engagements planned. As she seems perfectly clear about those foods that aggravate her condition and as she avoids them, I have no dietary advice to give her.

Working very gently

On the day of the first treatment Patricia is a little anxious. She tells me that she has already had an acupuncture treatment but that it was so painful that she couldn't stand it or continue with the course of treatment. I do my best to reassure her, and ask her to let me know if she feels any pain or discomfort. I explain that I will manipulate the needles gently and will stop immediately if she wants me to. Patricia cooperates very well and tells me that she finds the insertions and the manipulations easy to bear. I work very gently, and don't notice any particular reaction on the part of my patient except for a slight sweat. I put this down to Patricia's nervous tension and I concentrate on managing this by using a reassuring manner and keeping up a dialogue. On the whole, the first treatment session goes very well.

I decide to adapt for Patricia a personal variation of the acupuncture formula *wei tong fang* (Formula for Epigastric Pain).[4]

First treatment procedures

- P6 *neiguan*, bilaterally, to harmonise the Stomach, calm emotional tension and, together with ST36 *zusanli*, to stop acid regurgitation and treat epigastric pain.[5]

- REN12 *zhongwan*, the front *mu* point of the Stomach, is the main point for treating epigastric pain, especially when combined with P6 *neiguan* and ST36 *zusanli*. Together they resolve accumulation of food and harmonise the raising of the 'pure' and the descending of the 'turbid'. In the acupuncture formula *wei tong fang* (Formula for Epigastric Pain), this point is considered to be the 'Emperor Point'.

- ST36 *zusanli*, bilaterally, is the *he* sea point of the Stomach, and represents, together with P6 *neiguan* and REN12 *zhongwan*, the most fundamental formula for the treatment of epigastric pain. Furthermore, this point is used in cases when the pain radiates to the ribs.[6]

- LIV3 *taichong* helps to circulate the Liver *qi*, to control the invasion of the Stomach and Spleen by Liver *qi*, and to prevent the progression of the stagnation of Liver *qi* towards Liver Fire. This point also calms nervous tension, and soothes sleep when disturbed by dreams of conflict.

Needles: I use 25 mm x 0.26 mm needles for P6 *neiguan* and LIV3 *taichong*, and 37.5 mm x 0.26 mm needles for REN12 *zhongwan* and ST36 *zusanli*. These needles are inserted to depths of 12 mm, 8 mm, 20 mm and 20 mm respectively.

Needle technique: I obtain *de qi* and then disperse (*xie fa*) by methods of *ti cha* (raise and thrust) and *nian zhuan* (rotation), except for REN12 *zhongwan*, on which I use even manipulation (*ping bu ping xie fa*). I retain the needles for 10 minutes.

White tigers and green dragons

On the day following the treatment Patricia notices an improvement. On the day after this she feels quite well and doesn't have any pains, except in the evening, when the pains return. She comes for treatment the next day.

For the second treatment, I decide to continue along the same lines, modifying the formula only a little in order to take account of the underlying Spleen deficiency, which is quite clear on the pulse. I also decide to adjust the manipulation techniques to stimulate the production of *qi* and to restore the transporting and transforming functions of the Spleen.

I again use P6 *neiguan*, REN12 *zhongwan* and LIV3 *taichong* as before but for ST36 *zusanli* I use a 50 mm needle, inserting to a depth of 20 mm bilaterally, and mobilising the *qi* by using the needling method *bai hu yao tou* (the white tiger nods his head) which combines an action of dispersing and moving. I add SP6 *sanyinjiao* on the left, and use a 37.5 mm needle, inserting to a depth of 20 mm and mobilising the *qi* by using the needling method *cang long yao wei* (the green dragon wags his tail) which combines an action of tonifying and moving. This last point strengthens the Spleen (*jian pi*) and facilitates the transporting and transforming functions (*yun hua*).

Immediately after the treatment, the point REN12 *zhongwan*, which had been very tender to pressure, is much less sensitive, indicating that the stagnation of *qi* has been dispersed. For the rest of the day Patricia is pain free. On the following day, there is only a very mild attack, moderate both in duration and intensity.

Concentrating on the *ben* (root)

At the third treatment, 5 days after the first, I continue with another slight modification. Patricia does have less pain, but feels tired and lacks motivation. Her pulse is *xi* (thready) and *chen* (deep). I decide to concentrate my attention on the *ben* (root) of the condition, the *biao* (branches) now being less urgent since the excess of pathogenic *qi* seems to have been dispersed and that which remains is the underlying Spleen *qi* deficiency.

I decide to apply the techniques of coupling the front *mu* and the back *shu* point of the Stomach (REN12 *zhongwan* and BL21 *weishu*), in order to treat the retained pathogenic *qi* in the Stomach.

I combine with these two points the *luo* point of the Spleen and main point of the *chong mai* (SP4 *gongsun*), and needle bilaterally, to a depth of 10 mm. After obtaining *de qi*, I use the needling method *long hu jiao zhan* (the battle of the tiger and the dragon) which helps to circulate the *qi* in the channels. The action of this needling method alternates between tonification and sedation and is therefore very effective in treating pain. This helps to regulate the *chong mai* and the Middle Burner, and promotes the *yun hua* (the Spleen function of transporting and transforming).

Finally, I add the *xi* cleft point of the Stomach (ST34 *liangqiu*), and needle bilaterally, to a depth of 20 mm. After obtaining *de qi*, I use the needling method *bai hu yao tou* (the white tiger nods his head), which treats the chronic or persistent pain in the Stomach, regulates the Liver and dredges the Stomach channel of retained pathogenic factor.

No pain and no further attacks

Patricia is now entirely free of pain and has had no further attacks. A Chinese herbal decoction, based on a personal variation of the formula Rambling Powder *xiao yao san*, was prescribed for 2 weeks to stabilise the balance between the Liver and the Spleen. After 6 months, Patricia was questioned and reported that no new gastric symptoms had occurred.

Keys to success

A key to the success of acupuncture in this case was the identification of syndromes whilst understanding the condition to be one of mixed deficiency and excess. Also of importance was the selection of only a small number of points and the use of the correct technique of manipulation at these points. A further aspect of this case that I would like to emphasise is the timing of Patricia's treatments. The decision on when to treat was based on the needs of the patient rather than the needs of the practitioner. For the treatment of the *biao*, it is the patient's condition which will indicate when it is appropriate to treat again. The ideal timing of the treatment is when the benefits of the previous treatment are beginning to wear off, but before the patient's symptoms have returned. However, for the *ben*, it is the practitioner who decides the timing of the treatment. This approach to treatment requires the practitioner to be more attentive to the rhythms of change in the patient's condition and to make her or himself available on any day of the week in order to provide the best care for the patient.

NOTES

1 A 'bilious' temperament is one of the four temperaments in Hippocratic medicine, and is characterised by someone who angers easily, tends to have digestive problems, has an excess of bile, with a bitter taste, and has a yellow tongue coat.

2 Acid regurgitation reflects a disharmony between the Liver and the Stomach (*gan wei bu he*), rebellious Stomach *qi* (*wei qi ni*), and production of Heat in the Liver.

3 According to the Su Wen, Chapter 17, Mai Yao Jing Wei Lun (Huang Di Nei Jing 1960, 1982), sleep disturbances such as these can be associated with an excess condition of the Liver.

4 The acupuncture formula *wei tong fang* (Formula for Epigastric Pain) is described in the Zhen Jiu Zhi Yan Lu (Yang Rong Xuan & Yang Yi Fang 1965).

5 P6 *neiguan* has this action according to the Zhen Jiu Da Cheng (Yang Ji Zhou, various editions, undated) and the Qian Jin Yao Fang (Sun Si Miao, ancient editions, undated). Furthermore, this point also treats epigastric and costal pains in women.

6 ST36 *zusanli* is used in cases where the pain radiates to the ribs, as mentioned in the Ling Shu, Chapter 4, Xie Qi Zang Fu Bing Xing: 'In diseases of the Stomach the abdomen is distended, and there is epigastric pain radiating towards the costal region . . . one must needle *zusanli*' (Huang Di Nei Jing 1960, 1982).

REFERENCES

Huang Di Nei Jing 1960 Huang Di Nei Jing Su Wen Yi Jie. Dai Lian Guo Feng Chu Ban She, Taiwan
Huang Di Nei Jing 1982 Huang Di Nei Jing Su Wen. Ren Ming Wei Sheng Zhu Ban She, Taiwan
Sun Si Miao (ancient edition, undated) Qian Jin Yao Fang, China
Sun Si Miao (ancient edition, undated) Qian Jin Yi Fang, China
Yang Ji Zhou (various editions, undated) Zhen Jiu Da Cheng, China
Yang Rong Xuan, Yang Yi Fang 1965 Zhen Jiu Zhi Yan Lu, China

FURTHER READING

Huang Fu Mi 1989 Jia Yi Jing. Masson, Paris
Laurent P 1995 L'esprit des points. Bord de l'Oise, Paris
Marié E 1991 Grand formulaire de pharmacopée Chinoise. Paracelse, Vitré
Shang Han Lun Jiang Yi 1990 Ke Xue Ji Shu Chu Ban She, Shanghai
Shu Xue Xue 1983 Ke Xue Ji Shu Chu Ban She, Shanghai
Zhen Jiu Zhi Liao Xue 1990 Ke Xue Ji Shu Chu Ban She, Shanghai

■ Eric Marié

Eric Marié has been practising Chinese medicine for more than 15 years. His training was principally in the Far East, in China, Japan and Taiwan. He studied, on the one hand, within Chinese universities and hospitals and, on the other hand, he followed traditional masters, with whom he lived, sharing the essence of their experiences. As well as medicine, he has also practised many aspects of Chinese culture including painting, calligraphy and martial arts. A doctor of traditional Chinese medicine specialising in internal medicine (*nei ke*), he is a guest professor at the Jiangxi College of Traditional Chinese Medicine, Nanchang, China, where he lives for several months each year, giving lectures on specific aspects of Chinese medicine. He is also Director of Research in Internal Medicine at the Affiliated Hospital in Nanchang.

In Europe, he is President of the European Federation of Energetic Medicine, and Founding Director of L'Ecole Supérieure de Médicine Chinoise which is unique in being a full-time course taught by Chinese university lecturers. He also runs master classes as Director of Education Development at the Anglo-Dutch Institute of Traditional Chinese Medicine, at Ijmuiden in the Netherlands. He lectures to teachers in Germany at the Arbeitsgemeinschaft fur Klassische Akupunktur und Traditionelle Chinesische Medizine. He is the author of seven books including the *Grand Formulaire de Pharmacopée Chinoise*, and is the editor of the review *Médecine Chinoise et Médicines Orientales*.

Unwinding a volvulus to cure a migraine

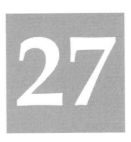

Satya Ambrose CLACKAMAS, OR, USA

When Ellen walked into my office I had no idea that she was in so much pain. She was 47 years old at that time and she carried her tall, thin frame erect and with dignity. She had an unusual complexion, very pale and yellowish. Her manner was very sweet and kindly, making it 'easy' to work with her. I felt her watching me to assess whether I could help her, but also, whether she could help me in any way. Our relationship unfolded easily and Ellen was open and accepting.

Downplaying of symptoms

Ellen relayed in a quiet, clear voice her three primary complaints: abdominal pain, headaches and chest pains. She seemed to downplay her symptoms as if she did not want to bother anyone. The following is her synopsis of these three problematic areas.

Abdominal pain

My digestion has always been poor. As a child, I remember terrible stomachaches, especially when I was at school. My stomach and head seemed to work together against me. Currently, I feel constant bloating. This gets worse with any food, and especially with foods containing any sugar. The pain is always dull and achey with periods of severe spasms which can last for hours, sometimes days. I've ended up in the emergency room with volvulus and intussusception.[1] They thought my gallbladder was the problem but once they had removed it they found that it was OK. They also removed over 3 m of intestines when I was suffering from one of my volvulus episodes. This made my pain worse. Now I think I have adhesions. I feel like there is a lead balloon in my stomach. (She prods her left periumbilical area.) It hurts when I press on it, but if I get in there and dig I can sometimes alleviate the pain. The sensation is also burning. I need a bulking agent to make my bowels move, otherwise they don't do anything. I have haemorrhoids from straining with stools. All of this got worse after the surgeries. It is also worse when standing.

Headaches

My headaches started when I began school as a child. No-one could figure out why. Glasses didn't help. I used to come home from school crying with pain. My headaches start at the front of my head and are dull, heavy, achey and throbbing. When they accompany my abdominal pain, they get really bad. They go to the right side of my head, from the root of my nose to just behind my hairline at the corner of my head. There's one spot that's especially painful. This is worse with white flour and oil, really bad with sugar, eating anything really, and when arising out of bed, with odours, chemicals, and fright.

She relayed to me that she would have to lie down in a dark room and would vomit if she moved. On a scale of 1–10 her pain would score 20. These headaches were daily when she first attended for treatment.

Chest pains

Ellen's chest pains had been present for the last 21 years and she suffered from them, on average, once a month. For some unknown reason they had recently become more frequent and intense, and she now experienced them weekly or even daily. These pains would 'move around in my chest, they were worse on the left side, radiating down my left arm, sometimes moving to the right, and were sharp and stabbing, coming on instantly and leaving immediately'. These pains were worse with exertion, fatigue and lack of sleep. They improved with ultrasound treatments.

Physical examination

During the course of the examination she exhibited weakness and lack of muscle tone but was cooperative and eager to assist. (For details see the box on Clinical Manifestations.)

Medical history

During her childhood she was quite prone to daily rages. This started after her father left without saying goodbye. Thus, there is a relationship between this painful past history and the advent of the daily headaches that she experienced from school-age. She remembered also having extreme abdominal pains from this time too. These symptoms became worse as a teenager. At the age of 27, she had a laparotomy and an appendectomy, with no relief of symptoms. A year later she had surgery with the removal of her gallbladder and her transverse and ascending colon. Over the next few years she had incidents where she experienced acute abdominal pain and was hospitalised. Her symptoms, although becoming less acute immediately, on the whole became worse. The medications that were tried caused violent reactions and they always made her worse.

Lifestyle

Emotionally, Ellen seemed quite at ease. Her religious beliefs supported very 'clean' living. Her life did not include harmful habits. She had no children. She had a great deal of support in her life and was married to a very nice, supportive man. She lived next door to her sister and mother, both of whom she loved dearly. She kept her home spotless and she devoted her life to her church. Her religious beliefs included the approaching apocalypse and the need to save people outside of her faith. This was quite stressful for her. She also rarely had time to exercise because of her low energy levels and also because of her devotion to her church.

Summary of clinical manifestations

Abdominal pain

- Constant, with episodes of acute abdominal pain and vomiting, without passing stools or gas.
- Sensation of 'lead balloon in the stomach'.
- Pain on pressure, alleviated with deep pressure, and sensation of burning.
- Particular areas of pain at periumbilical, left ST27 *daju* area and at McBurney's point on the right.
- Bloating and sensation of fullness coming on after food, especially after intake of sugar and fats.
- Acute symptoms worse for lying down.
- Constipation unless bulking agents used and unless manually pushing using hands.

Headaches

- Start frontally dull, achey, heavy and throbbing; move to right GB16 *muchuang* area, accompany abdominal pain.
- Worse with movement, odours, chemicals, fright, standing, light, food generally and oils, sugar and white flour in particular.
- Better for ice packs, lying down in a dark room and sleeping.

Chest pains

- Sharp stabbing, come and go.
- Palpitations, sometimes tachycardia.
- Worse with quick neck turn.
- Pains move around, are worse on left side and radiate down the arm.
- Worse with exertion, fatigue and lack of sleep.

Other symptoms

- Constant fatigue: starts feeling very low and then slowly builds, better by nightfall.
- Haemorrhoids with fissures, bleeding and sharp pain locally.
- Hair thin and brittle with hair loss.
- Skin colour pale, yellow.
- Rashes on the fingers and in the ears which itch, crack and weep.
- Bruises easily.
- Nails strong but brittle.
- Temperature: whole body always very cold.
- Eyes: vision weak.
- Ears: psoriasis or eczema in the ears with weeping, smelly, itchy discharge.
- Urine: frequent, 3–6 times per night; occasional bladder infections cause night-time urination to increase still further.

- Menses: painful, purple clots; headaches worsen; heavy bleeding.
- Breasts: fibrocystic lumps with painful, bruised feeling.
- Thirst: rarely.
- Sleep: difficulty falling asleep, awakens with abdominal distress at night.
- Emotions: anxiety due to pain and depression due to worries about her family's health and the future; hopelessness about the future; feelings worse in the dark; hates dust, spiders and anything out of place.

Physical Examination

- Tongue: greasy, white moss; pale, large with long fluted edges.
- Pulses: generally weak and slippery, somewhat slow, absent in the first left position, very weak in the third position both sides, and especially on the left. There was a 'twang' or tight sensation in the middle position, bilaterally.

- Breasts were tender with multiple fibrocystic-type lumps often along the stomach meridian below the nipple.
- Abdomen and pelvis: midline scar following the conception vessel both below and above the umbilicus.
- Neuromuscular: subluxations at thoracic levels T6, T10 and T11.
- Thoracic kyphosis at thoracic levels T1–T3.
- Left short leg prone and supine, musculoskeletal lumbarisation L5 to S1 with chronic low back pain and kyphotic posture.

Laboratory work

- Low RBC count.
- Low iron levels, ferritin (iron stores).
- Low total iron binding capacity (TIBC).[2]
- Electrocardiogram (ECG) normal.
- Mammogram shows fibrocystic changes.

Evidence for the patterns of disharmony

When I started seeing Ellen, her symptoms were fairly advanced, and she had many layers of disharmony. I found contradictory symptoms of hot and cold. I had never in my coursework or experience seen such a case before.

Kidney *yang xu*

- Extreme cold, whole body cold.
- Constant fatigue.
- Long-term weakness.
- Chronic low back pain.
- Frequent urination at night.
- Pale colouring.
- Pulses: very weak in the third position, slow.
- Tongue: pale.

Spleen *yang xu* and Damp

- Long-term cold sensations.
- Chronic bloating and indigestion.
- Food intolerances.
- Exhaustion, worse in the morning.
- Pale, yellow skin.
- Bruises easily.
- Dull, frontal headaches triggered by food.
- Lack of thirst.
- Lack of muscle tone.
- Tongue: pale and large with fluted edges.
- Pulse: slow, slippery and weak.

Liver *qi* stagnation, Liver *yang* rising:

- One-sided headache, accompanied by anger, often occurring after frontal headache.

- Headaches (Liver *qi* obstructed by Spleen Damp).
- Headaches worse premenstrually.
- Headaches with abdominal pain (Liver invading Spleen).
- Menstrual cramps, purple clots (Liver Blood Stagnation).
- Breast lumps.
- Depression.
- Weak vision.
- Brittle nails.
- Pulses: tight in the middle positions.

Qi and Blood stagnation in middle/ lower jiao

- Acute abdominal pain episodes.
- Specific areas of pain at ST27 *daju* area left, and McBurney's point on the right.
- Bloating, fullness.

- Pain with pressure; deep pressure alleviates pain.
- Constipation, manual stimulation of bowel movements required.
- Abdominal pain after eating.
- Abdominal symptoms worse for lying down.
- Pulse: tight bilaterally.

Heart *qi xu* and Heart Blood stagnation

- Chest pains come and go, worse with exertion and fatigue.
- Radiating pain on left chest and down left arm.
- Palpitations.
- Insomnia and anxiety (Heart Blood *xu*).
- Tongue: pale.

Aetiology and pathology

The aetiology of this case shows several factors. The underlying factor is Kidney *yang xu* and is due to family *jing* (genetic) weakness and the anger from abandonment affecting the Liver. Both these factors have weakened Ellen's Spleen function. Another Spleen/Liver weakening factor in Ellen's case has been the 'SAD' diet (Standard American Diet) and accompanying lifestyle of 'no exercise'. Furthermore, there are many food additives which can cause further damage if the digestive tract is already dysfunctional, thus causing 'leaky gut syndrome'.[3] In Oriental medicine this is called Spleen-Liver disharmony. Ellen had the symptoms of coeliac disease with additional food intolerances. I thought the volvulus and intussusception were related to adhesions binding her intestines. These, in turn, were a result of the surgeries to and inflammation in her peritoneum. During peristalsis, the areas of adhesions reacted strongly to her allergens, thus causing telescoping and twisting, blocking off normal bowel function.

The aetiology and pathology diagram (Fig. 27.1) illustrates the interrelationship of the syndromes in Ellen's case. It demonstrates how the underlying Kidney *yang xu* causes Spleen *yang xu*. This is aggravated by the overstimulation of the Liver *yang* by the emotions. Thus the Spleen *qi* is not facilitated to move and the Damp becomes stagnant in the middle and lower warmers, thus causing *qi* and Blood Stagnation. Eventually, the *yang*, Blood and *qi* of the Heart are compromised.

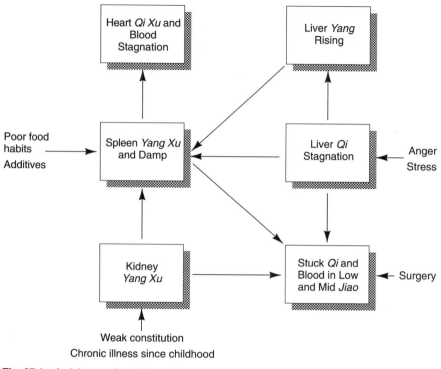

Fig. 27.1 Aetiology and pathology diagram.

Initial treatments

Initial treatments for Ellen were aimed at moving the stagnant *qi* and Blood, harmonising the Liver and Spleen and removing toxins. I felt over-whelmed by her myriad of symptoms, so I treated what was most pressing symptomatically. I merely tried points gently to see if they prompted any results. If they proved effective, I maintained and developed their usage. It was appropriate, I believed, to remove the top levels, thus exposing and allowing treatment of the underlying layers. In other words, I treated the stems and branches in order to reach the roots. If I had been too quick to treat the roots directly, this would have caused Ellen to have a very intense 'healing crisis' which would have been no small thing and could not be ignored.

Preceding the treatments, I explained to Ellen that her condition had several layers, beginning with a weak constitution that had been stressed by heavy emotions in childhood. This had also been aggravated by poor food habits and unrecognised food sensitivities. The final insult was her surgery, which had worsened her condition. Ellen agreed with my analysis.

Treatment procedures

TREATMENT PRINCIPLES

Treatment was specifically designed to:

- Move Stagnant Liver *qi* and Stagnant Liver Blood.
- Build Spleen *yang*.
- Move Damp stagnation, thus removing toxins.
- Assist the Heart *yang* and *qi* deficiency and move Heart Stagnation.
- Eventually tonify the Kidney *yang*.
- Support the Large Intestine functions to properly rid the impurities, thus clearing internal Heat and supporting the lower *jiao*.

POINTS

- ST36 *zusanli* builds Spleen and Stomach *qi* and Blood, transforms Damp, and 'cures a hundred ills'.
- ST37 *shangjuxu* moves Stagnation in the Large Intestines and helps malabsorption.
- SP10 *xuehai* builds Blood and supports the Spleen which holds the Blood in the vessels, thus helping haemorrhoids.
- SP6 *sanyinjiao* builds the Spleen and three leg *yin*.
- SP4 *gongsun* moves Damp stagnation and accumulation in the middle and lower *jiao*, resolves Stagnant Blood in the chest, and resolves conflict with ancestors (via *chong mai*).
- LIV3 *taichong* moves constraint in the Liver and subdues Liver *yang*.
- LI4 *hegu* opens the energy to the head, stops pain and assists LIV3 *taichong* in opening the gates for the smooth flow of Liver *qi*.
- REN12 *zhongwan* builds the middle warmer *qi*.
- REN6 *qihai* builds *qi* to move stagnation.
- REN4 *guanyuan* is the meeting point of Blood and *yin* and facilitates movement of the bowels and urine.
- ST26 *wailing* (left) is a local point for pain.
- ST27 *daju* (right) is a local point for pain.

- P4 *ximen*, a *xi* cleft point, resolves Stagnation of Blood in the Heart and is a special point for haemorrhoids and fissures (use moxa).

Important points used later

- *LIV8 ququan:* useful in resolving severe headache; light needle (thin Japanese).
- *KID1 yongquan* resolves cramps; very helpful for excruciatingly painful headaches.
- *DU1 changqiang:* local point for haemorrhoids.
- *ST25 tianshu:* smoothes intestine flow.

Needle technique: Free hand insertion was used except on the more painful points where a guide tube was utilised. Even method was used except on the abdominal points where strong *qi* stimulation was obtained aimed at dispersing stagnation.

Needles: Due to the use of so many points, a very fine gauge (36 gauge) was used on all points. 25 mm needles were used except on REN6 *qihai* and SP10 *xuehai*, where 40 mm needles were used, and except KID1 *yongquan*, LIV1 *dadun* and on the head points where 12.5 mm needles were used.

HERBAL MEDICINE

Ellen also tried various herbs, but was sensitive to most. We therefore decided to use single, local, organic, Western herbs because they could be easily obtained. These included: dandelion, hawthorn, witch hazel, phytolacca, burdock, grapefruit seed extract, and bilberry.

HOMEOPATHY

We also made use of homeopathic medicine which was very effective and had low toxicity. Ellen was very sensitive to 'energy' medicine and, as long as we stayed away from calcium lactose pellets and used dilutions in water, she did well. The homeopathics that seemed to serve her the best were Staphesagria, Bryonia, and Natrum Muriaticum.

Establishing a relationship of love and trust

I knew Ellen would require several years of treatment since her symptoms were more than 40 years old. Thus I estimated 40 or more months of treatment. I did not discuss this with her. I basically worked to establish a relationship of love and trust between us, believing that the rest would follow and would create a vessel in which our work could take place. We started with once weekly treatments. As I began to treat her, I told her the names of the different points and their purpose. She was very curious, relaxed and trusting. She stated that nothing could be as bad as the pain she had already experienced and other forms of medicine that she had taken. She was easily treated, experiencing little pain from the needles and reporting immediate relief from discomfort as well as a great euphoria. She said she could become addicted to the treatment! I find that if I can elicit an immediate relief from the acute symptoms when using an Eight Principles approach, it often indicates a positive potential outcome. I expected that her long-term symptoms would return after a few days, or that they might be somewhat less frequent and less intense, and this is what happened. At the end of each treatment I had her rest. This is particularly important with fatigued patients and seems to prevent most post-treatment exhaustion and disorientation.

Ellen found immediate relief from her headaches. They changed from a crushing pain headache every day to a milder pain headache once weekly. Then, after a series of five treatments, we introduced her first homeopathic remedy (Staphesagria) together with dandelion to encourage detoxification and stimulate the liver. This improved her digestive tract immensely. At this point, I requested that she modified her diet.

She removed all 'chemical additives', eating only organic food where possible, and followed a very strict elimination diet for a period of several months, thus eliminating all possible food allergens. She then reintroduced foods one at a time to check for reactions such as abdominal pain, headaches and palpitations. She was extremely compliant because of the great benefit she felt from being pain free. I also asked her to exercise regularly when she was physically able. This she was able to do some of the time. In addition, I encouraged her to attempt some stress reduction techniques to help reduce her anxiety and depression. These interested her less and so she did not utilise them as much as she did the other suggestions. This was also partly due to the fact that she was feeling much better emotionally because of the treatment.

We continued treatments and, on one occasion, I decided to needle the Liver meridian at LIV1 *dadun* and LIV8 *ququan* to help one of her severe headache episodes. These points were needled gently, together with LI4 *hegu*, KID1 *yongquan* and *ahshi*, or painful points, on her abdomen and head. This miraculously completely stopped her headaches for months, until she ate sugar again. She then did quite well as long as she stayed away from foods which caused her problems. On another occasion, I decided to use moxa to try to clear the Damp stagnation in her gut and to build her Kidneys. I did three direct moxa on REN4 *guanyuan*. After this, Ellen became very constipated, her haemorrhoids flared up and she developed very painful rectal fissures. I treated her several times a week with points to heal the rectal fissures: P4 *ximen* with moxa, SP10 *xuehai* with direct moxa and DU1 *changqiang*. These points were helpful and prevented her from having further surgery. I also found that the Pericardium meridian helped her palpitations. However, physical manipulation helped her cardiac symptoms more than anything else. She currently uses Vitamin E, Vitamin C and slippery elm daily. If she needs antibiotics she uses colloidal silver, and she uses free-form amino acids for her energy levels and to prevent her hair from falling out.

Experiencing trepidation

As we worked together, Ellen would call to say she was having a 'little' trouble and ask if I could treat her. I would question her regarding symptoms and she would say that she was experiencing an acute abdominal episode, with vomiting but without passing stools or gas. She would say that her pain and other symptoms were the same as those she had when she experienced her intussusception and volvulus episodes. I would try to refer her to the emergency room. However, she would calmly say that she did not want to go to hospital and that she just knew that acupuncture would work. I would therefore ask her to attend immediately for treatment and would keep her in my office for observation until I was confident that her intestines would 'unwind', reverse the telescoping of the intussusception, and start functioning normally again. During these acute episodes I would experience trepidation, but her acute symptoms would abate usually within 2 hours. Over the 9 years that I've been treating Ellen, I have never had to 'drag her off' to the hospital.

If Ellen needed more frequent treatments or was short of money, I would tell her that I was having a 'special' offer that month where treatments were three for the price of one, or whatever else I could do to encourage her to continue her treatment. I made it clear that she was never to stay away because of lack of funds.

Currently, I still see Ellen for 'tune-ups' once every few months or if and when she has a flare-up. She has rare headaches now and her digestive tract does well with the supplements she uses. If she starts to get a headache or an abdominal problem (usually caused by a dietary indiscretion), the symptoms are slight and usually go away by themselves or with a gentle treatment.

Valuing the process as much as the 'cure'

Ellen's case was so successful that I ended up treating her whole family as well as many of her friends from church. This allowed me see a different side of Ellen, which was helpful since patients do tend to downplay their symptoms.

I have come to greatly love and respect Ellen during the time in which we have worked together and I look forward to her occasional visits. In her particular case, I learned to value the process as much as the 'cure'. As time went on, treatment requirements became very clear and the treatment plan needed to have great flexibility. Ellen's faith and patience in me were inspiring and have stayed with me. When she now visits my clinic, I ask her what she has come to teach me today.

Summary of outcome

- Headaches are rare.
- Abdominal distress is very rare; eats a much wider range of foods.
- Palpitations occasionally.
- Sleep is deep and easy.
- Fatigue goes up and down, but never 'bone tired' exhaustion.
- Face colour is still pale but less yellowish.
- Urination now once nightly.

- Body temperature is chilly but not permanently freezing.
- Thirst has increased but is still low.
- Emotions are stable.
- Eyes are fairly strong.
- Breasts are still fibrocystic; regular mammograms are undertaken.
- Ears are still problematic: itchy and weepy.
- Bowel movements are regular with the daily use of slippery elm.

NOTES

1   Volvulus and intussusception cause an acute abdominal pain similar to appendicitis. Volvulus is a twisting of the intestines, causing necrosis of the bowel if it lasts for more than 24 hours. Intussusception is a telescoping of the bowels, which can also cause occlusion and necrosis. It too, is an emergency condition.

2   Total Iron Binding Capacity (TIBC) is the capacity of a liver-made protein to bring iron over the gut lining, thus allowing its absorption. Low levels of TIBC can indicate protein malabsorption, or the liver's inability to make the required proteins.

3   Leaky gut syndrome. In this syndrome, toxic substances which have not been properly transformed are absorbed and other, normally non-toxic molecules are absorbed whole. The human body is not able to effectively deal with these chemicals. This creates blood toxicity and allergic reaction (the Cantonese call this 'sup' which I believe is *tan yin* or Damp stagnation turning to internal Heat). These toxins tax the Liver because it has to detoxify them instead of undertaking its normal functions. Symptoms of Liver taxation (constrained and depressed Liver *qi*) are:
1   Emotional lability (the brain is also affected).
2   Immune dysfunction.
3   Hormone excesses resulting in PMS and dysmenorrhoea because the Liver is already dealing with toxic chemicals from the gastrointestinal tract.

Eventually, there is an abnormal bacterial build-up in the gut, thus creating more toxins and preventing absorption of required substances such as proteins and fat soluble vitamins like Vitamin A and Vitamin K. As a result, insufficient total iron binding capacity (TIBC) protein is made and inflammation is more frequent. In addition, the lack of Vitamin A and Vitamin K causes bruising. This occurs in many serious digestive diseases e.g. coeliac disease, ulcerative colitis and Crohn's disease.

FURTHER READING

Barrie S 1994 Putting the pieces together. Notebook and Text from the Great Smokies Laboratory, Asheville

Crook W G 1980 Tracking down hidden food allergies. Professional Books, Jackson

Pizzorno J E, Murray M T 1985 A textbook of natural medicine. John Bastyr College Publications, Seattle

Pizzorno J E, Murray M T 1990 Encyclopaedia of natural medicine. Prima Publishing, Rocklin

So J T Y 1977 A complete course in Chinese medicine. New England School of Acupuncture, Watertown

Advances in acupuncture and acupuncture anaesthesia 1977 The People's Medical Publishing House, Beijing

■ Satya Ambrose

I have been practising Oriental medicine for 17 years. I trained in biochemistry and psychology in Washington State at Evergreen State College. While working as a counsellor in a woman's clinic I noticed a correlation between people (patients) holding onto their painful memories and illness. During the same period, I worked in a medical laboratory where I was exposed to the concepts of Oriental medicine by the head pathologist and I was intrigued by its holistic approach. I chose to further my studies at the New England School of Acupuncture (NESA) where I studied with Dr Yin Tau So, Ted Kaptchuk and Kiiko Matsumoto. I was very fortunate to be hired there at a later stage to teach.

In my practice in Boston at that time, I combined my psychological background and bodywork, including acupuncture, with outstanding results. Many of the Jungian analysts in the area became my patients and this further influenced my work to delve deeply into the past as well as the present to help resolution of the mind/body.

The National College of Naturopathic Medicine asked me to come to Portland Oregon to start an acupuncture programme. I established the Oregon College of Oriental Medicine in 1982 of which I was both director and a faculty member. I then studied naturopathic medicine and graduated with my doctorate in 1989. I now enjoy my family, a wonderful husband and three children on my 23-acre farm, where I live and practise. I teach, give seminars, write and weed the garden in my spare time. I am also starting an environmental detox centre, which I hope will provide greatly needed healing at all levels to people and to our planet.

Epigastric pain

Lucio Sotte CIVITANOVA, ITALY

20 years of pain

One afternoon, 3 years ago, a charming woman, Anna, came to my clinic for a consultation. At that time, Anna was 41 years old, but looked younger. She was married to a doctor (an anaesthetist and colleague of mine) and had three children. She complained of epigastric pain, which had been diagnosed as 'ulcerous gastroduodenitis', and which was characterised by winter and summer improvement and a worsening in spring and autumn. She told me that the pain had begun more than 20 years ago and had progressively worsened over the last 2 years.

Her most recent attack had started 1 month before attending for acupuncture. When treated with Western drugs, her condition improved and the epigastric pain lessened. Her current medication included the antiulcer drug, ranitidine, and the antacid drugs, magnesium hydroxide, aluminium hydroxide and dimethicone. However, each time she stopped taking the drugs, the pain returned as bad as ever. In the most recent attack, these Western drugs had not succeeded in relieving the symptoms. With the agreement of her husband, she had decided to try Traditional Chinese Medicine.

Anna told me that the epigastric pain was dull all day and was more severe in the morning and in the late afternoon, and was worst before meals and with an empty stomach. The pain was accompanied by a sensation of burning and distension in the epigastric region. All the symptoms worsened with exposure to external cold, after eating raw and cold foods, and with emotional states such as anger or resentment. The symptoms improved when something warm was applied to the stomach area (a woollen blanket or a hot-water bottle). Sometimes the pain disappeared with local massage or after eating a little light and warm food. Some years earlier Anna had discovered that a drop of red wine before meals helped to improve both her general and stomach conditions, except when the epigastric pain was strongly burning. Nausea and vomiting of thin fluids occurred rarely, and then only when the pain was very severe or in the case of severe exposure to cold. Even though she complained of a burning pain, her condition improved with the application of warmth to the epigastric region.

An excellent cook who didn't eat much

Anna had a good appetite but, for the last few years, she hadn't eaten very much. In other words, she felt hungry and attracted to food, but when she ate too much her stomach would feel upset and full and she would feel sleepy. For this reason she had become used to eating only small amounts of food and avoiding fatty foods which she found difficult to digest. Some days, when her epigastric pain was severe, she preferred to eat nothing. It was such a pity that she couldn't eat because, at our second meeting, I discovered that Anna was an excellent cook and even a sommelier (wine-taster). She regretted the fact that her epigastric disease prevented her from attending both cookery courses and meetings with her fellow sommeliers. Moreover, she thought herself to be underweight but confessed to me that she could not complain about this to her female friends because they all had the opposite problem of being overweight and would not therefore understand.

Anna said that she had suffered from some stomach problems even during her childhood. She used to be constipated, but after three preg-nancies her bowel movements had become irregular with loose stools and sometimes diarrhoea. Sometimes she had abdominal distension and complained of haemorrhoids with a burning pain. During the last 10 years she had also suffered occasional headaches with two different types of pain. The first type was located behind the eyes, particularly the left eye, and was accompanied by sensations of distension and stiffness, with flash-ing lights and aversion to light and noise. It was aggravated by tiredness caused by work problems or overwork. The second type of pain started from the neck, mostly on the right in the area of GB20 *fengchi*. Sometimes the pain radiated to the shoulder, on the right at GB21 *jianjing*, and then to the temples, particularly to the *taiyang* point. This pain was accompanied by dizziness and a sensation of 'fullness in the right ear'. It occurred gen-erally after exposure to cold or wind-cold, and sometimes after exposure to damp. Anna said that she felt better during cold weather if she covered up GB20 *fengchi* and this was why she was used to tying up an elegant silk scarf around her head. This second type of pain was improved by the local application of warmth.

Anna's menstrual flow had been regular in recent years, although gen-erally excessive in volume and sometimes containing blood clots. She complained of premenstrual irritability, accompanied by a worsening of the epigastric pain, and tiredness after menstruation. She had had three pregnancies with the birth of her three children when she was aged 26, 30 and 34. For some months after each pregnancy she had suffered from tiredness, and 4 months after the second pregnancy she had had viral hepatitis.

In the last 4 years she had felt tired, especially early in the morning, with muscle weakness and general lassitude. She felt better in the evening, but in recent months had preferred to go to sleep early because she 'needed to sleep to recover her energy'. Three years ago she had experienced a period of severe tiredness accompanied by insomnia, dream-disturbed sleep, nightmares, mental restlessness, palpitations, anxiety and a poor appetite. At this time she had been successfully treated with Western drugs and Chinese herbal therapy.

Observations and impressions

Anna looked a little pale, with irregular brown spots all over her face, mostly in the frontal region. The spots had worsened after each pregnancy and also worsened during the summer when exposed to the sun. The tongue was pale and purplish, a little swollen, with tooth marks and some red spots on the sides and on the tip. It was covered by a thin, white coating. The pulse was empty in all positions and was wiry mostly in the Spleen position.

I can add that, after our talk, my impression of Anna was one of a very intelligent and self-reliant woman, satisfied with both her job and her family life. I thought she was a little stressed, but she didn't want to admit this. Before leaving, Anna asked me for the titles of some books on Chinese philosophy and Chinese medicine: it was her habit to enquire into everything she did.

Summary of clinical manifestations

Epigastric pain

- Dull all day.
- More severe in the morning and late afternoon.
- More frequent in spring and autumn.
- Accompanied by a burning sensation and distension.
- Worse with an empty stomach and with exposure to external cold and cold food.
- Worse with anger and resentment.
- Better with application of warmth, and with warm food.
- Nausea and vomiting of thin fluids (rarely).
- Good appetite but poor intake of food.
- Irregular bowel movements, loose stools and sometimes diarrhoea.
- Abdominal distension, haemorrhoids with burning pain.

Headaches

Type one: pain behind the eyes, particularly the left eye; sensations of distension and stiffness; flashing lights; aversion to light and noise; aggravated by anger or resentment.

Type two: pain in the temples, particularly at *taiyang*; starting from the neck (mostly the right side from GB20 *fengchi*) and radiating to the temples; accompanied by dizziness and a sensation of 'fullness in the right ear'; occurs after exposure to cold or wind-cold and sometimes damp; improves with warmth, and in the cold if GB20 *fengchi* is covered.

Menses

Premenstrual irritability, accompanied by a worsening of the epigastric pain and tiredness after menstruation; tiredness, especially in the morning.

General tiredness

General tiredness of 4 years' duration, especially in the early morning, with muscle weakness and general lassitude; better in the evening; needs early nights.

An episode of very severe tiredness 3 years ago was accompanied by insomnia, dream-disturbed sleep, nightmares, palpitations, anxiety and poor appetite.

Complexion: paleness with irregular brown spots on the face, mostly the frontal region; spots worse after pregnancy and during the summer when exposed to the sun.

Tongue: pale and purple, a little swollen, with toothmarks and some red spots on the sides and tip; thin white coating.

Pulse: empty in all positions, wiry mostly in the Spleen position.

Identifying the patterns of disharmony

At the time of consultation, the major presenting symptoms suggested predominant patterns of Liver *qi* stagnation and Liver invading the Stomach, with the development of Stomach Heat. However, this was only the *biao*. The background to these patterns (the *ben*) was a long-standing Spleen *qi* deficiency and Cold. That the background of deficiency was more long-standing was confirmed by the episodes of tiredness after pregnancy and the period of Heart *qi* deficiency 3 years earlier.

The good appetite was contradictory to the case of Spleen *qi* deficiency and Cold. My opinion was that the good appetite was connected to Stomach Heat, and that the poor intake of food and the epigastric pain were related to Liver invading the Stomach, Spleen deficiency and Cold.

Evidence for patterns of disharmony

Liver *qi* stagnation; Liver invading the Stomach with Stomach Heat

- Burning epigastric pain with anger and resentment.
- Nausea and vomiting of thin fluids (rarely).
- Good appetite (despite poor intake of food).
- Irregular bowel movements.
- Distending pain behind the left eye, worse with anger.

- Premenstrual irritability accompanied by worsening of the epigastric pain.
- Brown irregular spots on the face, mostly in the frontal region and worse during summer and after exposure to the sun.
- Pulse: wiry.

Spleen *qi* deficiency and Cold

- Dull epigastric pain; worse with an empty stomach, with external cold and with cold food; better with warmth and warm foods.

- Poor intake of food.
- Dull headache aggravated by cold and dampness and ameliorated by warmth.
- Loose stools and diarrhoea.
- Tiredness worse in the morning.
- Tongue: pale, swollen teeth, marked white coating.
- Pulse: empty.

Heart *qi* deficiency

- Insomnia.
- Palpitations.
- Dream-disturbed sleep.
- Anxiety.
- Tiredness.

Aetiology and pathology

Anna had a constitutionally weak Spleen which had been aggravated by the three pregnancies which, in turn, had consumed Spleen Blood and *qi*. Many external factors, such as work problems, family discussions and emotional tension around the children's health, had created a pattern of Liver *qi* stagnation overacting on the Earth. This had aggravated the Spleen *qi* deficiency. Liver invading the Stomach had caused a congestion of Stomach *qi* leading to the production of Stomach Heat (Fig. 28.1). The reason for the episode of Heart *qi* deficiency was chronic worry consuming Spleen *qi*, and because Fire is the mother of Earth, thereby weakening Heart *qi*.

At our second meeting Anna told me that her parents had always quarrelled a lot during her childhood and she had suffered as a result of the unstable situation. She yearned to provide her children with a happy family life.

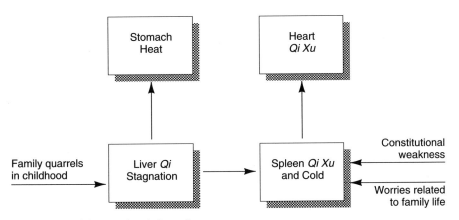

Fig. 28.1 Aetiology and pathology diagram.

Treatment issues

The *biao* principle of treatment was to soothe the Liver and regulate *qi*, and to clear Stomach Heat and restore the descending function of Stomach *qi*. The *ben* principle of treatment was to warm the middle and strengthen the Spleen. It was important to first resolve the Stomach and Liver pathology and then to fortify the Spleen (the background problem). I suggested to Anna that she continued taking Western drugs but reduced their intake as soon as she began to feel better and subsequently stopped them altogether.

I informed her that the treatment plan would comprise ten sessions of acupuncture, twice weekly for the first six sessions and once weekly for the last four sessions.

First treatment procedures

POINTS SELECTION

- LIV14 *qimen* to harmonise the Liver and Stomach.
- P6 *neiguan* to harmonise the Stomach, regulate Liver *qi*, calm the mind and subdue Stomach *qi*.
- ST21 *liangmen* to treat epigastric pain and stimulate the Stomach's descending functions.
- REN12 *zhongwan* and ST36 *zusanli* to stimulate Stomach *qi*.
- SP6 *sanyinjiao* to fortify the Spleen, protect Stomach *yin* and prevent injury by Stomach Fire.
- GB34 *yanglingquan* to soothe the Liver and eliminate stagnation.
- ST44 *neiting* to clear Stomach Heat.

Needling technique: Insertion of the needles was made with a guide tube.

For all the points, the *qi* sensation was obtained first. Reducing method was used on LIV14 *qimen*, P6 *neiguan*, ST21 *liangmen*, GB34 *yanglingquan* and ST44 *neiting*. Even method was used on REN12 *zhongwan*, ST36 *zusanli* and SP6 *sanyinjiao*. For all points 30 mm needles were used. Needles were retained for 20 minutes.

LIFESTYLE ADVICE

I suggested that Anna should eat slowly, avoid working and discussing business whilst eating and, most of all, avoid getting angry whilst eating. I advised her to avoid eating too much cold food, such as salad and fruit, and to eat rice.

After the fourth session, the burning nature of Anna's epigastric pain lessened. I eliminated from the therapy the use of ST44 *neiting,* and I added GB20 *fengchi* on the right (even method). I also began to use a moxa box on REN12 *zhongwan* and ST21 *liangmen*. GB20 *fengchi* on the right was used to eliminate Wind-Cold from the Gallbladder channel and to soothe Liver *qi* to treat the headaches.

After the first six sessions, the epigastric symptoms became less acute and the burning epigastric sensation ceased. After eight sessions, the epigastric symptoms completely disappeared. Anna's general condition had greatly improved — she experienced less tiredness, fewer headaches and less anxiety. At the end of the course of treatment the patient was completely recovered from the epigastric symptoms and her headaches and tiredness were ameliorated. I advised Anna to take Chinese herbal medicine, Free and Easy Wanderer *xiao yao wan* for 2 months to harmonise the Liver and Spleen.

Summary of outcome

- After the first six sessions, epigastric pain improved and the burning sensation lessened.
- After the eighth session, epigastric symptoms completely disappeared and the general condition of the patient improved with less tiredness, fewer headaches and less anxiety.
- After ten sessions, the patient had completely recovered from the epigastric symptoms and her headaches and tiredness were ameliorated.

Concluding remarks

During recent years I have treated an increasing number of patients with disharmony between Wood and Earth, as in this case. I think the reason this pathology is increasing in Italy is because of changes to the quality of the food which has become less digestible, less nutritious and less balanced than the traditional Mediterranean style of fresh food. In addition, people's mealtimes are no longer so in harmony with their physiological bio-rhythms. Fortunately, these people often respond well to treatment with acupuncture and Chinese herbal therapy.

In conclusion, I have been stunned by this case because I achieved such an excellent result in so few sessions, and because I knew the patient's husband. In Italy we say that the most difficult patients to treat are doctors and — particularly — doctor's wives!

FURTHER READING

Di Concetto G, Sotte L, Pippa L, Muccioli M 1992 Trattato di agopuntura e medicina Cinese. UTET, Torino

Muccioli M, Pippa L 1992 La farmacologia cinese, sostanze e rimedi naturali della medicina tradizionale cinese. Qiu Tian, San Marino

Sotte L 1988 Teoria e pratica del massaggio cinese, Civitanova Marche

Sotte L 1988 Rivista Italiana di Medicina Tradizionale Cinese No 3 'I catarri, classificazione e terapia'

Sotte L 1989 Rivista Italiana di Medicina Tradizionale Cinese No 6 'Le cefalee in medicina tradizionale cinese: agopuntura, farmacoterapia e massaggio'

Sotte L 1990 La farmacoterapia cinese: Manuale delle Prescrizioni. Qiu Tian, San Marino

Sotte L 1991 Rivista Italiana di Medicina Tradizionale Cinese No 1 'I principi generali della diagnostica cinese'

Sotte L 1992 Farmacologia cinese: la fitoterapia – principi, preparazioni ed uso dei rimedi vegetali. Red, Como

Sotte L 1994 Ricette naturali cinesi, Quaderni di Medicina Naturale, Civitanova Marche

Sotte L 1994 Massaggio cinese, edizioni mediterranee, Roma

Sotte L 1994 Il massaggio pediatrico cinese. Red, Como

Sotte L, Muccioli M 1992 Diagnosi e terapia in agopuntura e medicina cinese. Tecniche Nuove, Milano

■ Lucio Sotte

I work and live in Civitanova Marche, in the region of Marche, in central Italy. I graduated with an MD in Western Medicine at the University of Bologna in 1977 and specialised in anaesthesia and intensive care at the University of Trieste in 1980. At the beginning of my medical work (late 1970s) I was interested in acupuncture and its use in surgery for anaesthesia. I studied in France at the Centre d'Enseignement et de Diffusion de l'Acupuncture Traditionelle in Marseille and in Italy at the Italian School of TCM in Bologna. In 1981 I opened the first Italian public acupuncture service of the Italian National Health Service, in the hospital of my town. Practising reflexotherapy acupuncture, I continued my studies, receiving the Acupuncture Diploma of the Union at the School of Traditional Chinese Medicine in Switzerland, and making several visits to China, working under the supervision of famous Chinese teachers in the TCM Schools of Beijing and Guangzhou.

From 1983 I have been teaching acupuncture and Chinese massage at the Italian School of TCM in Bologna. In 1988, at the same school, I inaugurated the first Italian course of Chinese herbal therapy. Since 1990 I have taught acupuncture at the School of Medicine and Surgery at the University of Chieti, and Chinese herbal therapy at the School of Pharmacology at the University of Siena. I am a visited professor at the Guangzhou College of TCM.

Since 1990 I have been the editor of the Italian Journal of TCM (Rivista Italiana di Medicina Tradizionale Cinese) and I have been President of the Italian Society of Traditional and Chinese Herbal Therapy for 5 years.

When I began to study Chinese medicine it was impossible to find good publications on the subject in Italian. I worked with some of my friends at the Italian School of Chinese Medicine and, over the last 10 years, I have published, in Italian, more than 10 volumes concerning all the subjects of Chinese medicine.

Irritable bowel syndrome and a painful shoulder

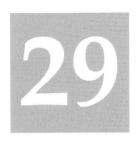

Bert Zandbergen ENSCHEDE, NETHERLANDS

A patient returns for acupuncture

When Jacob stepped into my office it was not the first time that he had consulted our clinic for acupuncture treatment. Three years before, he had come to seek treatment for occipital headaches of a deep and dull nature which radiated to the back of his head. His secondary complaints at that time were low back pain, asthmatic bronchitis and difficult evacuation of loose stools. My Chinese medical diagnosis at that time was of a Kidney and Spleen *yang xu* as the major pattern. After 12 treatments, the headaches disappeared, the respiratory problems subsided markedly and the stools became normal. All this crossed my mind when I shook Jacob's hand on this occasion. I noticed that it felt cold. This time he had been referred to our clinic because of a severely painful right shoulder, diagnosed as an inflammation of the supra-spinatus tendon and the subdeltoid bursa.

Jacob was a 52-year-old, tall, slim man, with a pale, sallow complexion and a lustreless face, who spoke in a toneless voice. Although he looked at me directly in the eyes, suggesting good communication, his eyes lacked lustre. My immediate feeling at that time was that Jacob was suffering from a *qi*, *yang* and Blood *xu* and a weakened *shen* or Spirit.

His chief complaint, the severely painful right shoulder, had started a couple of weeks before, quite suddenly, when he had woken one morning. The pain was present all the time and Jacob told me that cold and damp weather seemed to aggravate the condition. The pain covered the ventrolateral region of the shoulder and radiated down to the lateral side of the elbow. A hot shower did bring some temporary relief. Based on the good results of the acupuncture treatment 3 years earlier, he had decided to try acupuncture once again. I explained to him that I needed more information in order to understand the full nature of his complaint.

Depression and diarrhoea

He had been working for many years at a social security office, taking care of other people's affairs and worries. In a time of high unemployment, this obviously had been a demanding and stressful job, and had led to a period of overexertion, resulting in a period of mental depression about 3 years ago. As a result of his ill-health, he had been made redundant and an outplacement procedure[1] had been implemented. He now works for the Civil Servants' Union on a voluntary basis and he finds this rewarding and much less stressful.

At the time of his depression, he had suffered from acute diarrhoea for 5 weeks, for which his physician had found no specific cause. He had been prescribed medication and after a couple of days his defecation pattern returned to 'normal'. At the time of his consultation, his defecation was still normal although he experienced very difficult defecation once every 3 days. The first part of his stools was dry and hard, the second part very loose, containing undigested food particles. The biomedical diagnosis had been irritable bowel syndrome, complicated by diverticulitis. Therapy comprised a strict dietary regime of fresh and raw vegetables.

His situation now was that he evacuated his bowels once every 3 days only. On the first day after defecation he felt good but, starting during the second day and worsening during the third day, he suffered from difficult breathing, painful abdominal distension, occasional nausea and a stabbing, intermittent pain in the lower left quadrant of his abdomen. In general, he felt very tired, always cold and perspired spontaneously and profusely. In addition, he suffered from low back pain.

Physical examination

The physical examination revealed that his ankles were somewhat swollen and that, in general, Jacob felt sweaty and cold to the touch. Palpation showed that the epigastric and abdominal region was tense. A stabbing pain was elicited when I pressed the region ST29 *guilai* on the left side. REN12 *zhongwan* and ST25 *tianshu*, the front *mu* points of the Stomach and Large Intestine, were also painful upon palpation.

As a rule, I check the back *shu* points of my patients for tenderness and tension. In this case, BL25 *dachangshu* on the left side was very tense and the paraspinal muscles in that region were contracted and painful.

There was a marked tenderness of the ventrolateral region of the shoulder and there the skin felt cold to the touch. LI15 *jianyu* and the centre of the deltoid muscle reacted upon palpation as *ah shi* points. His tongue was pale, slightly swollen and a little wet. The edges were wetter, paler and covered with transverse cracks. In the centre was a deep and wide central crack which extended forward to just behind the tip. There was a thin yellowish coating at the root only. The pulses were deep, weak, fine and a little wiry. Both rear positions were weakest.

During these procedures Jacob remained calm and relaxed, as if he did not have enough energy to react to my hands-on examination. At the same time, I realised it could have been that he had confidence in me as a practitioner. This was a reassuring feeling for me, because it showed that we were really communicating which, in my opinion, is a prerequisite for a successful therapeutic intervention.

Summary of clinical manifestations

- Pain and tenderness at the ventrolateral region of the right shoulder, radiating down to the lateral side of the elbow; worse on exposure to cold and damp weather; sudden onset.
- Right shoulder cold to touch.
- Pale and sallow complexion, eyes lack lustre.
- Low energy, feels very tired and perspires spontaneously.
- Cold hands and feet, sweaty and cold to touch.
- Difficulty in evacuating stools, occurs once every 3 days; first part dry and the second part very loose with undigested particles.
- Periods of constipation accompanied by a feeling of abdominal distension, low abdominal fullness and a stabbing pain in the left lower quadrant of the abdomen, also asthmatic breathing and nausea; after every defecation these symptoms disappear.
- Low back pain and slightly swollen ankles.
- Tongue: is pale, slightly swollen and somewhat wet, with transverse cracks on the edges and a wide deep central crack, yellowish coating on the root only.
- Pulse: is deep, weak, fine, slightly wiry, both rear positions weaker.
- Palpation: pain at ST29 *guilai* left, REN12 *zhongwan*, ST25 *tianshu*; tension at BL25 *dachangshu*; paraspinal muscles contracted and painful; tenderness in the ventrolateral region of the shoulder, cold to touch; LI15 *jianyu* and the centre of the deltoid muscle react as *ah shi* points.

Identifying the patterns of disharmony

As far as the painful shoulder was concerned, the Chinese medical diagnosis seemed straightforward. The sudden onset and the severity of the pain suggested the presence of an external pathogenic influence, causing an obstruction of the flow of *qi* and Blood in the Large Intestine meridian, resulting in a local *shi* condition. As cold and damp weather seemed to aggravate the condition I diagnosed a Cold and Damp *bi* syndrome. However, the other relevant signs and symptoms denoted an internal disbalance of a much more chronic nature.

The low energy, the spontaneous perspiration, together with the pale, swollen tongue and weak pulse indicated a *qi xu* condition. The sallow complexion, the weakened *shen* Spirit and the fine pulse showed that there was also a Blood *xu* condition. The general feeling of cold and the wetness of the tongue denoted a progression toward a *yang xu* condition. In order to refine this internal picture I interpreted the swollen ankles, the low back pain and the weak rear pulse positions as pointing to a Kidney *yang xu*, whereas the loose stools, containing undigested food particles, were manifestations of a Spleen *yang xu*.

The Kidney and Spleen *yang xu* condition manifested as an internal deficiency of Cold, accumulating in the Large Intestine. The resulting slow bowel movement caused an accumulation of faeces, which after 3 days reached the point of a complete stagnation of *qi* in the Large Intestine. The Kidney *yang xu* was not able to grasp the Lung *qi* and keep it down and this, combined with a hindrance of the descending of *qi* in general, caused the asthmatic condition and the nauseous periods.

The *qi* and *yang xu* condition, together with the disturbance of the descending and spreading function of the Lung *qi* on the one hand and the internal Cold in the Large Intestine on the other hand, predisposed the Large Intestine meridian to an invasion of external Cold and Damp pathogenic influence.

So far, this way of reasoning seemed sound and logical. Still, I was puzzled by the yellowish coating on the root of the tongue and the wide central crack. I assumed that the accumulated Cold and the resulting stagnation were beginning to transform into Heat, which explained the yellow colour of the coating. As for the central crack, this could be because of a constitutional *yin xu* of the stomach. In particular, the combination of a wide central crack and transverse cracks on the sides of the tongue can be observed in a chronic Stomach *yin xu* and Spleen *qi xu*, also known as a Spleen *yin xu* (Maciocia 1987).

Obviously, the main shoulder complaint could be seen as the *biao*, whereas the internal disharmony, a composition of three patterns of disharmony, could be considered the *ben*.

Patterns of disharmony

THE *BIAO*

Cold-Damp *bi* syndrome of the Large Intestine meridian

- Severe pain of a rather sudden onset in the ventrolateral region of the shoulder, radiating downwards along the Large Intestine meridian.
- Shoulder cold to touch.
- Pain aggravated in cold and damp conditions.

THE BEN

Kidney and Spleen *yang xu*

- Low energy and spontaneous perspiration.
- General feeling of coldness.
- Swollen ankles and low back pain.
- Undigested food particles in the loose part of the stool.
- Sallow complexion and weakened *shen* Spirit.

- Tongue: pale, slightly swollen and wet.
- Pulse: deep and fine, both rear positions weaker.

Large Intestine Cold/deficient

- Slow bowel movement, defecation every 3 days.
- Difficulty in evacuation of stools, which are mainly loose and not smelling.
- Stabbing intermittent pain in lower left abdomen, relieved after defecation.
- Tongue: coating at the root.

Disturbance in the ascending/descending of *qi* and Lung *qi* deficiency

- Asthmatic breathing.
- Periods of nausea and epigastric fullness.

Stagnation of *qi* in the Large Intestine

- Intermittent stabbing pain in the lower left abdominal quadrant.
- Symptom relieved by defecation.

Aetiology and pathology

Emotions

The years of taking care of other people's worries and uncertainties, at a time of social insecurity and unemployment, must have caused pensiveness and worry, over time weakening Spleen and Lung *qi*. A weak Spleen means that, amongst other things, transformation and transportation processes in the body are not performed adequately, which, on a non-physical level, can cause mental depression. In addition, the Earth element, namely Spleen and Stomach, are not able to nourish Metal, namely Lungs and Large Intestine. Chronic Spleen *qi* deficiency progressed into Spleen *yang* deficiency. The close connection between Spleen *yang* and Kidney *yang* is the reason that chronic Spleen *yang xu* depletes Kidney *yang*. The outplacement procedure and the struggle against it obviously caused irritation and frustration. This rather acute type of emotion must have caused a stagnation of Liver *qi*, which attacked the already weakened Spleen *yang*, resulting in the acute diarrhoea. After losing his battle, he felt insecurity, fear and anxiety towards the future. These are emotions which damaged Kidney *qi* even more.

Dietary

The Kidney and Spleen *yang xu* is maintained or even worsened by the strict diet of raw and cold vegetables.

External pathogenic influence

When Kidney *yang* is weak, the *yang* of the whole body becomes weak, including the defensive potential of the body, the *wei qi*. Moreover, Spleen *yang*, together with Stomach *qi*, is responsible for the production of *qi* and

Blood, including the *wei qi*. The weakened Lung *qi* (Earth not nourishing Metal), is not properly spreading and descending. *Wei qi xu*, combined with insufficient spreading of Lung *qi*, makes the body extremely vulnerable to invasion of external cold and damp. In particular, the Large Intestine meridian, in this case, is easily invaded by cold, because Spleen *yang xu* and Kidney *yang xu* manifest as an internal deficiency of Cold in the Large Intestine. Finally, Kidney *yang xu* means that Lung *qi*, already not descending properly, is not sufficiently grasped and kept down. This, combined with the accumulation of faeces in the Large Intestine, causes a disturbance in the ascending and descending of *qi* (Fig. 29.1).

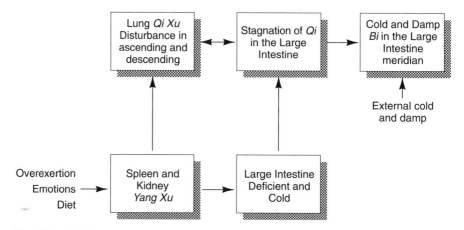

Fig. 29.1 Aetiology and pathology diagram.

Treatment issues

The treatment principles in order of importance were:

1 Remove the Cold and Damp from the Large Intestine meridian and restore normal circulation of *qi* and Blood in the meridian.
2 Tonify and warm Kidney and Spleen *yang*.
3 Restore the *qi* circulation in the Large Intestine.
4 Adjust ascending and descending of *qi*.

I decided first to focus on the shoulder pain because it was quite severe. However, based on the principle that acupuncture needs to have two actions, 'to fight the pathogenic *qi* and to support the anti-pathogenic *qi*', I would also tonify and warm the Kidney and Spleen *yang*. If this approach did not restore a normal circulation of *qi* in the Large Intestine and adjust the ascending and descending of *qi*, I could always focus on these imbalances at a later phase. I expected the shoulder problem to be resolved within ten treatments over 5 weeks, and I related this information to Jacob. As far as the other imbalances were concerned, I surely would need at least a further ten treatments. Even then I could not be sure that a complete restoration of the normal bowel function would be possible. The treatment costs would be reimbursed by the insurance company, and therefore money was not a major issue.

I told Jacob that his 'part of the deal' would be to practise abdominal breathing[2] for 10 minutes every day, to eat cooked vegetables, and to avoid cold food and beverages.

First treatment

Having explained to Jacob where I was going to insert the needles and the extent and nature of discomfort he might expect, I asked him to lie down on the treatment couch, in the supine position. He still seemed very relaxed, and so I first explained to him the procedure of abdominal breathing, which he mastered within 5 minutes.

After inserting a needle at LI4 *hegu* on the right side with an even needle manipulation, I selected LI15 *jianyu* on the right side and used a reducing needle technique. I then chose LIV3 *taichong* on the left side and treated with an even manipulation. Leaving the needles in place, I immediately inserted LU7 *lieque* on the left side. In order to scatter the Cold, I warmed LI15 *jianyu* with moxa on the needle.

Fifteen minutes later, I selected KID7 *fuliu* and ST36 *zusanli* on both sides, together with REN6 *qihai*. I burned moxa on the needles at ST36 *zusanli* and REN6 *qihai*. I removed the needles after 35 minutes. During the treatment I made sure that Jacob continued with his abdominal breathing. Immediately after the treatment he told me that his shoulder pain was much reduced.

First treatment procedures

POINTS PRESCRIPTION

- LI4 *hegu* alleviates pain in general; also, used as a distal point it removes obstruction from the meridian; as a *yuan* source point it stimulates the function of the Large Intestine; when used in combination with LU7 *lieque*, it stimulates the dispersing function of the Lung; and when used in combination with LIV3 *taichong*, it harmonises the ascending and descending of *qi*.
- LI15 *jianyu*: major point for *bi* syndrome of the shoulder.
- LIV *taichong*: promotes the free flow of Liver *qi* and removes stagnation in general and specifically in the lower burner when combined with REN6

qihai; together with LI4 *hegu* it adjusts ascending and descending.

- LU7 *lieque:* the *luo* point, connecting the Lung meridian to the Large Intestine meridian; in combination with LI4 *hegu,* it reinforces the Large Intestine meridian and at the same time stimulates the descending of Lung *qi,* supporting the evacuation of the stools; the combination with REN6 *qihai* promotes the grasping and holding of the Lung *qi* by the Kidneys.

- ST36 *zusanli:* tonifies *qi* and Blood, by tonifying the root of post-heaven *qi,* i.e. Spleen and Stomach; regulates ascending and descending of the central *qi,* thus supporting the adjustment of ascending and descending in general; tonifies Lung *qi,* because of the principle of 'Mother nourishing the Son'; regulates *ying qi* and *wei qi,* helping to push out the Cold and the Damp and regulating the sweating from deficiency.

- REN6 *qihai:* tonifies *qi* and *yang;* tonifies *yuan qi* and Kidney *yang;* moves *qi* in the lower burner, thus dispelling stagnation, especially in combination with LIV3 *taichong;* helps to keep down the Lung *qi,* especially in combination with LU7 *lieque;* the combination REN6 *qihai,* ST36 *zusanli* and LI4 *hegu* promotes the production and spreading of *wei qi.*

Needling technique: LI15 *jianyu,* REN6 *qihai* and ST36 *zusanli* were needled with 40 mm needles, gauge 30. The other points were needled with 25 mm needles, gauge 30. Where possible, given the patient's level of deficiency, I used unilateral needling so as to limit the number of needles.

Moxa: this was used on the needles at points LI15 *jianyu,* ST36 *zusanli* and REN6 *qihai.*

Adjusting the point combinations

After six treatments the shoulder pain completely disappeared, and Jacob perspired much less. Also, he felt less cold in general. However, the defecation pattern did not change, nor did the frequency and intensity of the asthmatic periods. So I adjusted the combination of points and decided to concentrate more on treating the accumulation of faeces and the circulation of *qi* in the Large Intestine, hoping that this would influence the descending of Lung *qi* as well. With a reducing needling technique, I started with ST25 *tianshu* and ST37 *shangjuxu* which are, respectively, the front *mu* point and lower *he* point of the Large Intestine. I combined these points with LI4 *hegu* and LU7 *lieque* on the left and right side respectively. I completed the combination with LIV3 *taichong* on the left side and REN6 *qihai.* I burned moxa on the needle at REN6 *qihai.* After 25 minutes I removed the needles and finished the treatment with a tonifying technique on BL25 *dachangshu* using needles only.

After this treatment I told Jacob to expect an increase in bowel movement. From this point onwards, treatment continued once weekly. After six further treatments, Jacob no longer perspired spontaneously, he defecated once daily and his asthmatic periods had disappeared. His shoulder pain never returned. However, the stools were still very loose.

We decided to continue the treatment, decreasing the frequency and adjusting the combination of points. Chosen points were SP6 *sanyinjiao*, ST36 *zusanli* and REN6 *qihai* combined with LU7 *lieque* on the left side, with removal of the needles after 20 minutes, followed by BL20 *pishu* and BL25 *dachangshu*. All points were tonified, including those on SP6 *sanyinjiao*, REN6 *qihai* and BL20 *pishu*. After another six treatments he still defecated once daily and the stools had gradually become firmer. All other symptoms had disappeared.

At this point we both were curious as to what would happen if we discontinued the treatment. So we did. After 4 weeks Jacob called to tell me that the intestinal problems had recurred, although they were not as severe as they had been previously. Since that point, Jacob received ten further treatments on a regular basis, with an average frequency of one treatment every 3 weeks. Once again he was symptom-free and we discontinued the treatment for a second time. A follow up consultation after 3 months has shown that he is still functioning very well without any complaints.

Summary of outcome

- No longer any shoulder pain.
- Feels good, no tiredness.
- No perspiration.
- Frequent bowel movement, daily evacuation of firm stools.
- No respiratory complaints.
- Is satisfied with the situation as it is.
- Pulse: stronger in every position.
- Tongue: normal shape and colour, still a wide central crack and a tiny little bit of yellowish coating at the root.

Creating a positive image

Although this case was not particularly unusual, there were several challenging and difficult aspects to it. First of all, Jacob's condition was rather chronic. Secondly, the internal disharmony clearly existed on more than just the physical level: it was caused by long-standing emotional stress which, in turn, caused the disharmony to persist. This implied that the therapeutic intervention should be based, not only on proper point selection and correct needling, but also on effective non-physical communication between the patient and myself.

The key to the successful outcome is the fact that acupuncture can be effective on the physical, emotional and spiritual level simultaneously. This effectiveness can only be achieved when there is a sound therapeutic communication between patient and therapist. As this was the case from my first session with Jacob, I allowed myself to express a positive prognosis from the start, and this was reinforced by his positive attitude towards treatment.

In a broad sense, as we create a positive image of the art of acupuncture, combined with a commitment to and respect for our patients, we are making a contribution to the spreading and acceptance of a wonderful healing system in our Western world.

NOTES

1 The outplacement procedure involves the employer, which in Jacob's case was the Government, hiring an external agency to help the ex-employee find another job, paying for the cost of retraining and, in the case of long-standing illness, ensuring admission to the social security system. In practice, this procedure can be used by the employer to evade problems with the Union to the disadvantage of the employee. Jacob felt that he was victimised when he was 'wasted and dumped' by his employer. So he struggled against the outplacement procedure, but in the end he was not able to beat the organisation. He still bears a grudge against his former employer.

2 Abdominal breathing has benefits at three levels.
   i. On the physical level it relaxes the diaphragm and, by so doing, regulates the Upper Burner. Furthermore, by facilitating the descending of Lung *qi* and connecting it with the *qi* of the Kidneys and Large Intestines, it assists in the expulsion of faeces. It also regulates the ascending and descending of *qi*.
   ii. On the mental level, the focus of the patient's mind is on REN6 *qihai*, thus connecting the *shen* (Spirit) to the *jing*, and the Upper Burner to the Lower Burner. Moreover, REN6 *qihai* works on the edge of the Spleen and the Kidney, thereby connecting the Middle Burner to the Lower Burner. All three burners are therefore connected.
   iii. On the spiritual level, REN6 *qihai* 'makes a person able to see the four directions, while being in the middle' (Kaptchuk T, personal communication, 1991). In other words, it creates vision and awareness because REN6 *qihai* enables the experiences of the preciousness of the moment (the virtue of the Lung meridian) to be transformed into wisdom (the virtue of the Kidney meridian).
   This understanding of REN6 *qihai* and its relation to abdominal breathing is based on an integration of my personal interpretation of material published by Matsumoto & Birch (1988), information gathered from discussions with T. Petzholdt (personal communication, 1993) and also on the ideas of Ted Kaptchuk (personal communication, 1991) concerning the spiritual aspects of traditional Chinese medicine.

REFERENCES

Maciocia G 1987 Tongue diagnosis in Chinese medicine. Eastland Press, Seattle
Matsumoto K, Birch S 1988 Hara diagnosis: reflections of the sea. Paradigm, Boston

■ Bert Zandbergen

Bert Zandbergen is an acupuncturist and Chinese herbalist in Enschede, the Netherlands, where he has practised since 1985. He graduated at the Anglo-Dutch Institute for Oriental Medicine in Haarlem, the Netherlands. He has lectured at the Anglo-Dutch Institute since 1987 and is presently the Director of Education at this Institute. He hopes to graduate with a Masters degree in psychology in the near future. He is especially interested in the mutual interaction of emotional disturbances and the condition of the *zang* and the *fu*. Having studied both Chinese medicine and psychology, he hopes to be able to contribute to the integration of both acupuncture and Chinese herbal medicine into our Western society.

During his acupuncture training, he was very much influenced by the publication of the book *The web that has no weaver* by Dr Ted Kaptchuk and *Zangfu, the organ systems of TCM* by Jeremy Ross. Later, in 1992, his style was influenced by Ted Kaptchuk's perspective on the emotional and spiritual aspects of Chinese medicine. Recently, he has returned to his roots, becoming increasingly interested in the hands-on style of acupuncture which has been brought forward by, among others, Dr Kiiko Matsumoto. During his 10 years of practice, he has become aware that we can learn most from our unsuccessful or partly successful cases, and the case study he has submitted falls into this category. Such cases demonstrate the deficits of our knowledge and confirm that the study of Chinese medicine is a lifelong profession.

An Achilles heel

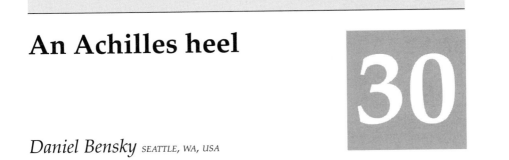

Daniel Bensky SEATTLE, WA, USA

Ms D was a 49-year-old, self-employed business woman. She appeared self-possessed and decisive. She had clearly come to our clinic as a last resort and had no previous experience of acupuncture or any other alternative therapies or treatments.

The first thing I do with any patient is global listening, which is a way of using one's hands to feel directly those part(s) of the body where there is some restriction or stagnation. In Ms D's case, this procedure led me to the liver and the right lower extremity. The area over the liver was warm. In addition the feet were cold, especially the right foot. Direct palpation of the channels revealed a sense of both constraint and deficiency in the Liver channels bilaterally throughout their course. The tongue was dark (most pronounced on the edges) and also pale; the pulse was wiry with a deficiency in the Liver position.

Recalcitrant Achilles tendonitis

Ms D had recalcitrant Achilles tendonitis of 4 years' duration. Originally in both ankles, she had received multiple types of conventional medical treatment including physical therapy, ultrasound, local cortisone injections, and an immobilising boot. The latter had helped the left ankle but she had resisted trying it on the right.

Until the onset of the problem, Ms D had run regularly and had also walked about 3 miles each day. Walking was very important to her as she used the time both to discuss her business and spend time with her husband who was also her business partner. While she continued to exercise, riding a stationary bicycle, she really missed the active time spent with her husband.

When she came to see me, her right ankle felt the weaker of the two and throbbed after any significant activity. Local application of ice and bandaging of the ankle were helpful. However, she had not been able to walk even a mile for a considerable period of time.

She described herself as impatient and stubborn. However, her challenging and sceptical attitude was clear and without animosity. I was immediately comfortable with her and felt that we could frankly discuss anything relating to her problem. While on the spectrum of possible health problems this was not a particularly severe disorder, I felt that it was a serious problem to Ms D.

Further history was mostly unremarkable. Her menstrual cycle was usually around 28 days with light periods of long duration. She reported no particular symptoms relating to her menstrual cycle. On further examination of the ankle areas there was diffuse dull tenderness around both Achilles tendons and discrete, tender nodules on the distal, medial aspect of the right ankle.

Clinical manifestations

- Right, painful Achilles tendon, worse with movement, better with rest.
- Diffuse, dull tenderness around both Achilles tendons.
- Nodule in the lower anteromedial aspect of the right Achilles tendon.
- Restriction at the liver.
- Restriction of lower right extremity; area over liver warm.
- Liver channel deficient and constrained.
- Feet cold.
- Self-directed, self-possessed and determined personality.
- Entrepreneurial lifestyle.
- Pulse: wiry, with deficiency in the Liver position.
- Tongue: dark and pale, with darker edges.

A diagnosis on three levels

When working with patients, particularly those with some clearly circumscribed chief complaint, I prefer to approach them on three levels. First, I try to gain an understanding as to the root (*běn*) of the problem. Sometimes I interpret the root using what I understand to be the Chinese perspective, i.e. the root is clearly and directly related to the symptoms. Sometimes I take what to me is more of a Japanese approach, where the root is something like the background or terrain over which everything else occurs and may not directly relate to the symptoms (Shudo 1990). Secondly, I look at the localised problems that brought the patient in and give a general diagnosis. Part of this process is choosing which theoretical system or filter to use. Finally, I try to gain a specific understanding of the particular problem in the particular patient. Often all three of these assessments of the patient are congruent; sometimes they are not.

In general, I use the most direct and quickest forms of diagnosis. The longer I spend in talking or thinking, the more likely I am to make up a diagnosis that appeals to me, rather than one that reflects the actual person. For this reason I favour first doing the palpatory examination and then taking a quick, focused history. This relates to my own strengths, weaknesses, and preferences. That is, I am quite weak visually, I do not particularly like talking to patients, and I have the benefit of a modicum of osteopathic training.

A root diagnosis

The primary osteopathic methods used in this case were developed by the French osteopath Jean-Pierre Barral. These are clear, quick, focused techniques which identify relatively important areas of the body with limited motion. A practitioner applying these techniques is actively engaged but receptive, like a good listener. Indeed, Barral calls these techniques 'listening' (Barral 1989, Barral & Mercier 1988). The listening is done before talking to the patient so that it is objective. In this case, I was drawn to the liver and the right ankle. I interpreted this as evidence that some liver-related dysfunction was contributing to the ankle problem.

The direct palpation of various flows in the channels is a technique that requires some imagination. It is done by touching important points on the 12 or 14 primary channels and imagining that one can tune into these channels. I have practised this technique for approximately 12 years and it has been helpful to me in about one-third of cases. In this case, what I felt was a hollowness of the Liver channel (equal bilaterally) together with an increase in tension (bilaterally but more on the right).

These findings were reinforced by the pulse (overall wiry with deficiency in the deep aspect of the left middle position) and the darkness along the edges of an otherwise pale tongue. These findings all suggested the presence of both deficiency and constraint in the Liver, a combination which, in my experience, is quite common. Unless it appears to be especially useful, I do not differentiate channels from organs from axes. If not merely facets of the same thing, they are extremely closely related. In this case, this diagnosis served as the root. The lack of significant menstrual disorder was not fully congruent with my interpretation but I simply ignored this fact.

A local diagnosis

The next step is to have a diagnosis for the chief complaint itself. Here we have a clearly localised musculoskeletal problem. I have recently learned the barrier point system for these types of problems as developed by the French Acupuncture Association (AFA) under the leadership of Jean-Marc Kespi and taught to me by Gérard Guillaume and Peter Eckman (Guillaume & Chieu 1990, Kespi 1982). One very useful part of this system is the application of the eight parameters *(bā gāng)* to local musculoskeletal phenomena. In Ms D's case this leads to a local diagnosis of *yin* deficiency. Why? *Yin* deficient pain becomes worse with motion, better with rest and immobilisation, and is helped by the local application of ice. This described Ms D's pain exactly. Notice that this is a purely *local* diagnosis and is not necessarily connected in any way with the patient's constitution or their systemic diagnosis. It is quite possible that a person who appears to have *yang* deficiency systemically could have *yang* excess type pain in a joint.

Once you have characterised the pain in the eight parameters, the barrier point system has a protocol for deciding which point on which channel should be used. According to this system, a *yin* deficient type pain in the ankle is a terminal *yin (jué yīn)* problem and should be treated by needling LIV6 *zhōng dū*. This served as my local diagnosis.

A specific diagnosis

When possible, I like to have a more specific diagnosis that allows me to think that I have a handle on what is going on with this person at this time. By this I mean some idea why this particular person developed this specific problem. For Ms D, I wanted to have at least a guess as to why she developed pain in the particular area and not somewhere else. This might also have given me a clue as to why her problem had been so recalcitrant.

As Achilles tendon problems involve the sinews which relate to the Liver, just treating the Liver or the Liver/Gallbladder system could be an attractive approach. I prefer to have a more specific link to problems, especially when I use herbs. In this case topography came to my rescue. The part of the tendon involved was clearly along the lesser *yin* or Kidney channel. This fine tuning directed me towards finding some lesser *yin* approach that would include the Liver.

My cursory and generalised impression of Ms D as a self-directed, self-possessed and decisive individual, together with her self-description of stubborness and impatience, did not go against the general tone of the diagnosis. I did not give too much thought to the aetiology in this case. Given the patient's nature, I assumed (without evidence) that after suffering some slight injury to her heel, she had continued to stress it beyond the point where it could heal itself.

This is the way in which I normally proceed as I like to meet my patients at the point at which they are. This involves learning all I need to know, and no more than I need to know, in order to treat them. I envisage acupuncture treatment to be a conversation or a call-and-response procedure. Once we start to work, the patient's response to treatment enables us to see whether or not our diagnosis is correct.

Evidence for patterns of disharmony

Root diagnosis: Liver deficiency/ constraint

- Restriction at liver, area over liver warm.
- Liver channel palpated as hollow (bilaterally), with increase in tension (bilaterally, but more on the right).
- Cold feet.
- Pulse: wiry with deficiency in the Liver position.
- Tongue: pale with darker edges.

Local diagnosis: Local *yin* deficiency

- Achilles tendon pain.

- Pain worse with movement.
- Pain better with rest.

Specific diagnosis: Lesser *yin* aspect of the Liver

- Symptoms and signs in the root diagnosis above.
- Pain focused on the medial aspect of the Achilles tendon.
- Pain originally bilateral.
- Recalcitrant problem.
- Cold hands and feet.

Keeping the first treatment simple

I usually keep first treatments as simple as possible. I first validated Ms D's concerns by explaining that our goal was to work together in order that she might walk again with her husband as soon as possible. I alluded to some possible lifestyle changes but did not talk about specifics. I told her that she could continue to apply ice to her ankle but for no more than 10 minutes per hour and only when and if the pain was acute. She was only to stretch carefully (I demonstrated the correct stretches for the soleus and gastrocnemius muscles) and to stop immediately if she experienced discomfort. I also told her the general outline of the diagnosis.

Relying on palpation

For acupuncture I used one point on each side of the body. As noted above, in the barrier point system, the point for this type of problem should be LIV6 *zhōng dū*, the cleft point. However, I have an inherent distrust of formulaic approaches to anything, acupuncture not excepted. Given my own strengths, I rely on palpation to decide what points to use and their exact location. I use three approaches. First, moving my hand quickly, I feel with my palm about 5 cm above the body around the area of concern, looking for areas that feel relatively hot. Secondly, with my eyes closed, I stroke along the channels in question, feeling for areas of increased resistance or 'stickiness'. If I have to press harder to feel the resistance, I will probably have to needle deeper. These two modes of palpation act as confirmation of each other. Finally, once I think I know where the point is, I needle it. If it is a correct point, then I will be able to feel the *qi* arrive. This is the golden standard of acupuncture. If I do not feel the *qi*, I stop and start the whole process again.

In this case, the point that was felt was LIV5 *lí gōu* on the right. Upon finding this point, I reflected and realised that the combination of deficiency and constraint in this case made appropriate the use of the collateral (*luò*) point. So, while I had used the barrier point system to allow me to focus on the foot terminal *yin* Liver channel, I let the palpatory examination guide me to the specific treatment. This involved switching the theoretical emphasis. The other point used was a reactive point on the left ankle, posterior to KID3 *tài xī*. I take this as a form of 'eccentric needling' (*miù zhēn*) as described in Chapter 63 of the 'Basic Questions' (*Sùwèn*).

Changes occurring during treatment

I subscribe to the belief that for acupuncture to make a change in a patient's condition, some changes must occur during the treatment. This is especially true if we treat people every 7–14 days instead of every 2–3 days. Of course it is necessary to be sure that all the needles 'connect' to the intended channel and that this connection goes as far as is necessary. In addition, it is a good idea to check all relevant signs after every needle or so.

Fortunately, in this case, once the needles were in place there was a significant positive change in the tongue and pulse, together with other positive findings. Needles were left in place until they could be pulled out easily. This is my common practice and is based on my understanding of the statement in Chapter 1 of the 'Divine Pivot' (*Língshū*) about the relation of needling to the arrival of *qi*. In this treatment the needles were ready to come out after about 20 minutes.

Chinese herbs

The combination of signs and symptoms of a Liver root and a lesser *yin* branch, together with the cold feet and warm hypochondrium, led me to use a modified version of Frigid Extremities Powder *sì nì sǎn*. This is a lesser *yin* stage formula which is generally used for Liver disorders in addition to its more classic use for hot-type collapse (*jué*). I added Fructus Chaenomelis Lagenariae *mù guā* for its effects on the sinews, especially of the legs, and substituted Herba Artemisiae Yinchenhao *yīn chén hāo* for Radix Bupleuri *chái hú* as I believed that the latter was too scattering and ascending for this particular patient. Herba Artemisiae Yinchenhao *yīn chén hāo* is a good herb to use for structural Liver complaints, including biomedically-defined liver disorders. I believe that this can be extended to such conditions as tendon problems with discrete nodules.

This formula was first noted in paragraph 318 of the 'Discussion of cold-induced disorders' (*Shang han lun jiang jie*), where it was placed in the section dealing with lesser *yin* disorders (Wang Qi et al 1988). Practising Oriental medicine has taught me that these confluences are not arbitrary and I use them assiduously whenever I observe them. In this case, they led to my working diagnosis of disruption of the lesser *yin* aspect of the Liver system which underlay Ms D's vulnerability to long-term problems with the medial aspect of her Achilles tendon.

First treatment procedures

ACUPUNCTURE

- LIV5 *lí gōu*, on the right. This point is on the foot terminal *yin* Liver channel and was chosen on the basis of palpation; it is also a collateral *(luò)* point.
- Point posterior to KID3 *tài xī*, a reactive point on the left ankle, and chosen as a form of 'eccentric needling' *(miù zhēn)*.

Needles: I used 34 gauge, 40 mm needles and treated the right side first (for no particular reason).

Retention: Needles were left in place until they could be pulled out easily, which was after 20 minutes.

CHINESE HERBS

A modified version of Frigid Extremities Powder *sì nì sǎn* was prescribed as it is a lesser *yin* stage formula often used for Liver disorders. The total dosage was 36 g which was ground into a fine powder. One teaspoon of herbs (less than 3 g) was taken as a draft (boiled with 1 cup of water for 10 minutes, strained, and drunk) once a day in the morning.

Enjoying the trip

When Ms D returned to our clinic a week later she told us that she had felt better immediately after the treatment and was able to walk 3 miles a day within a few days. She was stretching faithfully and had not used ice. She was encouraged as were we.

In addition, she remarked that she had felt like crying off and on during the first day that she had taken the herbs. Then she began to notice a change in some aspects of her outlook on life. Previously, when commuting or travelling, she had not enjoyed the journey because she was so focused on her destination. Now she noticed things along the way and began to enjoy her trips — she could 'smell the roses along the path'. This change, whilst very welcome, was surprising to her as previously she had not noticed this aspect of her being or thought its absence a problem. We took this opportunity to talk with her about her life, what it means to express oneself, and how that fits in with the traditional Oriental concept of the Liver.

While I had expected some significant improvement and a subtle light-ening of her disposition, I was somewhat surprised by the extent of the change. I have observed that 'Wood' people can respond intensely to treatment, and with luck that response can be positive. There was also significant improvement in Ms D's tongue and pulse, and there were other positive signs: more energy, more even temper, finding it easier to breathe.

We saw Ms D three more times in the ensuing 6 weeks, continuing the acupuncture treatment of 2 to 4 needles per session. As she improved, the wiry aspect of the pulse dissipated, the darkness went out of her tongue, and the palpatory findings also improved. The third treatment, however, was a little too similar to the earlier treatments and I had not detected that whilst the constraint had improved, the deficiency had become more marked, even though this is a common occurrence. Hence, Ms D had a day of increased pain after this treatment. At the next treatment I modified both the acupuncture and herbal remedy, adding LIV8 *qū quán*, KID10 *yīn gǔ* and Sclerotium Poriae Cocos *fú líng* and this reaction did not occur a second time.

Ms D continued to walk and began exercises to strengthen the muscles of both plantar flexion and dorsiflexion. By the fourth treatment the pulse was no longer wiry, the tongue was a normal colour and slightly scalloped. At this point we recommended that she attended a follow-up visit at the clinic every month for 2–3 months as she regained normal strength and flexibility. At her 1-month follow-up she continued to show improvement with increased walking ability with little or no pain.

Summary of outcome

- Now walking 3 miles a day with little or no pain.
- Appreciating journeys, no longer focusing exclusively on her destination.

- Palpatory findings improved.
- Pulse: no longer wiry.
- Tongue: normal color, slightly scalloped.

Therapeutic minimalism

I enjoyed this case immensely. First of all, I had the chance to work with my favourite type of patient — an intelligent, focused, and sceptical indivi-dual. Secondly, I was able to indulge in one of my favourite approaches, that of therapeutic minimalism. I really get a kick out of having a positive impact on someone's life by simply using a couple of acupuncture points every week or so and about 3 g a day of ground herbs. This supports my belief that the appeal of any type of natural medicine is its ability to encourage and direct the body's own healing mechanisms. Here, as is often the case, I pick and choose from among various Oriental medical theories. The one I decide to use generally depends upon my palpatory findings together with certain aspects that strike me about the patient.

REFERENCES

Barral J-P 1989 Visceral manipulation. Eastland Press, Seattle
Barral J-P, Mercier P 1988 Visceral manipulation. Eastand Press, Seattle
Guillaume G, Chieu M 1990 Rhumatologie et médicine traditionelle chinois, La Tisserande, Paris. English-language edition 1996. Eastland Press, Seattle
Kespi J-M 1982 Acupuncture. Maisonneuve, Paris
Shudo D 1990 Japanese classical acupuncture: introduction to meridian therapy. Eastand Press, Seattle
Wang Qi, Zheng Qizhong and Yan Yanli 1988 Explanation of the discussion of cold-induced disorders (Shang han lun jiang jie). Henan Science and Technology Press, Xinxiang

FURTHER READING

Ren Y-Q 1986 Huang di nei jing zhang ju suo yin (Yellow Emperor's inner classic by chapter and sections with index). People's Medical, Beijing

ACKNOWLEDGEMENT

This case came about as part of the observational clinic at our school. I would like to thank all of the students involved for giving me the opportunity to work with them.

■ Daniel Bensky

I have a Diploma in Chinese Medicine from the Macau Institute of Chinese Medicine (1975), a Bachelor of Arts in Chinese Language and Literature from the University of Michigan (1978), and a Doctor of Osteopathy from the Michigan State University College of Osteopathic Medicine (1982). Currently I have a private practice in Seattle, Washington, am a director of the Seattle Institute of Oriental Medicine, and also am a medical editor at Eastland Press. Over time I have been fortunate enough to have opportunities to study with many wonderful teachers who have had great insight. Perhaps the first and foremost among my influences in acupuncture was Regina Ling, originally from Shanghai, who was kind enough to teach me in Taiwan. She impressed on me the importance of paying attention and that for acupuncture to be successful, the practitioner needs to obtain the desired sensation through the needle. I must admit that I was 'rotten wood' for her at the time, but believe that some of what she tried to teach me has percolated through my consciousness over the last 20 years. The Japanese practitioner, Shudō Denmei, whom I was fortunate to learn from while editing the English-language edition of his book, also made a lasting impression on me. Working with him reinforced my commitment to palpation, reading and studying the classics, remaining focused on the work itself, and not falling into any type of dogmatic thinking.

Coffee, marijuana and back pain

Arya Nielsen WOODSTOCK, NY, USA

Resisting my judgements, listening to the patient

The patient was referred for acupuncture by his Rolfing practitioner. A male athlete, 35 years old, he appeared in excellent physical shape. He excelled in downhill bump skiing, wind surfing, and mountain climbing. He was a well-known wildlife photographer, trekking deep into the wilderness with the weight of his gear on his back for that special shot. This required physical stamina as well as a creative eye.

He presented with back pain that sheared into his left hip, groin and thigh, down to his foot. The top of his left foot was numb. He was diagnosed by a neurologist as having disc herniations at the fourth and fifth lumbar vertebrae. Disc problems are sometimes difficult to treat and athletes are often the worst patients because they refuse to rest. I resisted my judgements in favour of listening to this patient. It seemed a logical conclusion that his pain was a result of the disc herniations until I learned more about his case.

He admitted to becoming cold easily. Where his hands and feet had never chilled, they now became cold quickly in cold weather. He tired easily. Climbing positions he normally sustained would now cause pain. His muscles, especially his legs and hips, would cramp, tighten, contract or give out. When clinging to the side of a mountain, this was more than inconvenient.

His tongue was slightly pale, scalloped, with a white coating and slightly reddened rim and tip. His pulse was thin. His Kidney pulses were deep and weak. His Spleen pulse was tight. His Liver pulse was wiry and thin. His Heart pulse was empty.

I learned that his stools were loose and his urine more frequent when active. His sleep was light. He did not remember his dreams. This led me to ask about his diet and daily habits. Something was compromising his Kidney and Spleen *yang*, and I was curious to discover what it was.

Typical of many Americans desiring to 'get up and go', he drank coffee for breakfast, most often without food. Throughout the day, when he wasn't drinking coffee, he was drinking cold fruit juice. The sugar in the fruit juice gave quick energy with a light belly. He didn't take time to eat and digest his meals. He ate his largest meal at night, also typical of most Americans. He used marijuana daily to expand his creative eye, and at night to relax.

Summary of clinical manifestations

- Pain at lower back. Shears into the hip, down thigh and leg into the foot.
- Numbness at top of the left foot.
- Disc herniations at the vertebrae L4 and L5.
- Very developed musculature.
- Tight at neck, shoulders and back.
- Muscle cramping with exertion such as climbing.
- Pain at the sinews.
- Chills with exposure, especially at hands and feet.
- Fatigue with exertion.
- Sinus congestion.
- Frequent urine with exertion.
- Abdominal distension.
- Loose stools.
- Craves sweet foods, takes a lot of fruit juice and sugar.
- Drives self physically in work and sport.
- Has difficulty calming down.
- Sleep is light, unable to remember dreams.
- Creative vision obscured.
- Smokes marijuana to stimulate creativity in work and to relax.
- Drinks coffee to wake up and for energy.
- Tan but pale-coloured skin.
- Tongue: is pale, scalloped, slightly red tip and front rim with white coat.
- Pulse: is thin; Stomach and Spleen pulses are tight; the Blood and Kidney pulses are weak; the Liver pulse is wiry; the Heart pulse is empty; and the sinus pulse on the right is quite full.

Patterns of disharmony

I recognised that this patient was suffering from depleting behaviours. He was overactive, which depleted the *yang*. Coffee and fruit juice had become a substitute for food. He had become undernourished, which had depleted the Blood and *yin*. Repeated exposure to cold with compromised *yang* had allowed penetration of Wind-Cold-Damp at the Exterior: his back was tight, achey and cold, with palpation revealing the presence of *sha*.

Sha is a term used to describe external factors having penetrated the exterior of the body, obstructing the *qi* in the channels and congealing Blood in its minute vessels. *Sha* is evidenced by characteristic blanching of the flesh from palpation. This is apparent to the practitioner who observes her/his finger marks immediately after pressing the patient's flesh. The practitioner's finger pressure displaces the blood in the tissue. Finger marks that linger indicate the blood is slow to return due to obstruction in the tissue.

Gua means to scratch or friction. *Gua sha* is the technique applied to release *sha* at the surface. As *sha* is released, it appears as small petechiae or ecchymotic patches. The term *sha*, then, is also used to describe the petechiae of extravasated blood that results from applying *gua sha*. *Gua sha* releases the Exterior, moves obstructed *qi* and congealed Blood. This results in nourishing the tissues of the Exterior and Interior, and affords immediate relief of pain.

The predominant pattern of this patient was Spleen *yang xu* with Damp and Kidney *yang xu*, with secondary Kidney and Liver *yin xu*. There was disturbance of the Heart *shen*, Liver *hun* and Spleen *yi*. The box below lists the patterns of disharmony.

DOMINANT PATTERNS

Spleen *yang xu* with Damp

- Abdominal distension.
- Loose stools.
- Craves sweetness (from fruit juice and sugar).
- Sinus congestion.
- Muscle fatigue and cramping with exertion.
- Creative vision obscured.
- Smokes marijuana for creativity.
- Pulse: Sinus pulse on the right is quite full, Stomach and Spleen pulses are tight.
- Tongue: pale and scalloped.

Kidney *yang xu*

- Chronic back pain with disc herniation.
- Cold hands and feet, especially in cold weather.
- Fatigue with exertion.
- Paleness.
- Drinks coffee for energy.
- Climbing positions cause back pain.
- Frequent urination with exertion.
- Tongue: pale with white coat and scalloped.
- Pulse: Kidney pulse weak.

Invasion of Wind-Cold-Damp at the Exterior

- Back chill and achiness, especially with exposure.
- Back tight and cold.
- Leg pain, foot pain and numbness.
- Palpation indicating penetration of *sha*.

SECONDARY PATTERNS

Kidney-Liver *yin xu* with Fire, Liver-Heart Blood *xu*, disturbance of Liver *hun*, Heart *shen* and Spleen *yi*

- Back pain.
- Muscles cramping, pain at the sinews.
- Has difficulty calming down.
- Uses marijuana to relax.
- Overactivity, unable to rest.
- Light sleep, unable to remember dreams.
- Dulled creative vision.
- Tongue: red at tip and front rim.
- Pulse: is thin, Liver pulse wiry, Heart pulse empty.

Aetiology and pathology

In 19 years of practice I have found that the two most Kidney-compromising behaviours in our culture are overwork and coffee drinking. I consider both to be leaking behaviours. Overactivity leaks *yin* and *yang*. When moderated the vessel is contained and reserves allowed to build.

Coffee is a herb that is a diuretic and stimulant. As a diuretic, coffee stimulates urination, overworking the Kidneys, and depleting the Fluids and *yin*. Eventually the Kidneys weaken causing frequent urination, night urine, weakened back and knees. Western studies have shown coffee to leech out water soluble nutrients, such as vitamin C, B-complex, calcium and magnesium. Considered aspects of *yin* in Chinese medicine, these nutrients are essential in nourishing the muscles, allowing for appropriate flexion and relaxation, reducing inflammation and repairing normal microtears. Repeated use of diuretics causes continued leaking of nutrients so that they are not readily available to the body and are difficult to replace with vitamin pills.

Coffee also acts as a stimulant, arousing the *qi* and *yang*. A person immediately feels awake, warm and energised. However, there is a backslide when the stimulation wears off. Eventually the *qi* becomes depleted. The stimulation also disrupts the harmony of Liver *qi* eventually causing constraint. More coffee will temporarily relieve the constraint and again arouse already depleted *qi*. This then leads to habituation. This patient's constrained Liver *qi* was not an apparent pattern due to the deconstraining nature of his physical activity.

Fruit juice is often taken cold, and is by nature cooling. This chills and dampens the Spleen, weakening digestion and causing the stools to be loose and the abdomen to be distended. It also contributes to congestion and mucus from the nose, since the Spleen owns the nose, and is associated with any concentration of Damp or Phlegm.

In addition, the patient used marijuana daily to relax and to stimulate creativity. Marijuana is a herb that deconstrains the Liver *qi*, and expands the inner vision. It stimulates appetite and desire and increases urination. Over time it depletes the *yin* and the *yang*, unroots the Liver *hun*, weakens the Heart *shen* and fogs the Spleen *yi*. Marijuana smokers can also experience chill, hunger and sometimes fear or paranoia, reflecting weakening of the Spleen *yang* and Kidney *yang*.

Dr Lum Tai Cheng, now deceased, associated creativity with Kidney *jing* and thought marijuana stole a person's creativity by overstimulating it (Cheng L T, personal communication, 1978). The creativity can bubble to the mind's eye; no longer channelled it floats away, inspired but not manifested. Studies have shown that men who use marijuana regularly have decreased sperm count (Nelson 1992). According to Chinese medicine this represents a compromise of the Kidney *jing*.

In this case, the symptoms of chill, cramping and loose stools are typical of deficient Spleen *yang*. Chill, frequent urination, back pain and back injury are typical of deficient Kidney *yang*. Inability to relax without a substance, typical of habituation, reflects Liver constraint.

Inability to remember dreams is common to those who use marijuana. This patient's sleep patterns indicated a disturbance in the *hun* and *shen*, and his dulled creative eye a disturbance of the *shen*, *hun* and *yi*. The diagram in Figure 31.1 shows the relationship of the Organs, and their aspects in disharmony.

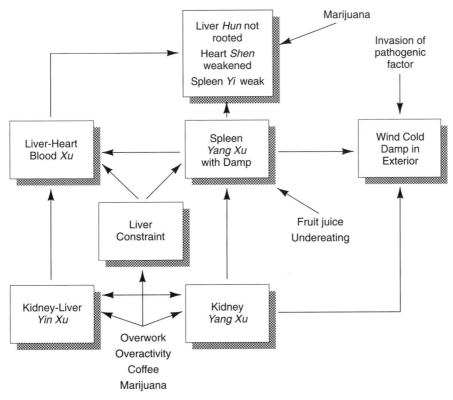

Fig. 31.1   Aetiology and pathology diagram.

Treatment issues

If the vessel is leaking, first stop the leaks. Before I began my treatment, I explained to this patient how his lifestyle was weakening him. In his case, only he could stop the leaks. He was excited that there might be a way in which he could not only recover but also continue to enjoy his body, nature and his work.

In my treatment, I chose to follow the wisdom of *xian biao hou li* meaning 'first treat the Exterior, then the Interior' (*Jinkui yaolue fanglun* 1987). I wanted to release the Exterior and move the *qi* and Blood that was obstructed by the invasion of Wind-Cold-Damp. Pressing and blanching, together with the patient's muscle tightness, achiness and chill, all indicated that he had *sha*. As is often the case with first treatments of chronic pain, I needled aggressively, arousing the *de qi* and then applying *gua sha* (Nielsen 1995). *Gua sha* is used widely in Asia, and is a special technique of classical Chinese medicine as taught by Dr James Tin Yao So (So 1987). If my diagnosis and treatment were correct, my patient would have immediate relief.

My second intention was to tonify the Kidney *yang* and Spleen *yang*, and to open the *dai mai* which is so often involved in back pain. The latter is accomplished using SJ5 *waiguan* and GB41 *zulingqi*. The former is accomplished by using points such as KID3 *taixi*, BL23 *shenshu*, BL20 *pishu*, and by recommending changes in daily habits in order to reduce the compromise of the *yang*. Only by enlisting the patient's help and interest could there be complete recovery.

I explained my diagnosis and treatment approach in detail. He understood completely. He was surprised that he had not noticed the cause of his gradual decline.

First treatment

I palpated and massaged the back area to discover *ah shi* or trigger points at the areas of tightness, pain or referral. I then needled to disperse and congest the *qi*, and then applied *gua sha* to release the Exterior and move *qi* and Blood obstructed at the surface by penetration of Wind-Cold-Damp. The same approach was applied to the lateral lower body for the leg pain, foot pain and numbness. Both local and distal points were used. The *dai mai* was opened with bilateral SJ5 *waiguan* and GB41 *zulingqi*. The Kidneys and Spleen were supported with BL20 *pishu*, BL23 *shenshu*, and KID3 *taixi*. I recommended weekly treatments but the patient was able to come bi-monthly at most.

I asked that he stop coffee, fruit juice and marijuana, eat warm cooked food regularly to build the Blood and *qi*, and moderate his activity in order to stabilise the *yin*, and allow the Blood to nourish the sinews. A tincture of Jade Pharmacy's 'Meridian Passage', based on *sheng tong zhu yu tang* plus *mo yao xiang sheng dan*, and "Meridian Circulation", based on *du huo ji sheng tang*, were given for his back (Jade Pharmacy Product Guide, 1990). Details of the first treatment are outlined in the box.

First treatment procedures

ACUPUNCTURE AND GUA SHA

Prone position

BL60 *kunlun,* pain at entire back, neck and legs.

BL40 *weizhong,* back pain and weakness, leg weakness.

BL23 *shenshu,* back pain, tonifies Kidneys.

BL25 *dachangshu,* abdominal distension, loose stools, back pain.

BL20 *pishu,* tonifies Spleen, local point for pain.

Ahshi point near left BL20, trigger referral point for pain.

DU14 *dazhui,* all *yang* channels meet at this point, piques the *yang,* treats backache and chill.

Gua sha to back, releases Wind-Cold-Damp from the Exterior, warms by moving the *qi* and *yang* to the surface, extravasates stagnant Blood at the surface allowing new Blood to nourish the muscles and sinews beneath, and stimulates production of new Blood by resolving stagnated Blood.

Lateral position, left side up

GB30 *huantiao,* treats pain in lower back, hip and leg.

GB31 *fengshi,* treats pain of the leg.

GB34 *yanglingquan,* treats numbness and pain of the lower extremity.

GB37 *guangming,* treats pain at the lower extremity.

Gua sha to left GB30 area releases the Exterior, moves *qi* and Blood to treat the obstruction in the leg.

Supine position

KID3 *taixi,* tonifies Kidney *yin,* treats low back pain and sleep.

SJ5 *waiguan,* opens the *yangwei mai.*

GB41 *zulinqqi,* opens *dai mai,* treats back pain through *dai mai.*

Later alternated with:

SI3 *houxi,* opens the *du mai.*

BL62 *shenmai,* opens the *yangqiao mai,* treats backache, leg pain, sleep.

Needle and Gua Sha technique:

Needling was undertaken with a guide tube. *De qi* was obtained at each point. Strong *de qi* was obtained at the back points. Back needles were not retained. *Gua sha* was applied to the entire back area, releasing the Exterior, decongesting the obstructed *qi* and Blood at the surface. The patient had a lot of *sha* which was red and slightly purple, indicating it was old.

Points at the lateral body were dispersed, with needle retention for 10 minutes, then *gua sha* applied. Points at the dorsal body were needled using the reinforcing method and needles were retained for 15 minutes.

Needles Seirin #5 (25 x 30) for all points except GB30 where I used Seirin #8 (30 x 50).

RECOMMENDATIONS

Lifestyle changes

- Stop coffee, fruit juice and marijuana.
- Eat regularly, warm cooked food.
- Eat 50–100 g of concentrated protein twice per day.
- Avoid cold food and drink.
- Moderation in activity.

CHINESE HERBS

Tincture given of Jade Pharmacy's 'Meridian Circulation' *du huo ji sheng tang* and 'Meridian Passage' *shen tong zhu yu tang* plus *mo yao xiang sheng tang.* Later a modified Ginseng, Poria and Atractylodes Powder *sheng ling bai zhu san* was given in decoction, then as a powder.

Recovery of stamina and vision

Upon leaving the table after the first treatment the patient's back pain improved and he immediately felt warm. This confirmed the diagnosis that at least part of the cause of his pain was Wind-Cold-Damp obstructing the *qi* and Blood. He was pleased, and I was heartened.

He received a total of six treatments. The second was 2 weeks after the first. Stopping fruit juice helped his stools and stopping coffee helped relieve his fatigue, urine frequency, back and muscle weakness and sinew pain. It was difficult for him to give up the marijuana so I prescribed a modified version of Ginseng, Poria and Atractylodes Powder *sheng ling bai zhu san* (Bensky & Barolet 1990).

Overall the formula strengthened the Spleen and Kidneys and clarified his creative vision, making it possible for him to give up the marijuana which injured his creativity and thinking. He was ecstatic to have the experience of working while using the herbs. He doubled his photographic images and boasted at the superiority of the work. He changed from a decoction to a powder for ease of travel.

By the sixth session, I needed to merely tune up his back and treat his sinus pain which had been exacerbated from water rushing up his nose during 5 days of wind surfing.

As the box below indicates, this patient completely recovered from his presenting complaint through the careful application of Chinese medicine; acupuncture, *gua sha*, diet recommendations, lifestyle changes as well as herbs. He was delighted to learn of ways that he could improve and maintain his health. I don't know whether a post-treatment magnetic resonance image (MRI) would have revealed the same disc herniations as before. What I do know is that this patient was happy not only to have recovered from his back pain but also to have increased his stamina and vision. I referred him back to his Rolfing practitioner (Rolf 1977) to continue his work of fascial awakening for increased flexibility.

Summary of outcome

- Immediate pain relief at the back from first treatment.
- Patient felt warm at the back and extremities.
- His stools were well-formed.
- Abdominal distension resolved.
- His muscle cramping and fatigue improved.
- Urination became normal.
- He maintained his body temperature with exposure.
- He resumed physical overactivity and presented two more times with slight numbness in the foot, which improved after treatment.
- The pain and numbness at the foot,

typical of disc herniations, became a whisper of discomfort, and had stopped completely by the sixth session.

- His sleep became deep with normal dreams and dream recall.

- His creative vision in photographic work improved and, to his surprise, he both increased and improved the number and quality of his images.

A reminder to remain open

Two years later I read an interesting article on back pain (Jenson 1994). In the United States, back pain is the leading cause of work-related disability and the second leading cause of visits to the doctor. Magnetic resonance imaging (MRI) as well as other non-invasive technologies can examine the spine in detail allowing diagnosis of fractures, disc problems or tumours. However, this study at Hoag Memorial Hospital in Newport Beach, California, questioned the usefulness of such technologies, especially when they were used to set in motion medical interventions to treat back pain. In the research study MRI was done of 98 participants who were symptom free and without history of any back pain. Remarkably, 64% had disc abnormalities, more than 50% had a bulge in at least one disc, and 27% had at least one herniation. Both this research study and my case study remind me to remain open, to listen and to apply the principles of Chinese medicine.

REFERENCES

Bensky D, Barolet R 1990 Chinese herbal medicine: formulae and strategies. Eastland Press, Seattle
Jade Pharmacy Product Guide 1990 East Earth Herb Company, Eugene
Jenson M 1994 Magnetic resonance imaging of the lumbar spine in people without back pain. New England Journal of Medicine 331 (2)
Nelson H 1992 Paternal-fetal conflict. Hastings Center Report, vol 22 no 2 p 3
Jinkui yaolue fanglun (Synopsis of the golden chamber) 1987 (first published 220 BC). New World Press, Beijing
Nielsen A 1995 *Gua Sha,* a traditional technique for modern practice. Churchill Livingstone, Edinburgh
Rolf I 1977 Rolfing, the integration of human structures. Harper & Row, New York
So J T Y 1987 Treatment of disease with acupuncture, Vol 2. Paradigm Press, Brookline

FURTHER READING

Foreign Language Press 1980 Essentials of Chinese acupuncture. Beijing
Shanghan Lun Treatise on febrile diseases caused by cold 1986 (first published 220 BC). New World Press, Beijing

■ Arya Nielsen

Arya Nielsen was born in 1949 in Wisconsin USA. She received her BA from the University of Wisconsin in 1971, her MA from Queens College in 1974, and declined acceptance to Tuft's University Medical School in 1976 in order to continue her study of acupuncture. She graduated from the New England School of Acupuncture in 1977 in the first graduating class of the first licensed acupuncture school in the United States. She studied and apprenticed with Dr James Tin Yao So, a classical acupuncturist, and Dr Ted Kaptchuk, OMD.

She is National Board Certified in Acupuncture and Chinese Herbology (NCCA, National Commission for Certification of Acupuncturists), a Fellow of the National Academy of Acupuncture and Oriental Medicine, and Chair of the New York State Acupuncture Board. Arya is a Doctor of Acupuncture licensed by the States of Rhode Island, Wisconsin, and New York. She has been in private practice since 1977, currently in Woodstock, New York. She is a Senior Clinical faculty member at the Tri-State Institute of Traditional Chinese Acupuncture in New York City and is author of the book **Gua Sha**, a *Traditional Technique for Modern Practice*, published by Churchill Livingstone in 1995.

A crushing pain in the chest

Mark Seem NEW YORK, USA

A possible heart condition

Nearing my office one morning I ran into a store clerk I often encountered on my way to work. He approached me with a look of concern, asking for some advice about his condition. He was a man in his mid 40s, of medium height and quite powerful in stature. He looked quite shaken and proceeded to tell me of a crushing pain in his chest that he had been experiencing frequently for several days, with discomfort and 'strange sensations' down the inner aspect of his left arm. He wondered if acupuncture might help, and displayed a clear fear of orthodox medicine and physicians. I explained that symptoms such as his had to be checked out by an internist or cardiologist to rule out a possible heart condition, and assured him that if, as I suspected, his medical examination proved negative for such a condition, acupuncture probably could help a great deal.

I always send a patient with such symptoms to a physician to rule out serious pathology. In this case I was dealing with someone who had an exaggerated fear of doctors. He needed, however, to see that his probably slightly hysterical overreactions to his symptoms did not mean he could afford to ignore them for days on end. After all, it was possible that he had a very serious heart condition indeed, and the fear that led to his avoidance of physicians was not healthy in any case. Since he knew no physicians and rarely visited the doctor's office, I referred him to a local cardiologist, asking him to call me once he had seen the doctor.

He called me the next day greatly relieved, since extensive cardiovascular testing had proved negative, and the cardiologist felt the condition was due to some sort of muscular strain. The doctor prescribed a pain killer, which failed to relieve the chest pain and other symptoms.

When I examined the patient at his first visit to my office, he was greatly relieved by his doctor's findings, but still in severe pain and discomfort. This pain, which he described as 'crushing', extended from right over his heart to his armpit and produced a tingling, uncomfortable sensation down the inner aspect of his left arm to the last two fingers. He experienced frequent difficulty breathing and could not work as hard as he was used to. I asked if he had to lift heavy things at work, and he explained that indeed he had to lift rather heavy boxes, but the real problem was that they were awkwardly shaped and he often felt strained when lifting them. He could not, however, remember any specific incidents that preceded his condition, and he had never suffered from such chest pain before. Knowing the man, I also knew that he tended to appear always more optimistic than warranted and was actually under a lot of financial stress putting his daughter through college, with a son also ready to go to college in a few years time.

Palpating his chest

I explained to him as he was taking off his shirt that I had seen several cases exactly like his, which had turned out to be severe muscle spasms and had yielded quickly to acupuncture therapy. As I said this, I began to palpate the area he had pointed to when I initially asked him to locate his chest pain. I probed for possible muscular constrictions and trigger points in the pectoralis muscles which I knew could, according to the pioneering work of Dr Janet Travell (Travell & Simons 1983, 1992) and to my own experience, cause exactly such crushing pain and radiating sensations down the arm. After a few moments I hit upon a large muscular knot that, when pinched, caused the patient to blanch and yell in pain. This palpation was causing his precise symptoms and the longer and harder I pinched the knot, the more severe the pain and spreading sensations became. I expressed delight because this meant, in my experience, that the problem was primarily muscular. I told him that if we could get the knot to release, the problem should start to improve.

His pulse was slightly wiry in general, but basically quite normal, and his tongue was quite normal except for a touch of purple. Palpation for tight, tender spots along the meridians revealed extreme reactivity and sensitivity at points near LIV3 *taichong,* LIV5 *ligou,* LIV6 *zhongdu* and LIV9 *yinbao,* and P1 *tianchi,* P4 *ximen* and P5 *jianshi,* all on the left, as well as KID22 *bulang,* KID23 *shenfeng,* KID25 *shencang* to KID27 *shufu,* and H1 *jiquan* on the left. Slight pressure on REN18 *yutang* was unbearable to the patient, and a careful evaluation of the pectoralis muscles revealed several exquisitely tender trigger points that also recreated aspects of his spreading sensations and discomfort.

I explained to him that these knots were long-standing from the feel of them, and that in my experience they constituted a kind of *holding pattern,* a particular way in which he held stress, or reacted to stresses and strains from his everyday life. The repeated lifting of awkward heavy objects, coupled with the financial strains of sending his daughter to college, could exacerbate such a holding pattern, causing the sorts of symptoms he was experiencing.

Connecting with the patient

The job of an acupuncturist, I told him, was to become familiar with the various holding patterns which people develop, and to connect with the pattern most strained by an individual. In this way the acupuncturist enables the patient to become aware of his 'muscular straight-jacket' as well as prodding the body to release some of the constriction, thereby freeing up energy to flow more normally in the body-mind. I believe, after a decade and a half of treating patients, that these holding patterns are what the ancient acupuncturists perceived and charted as the meridian system. It is this complex meridian system that should serve as our guide as we explore the terrain of the patient's palpable body. In so doing, we often come very close to a person's actual lived experience of illness, because we are connecting, without interpretation, directly with a major aspect of this experience: the holding pattern itself.

Rather than search for a diagnosis, which separates patient from practitioner while establishing the unequal authority of the latter, I seek simply to *connect* with the patient at the point where he or she is 'stuck'.

This was the point in case for my store clerk, for the mere palpation of his tight chest muscles set off a sigh of relief as he explained that this was exactly where his problem was: his body recognised the block, the first step toward clearing it.

I explained again to the clerk that his referral to the cardiologist had been a necessary precaution, and now that we knew a cardiological condition was unlikely, and after finding these tight knots in his chest muscles, I was quite sure that acupuncture would be of rapid help.

I told him that in my experience men hold far more tension than women do in the left chest muscles, and that whenever I find such constriction over the heart I try to relieve it to prevent a holding pattern from becoming too constrictive in this crucial area. I cautioned him against lifting any awkward or heavy objects and suggested we treat once weekly for the next 3 weeks.

Summary of clinical manifestations

- 'Crushing' pain in chest, severe pain.
- Discomfort and 'strange sensations' down the inner aspect of his left arm to his last two fingers.
- Frequent difficulty breathing and couldn't work as hard as he was used to.
- Felt strained lifting heavy boxes.
- Tended to be more optimistic than warranted.
- Pulse: slightly wiry in general.
- Tongue: normal except for a touch of purple.

Palpation

1. There were tight tender spots at LIV3 *taichong*, LIV5 *ligou*, LIV6 *zhongdu* and LIV9 *yinbao*, P1 *tianchi*, P4 *ximen* and P5 *jianshi*, KID22 *bulang* to KID23 *shenfeng*, KID25 *shencang* to KID27 *shufu* and H1 *jiquan*, all on the left.

2. The patient also had several exquisitely tender trigger points in the pectoralis muscle that also recreated aspects of his spreading sensations and discomfort.

3. Palpation of the tight chest muscles set off a sigh of relief.

The three energetic levels

Identifying a pattern of disharmony, which I understand as a *reaction pattern* or *holding pattern*, is not really the same as that meant by most Oriental medical practitioners when making a diagnosis. From a meridian perspective, acupuncture treats at three different levels:

1 The surface energetic *wei* level, where myofascial constrictions, called '*kori*' by Japanese acupuncturists, can be found by palpation of the surface itself.

2 The functional energetic *ying* level, so well articulated physically as the *zangfu* organ functions by Traditional Chinese Medicine, and psycho-spiritually as the Twelve Officials by J R Worsley.

3 The core energetic *jing* level where genetics and early predispositions work their effects on the body-mind-spirit of the individual.

In my approach (Seem 1993), I aim to treat at least two, and often all three of these levels, focusing at first on clearing away the myofascial constrictions and blocks in the surface level. So rather than make a diagnosis, in this case, I just noted the constrained *qi* in the *jueyin* pathways of the ventral aspect of the body, essentially in the left chest where Liver and Pericardium energies converge.

Revealing the true aetiology

It appeared to me that the clerk probably always held a lot of tension in this area of the chest, and that an extra strain caused by lifting coupled with undue financial burdens lead to his symptoms: the straw that broke the camel's back. However, I have learned that the true aetiology of such conditions reveals itself, like an onion, with ever more layers under the one currently being treated. Therefore, I tend to wait for a clearer aetiological sense to emerge after treating several times and watching the developments from each treatment.

Deconstraining the *qi*

My treatment principle is to deconstrain *qi* where it is currently blocked, focusing on the immediate area of the patient's distress (surface energetic *wei* level), whilst at the same time treating the functional and core levels, wherever appropriate. In this case, as in most cases I treat, I suggested treatment once weekly for 3–4 weeks, followed by a break of 1 month to monitor whether the patient continued to improve on his own. In chronic conditions, I might then see someone once monthly, or perhaps only on an 'as needed' basis if progress was good. I prefer to treat as little as possible because I have developed an enormous faith in a person's capacity to heal himself once acupuncture has acted as a catalyst to release the myofascial blocks and promote change. The body-mind-spirit knows how to do the rest.

In this case, treatment focused on releasing the myofascial constrictions in the left pectoralis muscles. Points found to be reactive on palpation were released by needling with a pecking motion, with 30 mm 3 gauge Seirin Japanese-style disposable needles, until the pecking encountered a rubber-like resistance, which Kiiko Matsumoto calls 'gummies', like the rubbery sensation of needling into an eraser (personal communication, 1993). Generally in such tight spots of *kori* I remain at the depth where this resistance is encountered, usually only 6–13 mm deep, and begin again to peck once per second towards the resistance, until the muscle reacts. Usually the muscle begins to grab around the needle tip, experienced as a grasping in of the needle, and then gives a little shudder, which can be felt with the index and middle fingers of the left hand (on a right-handed practitioner) which straddles the spot being needled. Sometimes the muscle fasciculates several times, and I stop stimulating when this reactivity begins to wear down or cease altogether, and then leave the needles in situ for 10–15 minutes. I explain to the patient that these reactive areas are being released, and that the area or spots might feel quite tender or sore, much like postexercise achiness, and that a hot shower on the area, or a hot Epsom Salts bath can help for the first night or two, as can drinking more water to flush the tissues.

The first treatment

I treated the clerk in this fashion at tight spots near KID22 *bulang* to KID23 *shenfeng*, KID25 *shencang* to KID27 *shufu*, ST13 *qihu* to ST15 *wuyi* and P1 *tianchi* to GB22 *yuanye* with major fasciculations at a couple of these spots in the pectoralis muscles.

This front aspect of the body is the *yangming* zone, a cutaneous region, which is why I needled the tight points along the foot *yangming* Stomach channel in the chest. I generally also treat distal reactive points along the pathways where the local constrained *qi* is located, in this case ST36 *zusanli*, ST37 *shangjuxu* and ST39 *xiajuxu* on the leg, and the hand *yangming* LI10 *shousanli* to LI12 *zhouliao* area on the forearm.

For the functional energetic *ying* level, I was concerned about the Kidney and Pericardium which, in my experience, often become constricted and overly irritated under unabated stress. I therefore treated KID22 *bulang* to KID23 *shenfeng* where tight and angled towards P1 *tianchi*, which I also needled. I see these as kinds of '*mu*' points in the upper heater for the Pericardium and Kidney functions according to the Entry–Exit strategy taught by J R Worsely (Seem 1993). This is an excellent strategy in my experience for moving blocked energy at the functional level which often then leads to greatly improved organ function and clarity in the Officials involved. I also treated tender spots just below KID16 *huangshu*, as taught by Kiiko Matsumoto, which I have also found to be associated with aggravated adrenal function. This is also a sort of '*mu*' point and the total combination of points is treated according to triple heater regulatory strategies. Again I always combine local with distal points and, in this case, added the *ying* and *shu* points of the Kidney, namely KID2 *rangu* and KID3 *taixi* according to the Neijing strategy of treating 'yin of yin' (the yin organ functions) (Faubert 1977).

Since I was not sure whether my patient's problem had a chronic, or even deep-core energetic *jing* aspect, I decided to consolidate the treatment by utilising an eight extraordinary vessel strategy to treat the ventral *yangming* zone at the deepest energetic level. The extraordinary vessel pairs that traverse the ventral zone are either *renmai* and *yinqiaomai*, opened with LU7 *lieque* and KID6 *zhaohai* respectively, an excellent combination when Kidney and Lung *qi* do not communicate as in asthma, or *chongmai* and *yinweimai*, opened with SP4 *gongsun* and P6 *neiguan*. Since *yinweimai*'s chief complaint when constrained is chest distress, and since *chongmai* is ideal in relieving *jueyin* constrained *qi* in general, I selected the second combination, needling P6 *neiguan* on the left, as a distal point for the left Pericardium channel, and SP4 *gongsun* on the right, as I had learned from Van Nghi's French acupuncture approach (Van Nghi 1977). I completed the first treatment by needling the Root and Node points (Seem 1990) of *jueyin*, LIV1 *dadun* and REN18 *yutang*, since the area of REN18 *yutang* had been very tender on palpation and this was another core treatment for *jueyin*.

First treatment procedures

POINT SELECTION

Local points (*wei level*) at tight local spots near:

- KID22 *bulang* to KID23 *shenfeng* (angled towards P1 *tianchi*).
- KID25 *shencang* to KID27 *shufu*.
- ST13 *qihu* to ST15 *wuyi*.
- P1 *tianchi* to GB22 *yuanye*.
- REN18 *yutang*.

Distal points (*wei* level)

- ST36 *zusanli*, ST37 *shangjuxu*, ST39 *xiajuxu* (distal reactive points on the leg).
- LI10 *shousanli* to LI12 *zhouliao* area (distal reactive points on the arm).

Organ function points (*ying* level)

- KID2 and KID3 (the *ying* and *shu* points of the Kidney according to the Neijing strategy of treating the '*yin* of *yin*') (Faubert 1977).
- KID16 *huangshu*.

Core energetic points (*jing* level)

- SP4 *gongsun* (left), P6 *neiguan* (right) (utilising *chongmai* and *yinweimai*).
- LIV1 *dadun* and REN18 *yutang* (Root and Node points of *jueyin*).

Releasing the blocks

As often happens in treatment, things are not quite as simple as they first appear. In this case, the patient returned for his second treatment a week later expressing delight that his chest pain was much relieved, but concern that he now had even more severe discomfort under the armpit and down the inner upper arm along the Heart and Pericardium pathways, in the area near LU1 *zhongfu* to SP20 *zhourong*. Local needling of this trigger point in the pectoralis muscle, along with an incredibly tender spot near P3 *quze* on the left resulted in much more significant release of the pectoralis muscles. The treatment otherwise was much as before, adding in SP21 *dabao* on the left, and LU7 *lieque* distally, for this *taiyin* zone. In the third and fourth treatments, again spaced a week apart, the patient reported almost total relief from the chest pain and improvement of his inner arm pain, although this kept reappearing further down. Local treatment of the P3 *quze* and L5 *chize* areas in the third and fourth treatments essentially eradicated all presenting signs and symptoms. The various points treated corresponded with Travell's trigger points for the brachialis and brachio-radialis muscles (Travell & Simons 1983, 1992) and the chest discomfort never returned. I suggested to the patient that we take a break of 1 month, and at his next visit he reported that his symptoms had never returned and that he was quite relieved overall. He now paid much more attention to the way in which he lifted things at work and was considering a yoga class for stress reduction at the local gym.

Summary of outcome

- Chest discomfort never returned.
- All signs and symptoms essentially eradicated.
- Symptoms did not return after 1 month.
- Now paying attention to the way in which he lifted things at work.
- Was considering a yoga class for stress reduction at the local gym.

Free to heal

My treatment approach focuses heavily on the surface energetic-myo-fascial-level and constitutes acupuncture as a sort of laying-on-of-hands — essentially acupuncture osteopathy. In an acupuncture osteopathic or meridian acupuncture approach, the key to treatment is to meet the patient at the place where she or he is blocked, and to use treatment to release the block so that the patient is then free to heal her- or himself. I believe acupuncture serves as an excellent means of communicating with a patient's holding patterns, and that our simple interventions into naked flesh serve to correct short-circuits, thereby enabling more normal functioning to be restored. Such an approach must, of course, have enormous faith in people's capacity to heal themselves, and in the ingenuity and awareness of the ancient Chinese meridian system which is essentially a detailed map of the various holding patterns of human beings, with simple and safe methods for releasing those patterns of distress.

REFERENCES

Faubert A 1977 Traité didactique d'acupuncture traditionnelle. Guy Trédaniel Editeur, Paris

Seem M 1990 Acupuncture imaging. Healing Arts Press, Rochester

Seem M 1993 A new American acupuncture: acupuncture osteopathy: myofascial release of the body-mind's holding patterns. Blue Poppy Press, Boulder

Travell J, Simons D 1983, 1992 Myofascial pain and dysfunction: the trigger point manual. Vols. 1 and 2. Williams & Wilkins, Baltimore

Van Nghi N 1977 Pathogénue et pathologie énergétique en médecine chinoise. Dom Bosco, Marseille

■ Mark Seem

Mark D Seem received his doctorate in French Studies from the State University of New York at Buffalo, where he studied with Michel Foucault and wrote a dissertation on the Nietzschean concepts of power and force in modern French philosophy. While cotranslating Deleuze and Guattari's *Anti-oedipus: Capitalism and Schizophrenia*, he trained at the innovative La Borde clinic in France. Subsequent to finishing his dissertation, he worked with the mentally ill and retarded, taught psychology, and trained mental hygiene therapy aides in a state institution, while beginning his formal study of acupuncture. He trained at the Quebec Institute of Acupuncture in Montreal and at affiliated centres in New York City.

Dr Seem is founder and director of the Tri State Institute of Traditional Chinese Acupuncture and is a frequent lecturer at other acupuncture institutes and conferences. He is a past-president of the National Council of Acupuncture Schools and Colleges and a former commissioner on the National Commission for the Certification of Acupuncturists, from which he is a Board Certified Diplomate in Acupuncture. He has written several articles on acupuncture education and is the author of *Acupuncture Energetics, Body-mind Energetics, Acupuncture Imaging*, and *A new American Acupuncture*. Dr Seem has an acupuncture practice in New York City.

Unresolved shock

Holly Guzmán SANTA CRUZ, CA, USA

An unbearable pain

Sara sought acupunture treatment because she had right shoulder pain of such severity that she could neither sleep nor function in daily life. The pain had been ongoing for more than a year, and remained unbearable despite regularly using chiropractic and physical therapy treatments.

Sara had worked as a teacher of emotionally and physically challenged children. While working with a severe case she had been slammed in the shoulder by a ball — a frightening assault after which her shoulder pain began. She had seen me for acupuncture and herbs to resolve some gall-bladder irritation 3 years prior to the assault, then she had moved to Hawaii for over 2 years.

Sara was 49 years old and was large in a comfortably pleasing way, with a broad and open face and a general air of self-realisation. I had experienced her as an easy-going, relaxed and joyous person. She now complained of sleep disorder, fatigue, anxiety, low self-esteem, short atten-tion span, and short-term memory loss. She seemed to feel distraught because, whilst generally a very relaxed and accepting person who was able to spiritually transcend personal difficulties, in this instance she was unable to comfort herself or resolve her pain. Her tongue was pale with a red tip, and all her pulses were rapid, soft and sinking.

Clinical manifestations

- Ongoing shoulder pain for over 1 year, resulting from a severe blow.
- Extreme pain in shoulder preventing sleep at night.
- Lack of mobility at the shoulder.
- Fatigue, exhaustion.
- Anxiety, ongoing stress and fear.
- Low self-esteem.
- History of low back pain ('disintegration' of lumbar vertebrae L4 and L5).
- Short attention span.
- Short-term memory loss.
- Disorientation.
- Tongue: pale, red tip.
- Pulse: soft, sinking and rapid.

Medical history

Sara's medical history included an extreme blood sugar imbalance which she controlled by avoiding intake of refined sugar. (She fainted from low blood sugar 4½ hours into a glucose tolerance test.) She said her vertebrae had 'disintegrated' 25 years ago. She underwent two near death experiences when she reacted to the anaesthesic during surgery to her back to fuse the vetebrae at L4 and L5. The surgery was fairly successful, since which she had enjoyed a relatively active life.

Patterns of disharmony

Kidney *yang xu*

- History of low back problems ('disintegration' of L4 and L5).
- Short-term memory loss.
- Short attention span.
- Fatigue.
- Tongue: pale (red tip shows some Kidney *yin xu*).
- Pulse: soft and sinking.

Kidney *yin xu*

- Anxiety.

- Insomnia.
- Ongoing stress and fear.
- Tongue: pale with red tip.
- Pulse: rapid.

Channel blockage

- Extreme shoulder pain on right side.
- Lack of mobility at shoulder.
- Sudden onset at the time of injury.
- Duration of shoulder pain for 1 year, without ability to heal.

Aetiology and pathology

A severe fright or shocking experience can manifest itself in a reaction commonly known as 'the fright, fight, flight mode', and this is what happened in Sara's case. In Western medicine this syndrome is known as a sympathetic nervous system dominance in which the adrenals become very active, supplying the body with a high level of adrenaline. This adrenaline uses up Kidney *yang* so, if the body is unable to resolve the shock and move out of this mode, Kidney *yang* becomes depleted. A common term for this is 'adrenal exhaustion'. Long-term pain, especially physical but also emotional, also overstimulates the adrenals and therefore creates Kidney *yang xu*. The activated state does not allow for relaxation, so sleep is poor and the Kidney *yin* will also become depleted (Fig. 33.1).

According to Dr Nagano,[1] a famous Kiyoshi Japanese acupuncturist, when the body receives a shock which it perceives to be life-threatening, it will contract inwards in a motion energetically similar to the fetal position. The navel can be compared to a pull-chord at the centre of a web or parachute which, when contracted, causes shortening and tightening all

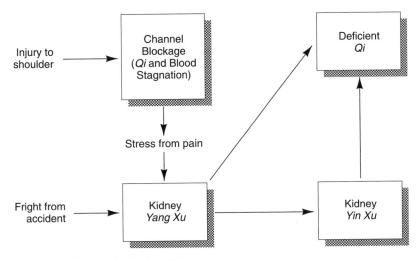

Fig. 33.1 Aetiology and pathology diagram.

the way out via energetic spokes to the extremities. Until the centre is released, it is very difficult to achieve normal relaxation in other areas of tension (such as the pelvis, neck or shoulders). Shock initially impacts the adrenal system, also considered to be the Kidney *yang*.

The shock itself causes a contracted tension, comparable to the body's response to physical pain by clenching. The body will respond to fear or emotional pain by clenching also, especially in the Kidney *yang* itself. The action of clenching itself creates a blockage preventing smooth internal communication. Once communication is blocked, a message to relax may never properly be received. In addition, if the pain is ongoing, the stress will overload the nervous system. The body will lose its ability to be either completely asleep or fully awake. This leads to further exhaustion of both the *yang* and *yin*. If the body is exhausted, it will be unable to appropriately function and the healing process will be impaired. In Sara's case she had been injured for more than a year, but was unable to resolve the injury to her shoulder. Her case is classic for many people who experience a shocking physical or emotional incident and then cannot get back to normal.

Opening the Kidney meridian

To nourish and release the adrenals/Kidney *yang* which had been impacted by the fright of the accident, I used Dr Nagano's treatment pattern for adrenal exhaustion.[2] This consists of the following points: KI6 *zhaohai*, KID27 *shufu* and two extra points around the navel called 4:00 and 8:00.

These extra points are located about one unit out from the navel at the positions of 4 o'clock and 8 o'clock, where 12 o'clock is located just above the belly button towards REN9 *shuifen*.

By connecting the Kidney meridian, bottom to top, and focusing on releasing the centre of the implosion using the two points by the navel which correspond to the *ming men* and the adrenal energy (4:00 and 8:00), the Kidney meridian is fully opened again. In cases where the Kidney meridian is impacted by shock and the meridian is not full, there will be soreness towards the top of the meridian, sometimes at KID27 *shufu* and sometimes a few points below this at KID26 *yuzhong* or KID25 *shencang*. As this area is needled, warmed, or rubbed by the patient, the Kidney energy extends into the region, the tenderness is resolved, and the long-term manifestations of shock such as sleeplessness and disorientation lessen. During the treatment, Sara fell into a very deep sleep, and awoke feeling transformed.

First treatment procedures

POINT PRESCRIPTION

The following combination of points opens and fills the Kidney meridian, reversing the impact of an unresolved shocking experience:

KID6 *zhaohai* is needled superficially towards the tip of the heel.

KID27 *shufu* is found by palpating in the region of the end of the Kidney meridian until distinct tenderness is noted; then it is needled with minimal stimulus, superficially, towards the sternum.

4.00 and 8.00 are points which correspond to Kidney *yang*, adrenals and *ming men*. The points are located in typical clock positions around the navel at 4 o'clock and 8 o'clock respectively, about one unit out from the navel. They are needled approximately 12 mm away from the navel, at a 45° angle towards the centre of the navel and at a depth of about 18 mm, or as deep as necessary to contact a gummy resistance in the tissue which is then gently stimulated with a few thrusting motions.

Needles: Japanese #1 gauge needles are used.

Vitamins: Vitamins B5 and B6, in a ratio of five B5 to one B6 were prescribed to help restore the adrenal cortex.

Promoting healing

One week later Sara returned saying that she felt better than she had in a whole year and that she was more oriented and felt somewhat grounded. However, her shoulder pain was still severe enough to interfere with her sleep. Diagnosis at this point took into account general exhaustion which had depleted the *qi*, and prevented the normal healing process. If the shoulder had been treated directly, the body would probably have had insufficient *qi* to respond favourably. So a famous formula of points to tonify *qi*, as developed by Miriam Lee, was implemented. Miriam Lee has written extensively on the theory and usage of this point group (Lee 1994). The points are ST36 *zusanli*, SP6 *sanyinjiao*, LI11 *quchi*, LI4 *hegu* and LU7 *lieque*. This group was needled, and 4:00 and 8:00 were added to reinforce the adrenal tonification of the previous treatment. A single Chinese herb, Schefflera Arboricola Hayata *qi ye lian*, was prescribed in patent form (five pills three times a day for 5 days) to resolve stagnant Blood and *qi* from the injury in the shoulder and to promote healing.

In the next session, 10 days later, Sara reported that after her last treatment she had experienced her first pain-free night in over a year. Treatment to directly affect the shoulder itself was now introduced. The body's energy was sufficiently balanced to tolerate the stimulus of working on the damaged joint. Prior to this time, any pain or stimulus would most likely have been poorly received, possibly aggravating Sara's entire system which was very overwhelmed, sleep deprived and hypersensitive. This point had been clearly illustrated by Sara's lack of response to both chiropractic and physical therapy.

Local treatment with acupuncture was now administered by needling three points on the shoulder, called the shoulder triangle, as used by Miriam Lee (1994) and a point behind GB21 *jianjing* as used by Kiiko Matsumoto (personal communication, 1993). The shoulder triangle is a general formula for shoulder pain, especially if it is aggravated by lifting the arm, as in this case. Its first point is located one unit below LI15 *jianyu*, its other two points are on either border of the deltoid muscle, forming an equilateral triangle with the first point. The point behind GB21 *jianjing* is specifically used when there is jaw tension aggravating the shoulder pain, and it is located directly behind GB21 *jianjing*, just off the muscle body. Cups were applied locally once the needles were removed, to move and resolve stagnant Blood from the site of injury. Siberian ginseng (Euletherococcus) in tincture form was given to nourish the Kidney *yin* and *yang*.

Release from pain

After direct treatment to the shoulder, Sara reported a 50% reduction in her shoulder pain. Local treatment was continued, with some interludes to deal with a common cold, some menstrual issues and urinary frequency. There were setbacks with tiredness, and two brief episodes that included disorientation and fatigue, although these were not as debilitating as they had been originally. Some 3 months after her initial visit, Sara said that she knew her life was coming together, although she still experienced some soreness in her right shoulder. Overall, her shoulder mobility had improved dramatically and she felt more like herself, regardless of the occasional irritation in the joint.

I have chosen to present this case not because it is dramatic, but because it is so common. Countless patients seem to remain emotionally paralysed in an injured state. This particular case shows a progression of treatment that is commonly appropriate. The treatment timespan is also average, although numerous times a single treatment using KID6 *zhaohai* and KID27 *shufu* is sufficient to catalyse dramatic healing and relief from pain. Most frequently, a single treatment for shock will facilitate access to the next level for change. From here steady progression can be expected, with some temporary setbacks.

Body and spirit

Although this case may seem ordinary to others, for Sara, in her own words, the treatment was life-saving and therefore profoundly dramatic. Her self-perspective radically changed. Prior to her shoulder pain, she had believed that she could transcend her bodily issues through spiritual practice and awareness. As a result of her trauma, not only was she unable to do this, but also her pain blocked her ability to contact her spiritual self at all. Her spiritual self became imprisoned by the pain in her body. Recontacting herself through her body showed Sara an important link between her body and her sense of connection with her spirit. After treatment, her relationship with her body became much more important than it had been previously. She knew, as she had done prior to the incident, that she could have pain and yet still be in contact with her spirit, but also that if she was out of contact with her spirit, then she could work with the blockages in her body to help her reconnect with her spiritual self.

Progress and outcome

- She felt more like herself.
- She knew her life was coming together.
- Shoulder mobility.

- Some soreness in her left shoulder.
- Her relationship with her body became much more important.

NOTES

1 Dr Kiyoshi Nagano is a Japanese acupuncturist who was born in the 1930s. He is a senior teacher of Kiiko Matsumoto and lives in Oita in southern Japan. While he is well published in Japan, his books have yet to be translated into English. His understanding of the effects of shock were communicated to me by Kiiko Matsumoto around 1988.

2 I was originally introduced to Dr Nagano's treatment for adrenal exhaustion by Kiiko Matsumoto around 1988.

REFERENCES

Lee M 1994 Insights of a senior acupuncturist. Blue Poppy Press, Boulder

■ Holly Guzmán

Holly Guzmán was introduced to acupuncture in Afghanistan at the age of 13 by the Chinese Embassy's acupuncturist. By 1974 she was studying in San Francisco with one of the first graduates of Worsley's acupuncture programme, Efrem Korngold. In 1976 she went to China and observed commune hospitals, herbal pharmacies and herb farms, acupuncture anaesthetics and an acupuncture programme to treat deaf mute school children in Guang Zhou. She attended the New England School of Acupuncture's first 2-year programme, and studied there with Dr Tin Yau So and Ted Kaptchuk. She helped to start an acupuncture pain and stress programme at the Lemuel Shattuck State Hospital with Ted Kaptchuk in 1980. She was also heavily influenced by a Japanese acupuncturist, Kiiko Matsumoto, whom she met at that time and has continued to study with since.

Holly moved to California and studied Chinese herbology with Yat Ki Lai in the first class of the American College of Traditional Chinese Medicine, and also took up a tutorial with Miriam Lee. Since then she has returned to the Orient to study paediatrics in Japan, to visit Kiiko's teachers, and to study in Chinese hospitals with a focus on epilepsy. Her private practice of the last 12 years in California specialises in pregnancy, childcare, and family health.

Surrender or control?

Jürgen Mücher BREMEN, GERMANY

A migraine out of control

Barbara was a small, energetic woman in her mid-30s who ran a successful business as a landscape architect. Briskly, she entered my office and immediately came to the point.

> *My migraine has got out of control and I don't want to get addicted to pain killers. I have heard good things about acupuncture but I also have doubts as to whether it can help in my case. I have already tried homeopathy and that did not have any effect on me.*

Her statement was determined, but at the same time sceptical. Her demeanour also gave me the impression that there were conflicting forces at work in her. Her movements were forceful but restrained and the liveliness of her face was restricted by the pronounced tightness of her jaw muscles.

I asked her to tell me what she thought was important about her problem. She replied:

> *I had my first migraine attacks when I was about 12. They used to occur just prior to my menstruation, but throughout the last year they have become more and more frequent. Now I have them almost every weekend.*

She added that the headache usually started in the morning with a pulsating pain in the whole right side of her head. It reached its climax around noon, when it concentrated behind the eye, and cleared up during the following evening. At the beginning of the migraine she had very cold hands and also felt nauseous.

When she was under stress, she frequently suffered from attacks of mouth and tongue ulcers and these had been diagnosed as aphthous stomatitis.[1] Other stress-related symptoms included an unpleasant awareness of her own heartbeat upon going to bed and waking up in the middle of the night with a feeling of restlessness.

Her energy level was good and her temperature regulation was normal except for the cold hands associated with the migraine. She had no digestive problems and no significant menstrual irregularities except for a rather pronounced premenstrual breast pain. She also had a white, watery leucorrhoea in the second half of her cycle.

Her pulse was wiry and a little weak in the proximal position. Her tongue was normal except for some redness at the tip.

Palpatory diagnosis

When I asked Barbara to undress for the palpatory diagnosis I was surprised to see the discrepancies between different parts of her body. Her head was rather large and well energised, whereas her chest looked somewhat tight and constricted. Below the waist, the forms of her body softened and expanded to a full pelvis and large, somewhat flaccid hips and thighs, giving an impression of heaviness.

Upon superficial palpation, her body felt warm except for some coldness in the area from BL17 *geshu* to BL19 *danshu* and in the sacral area. Going deeper, there was a lack of tone in the connective tissue at BL13 *feishu*. The musculature above the waist felt quite tense, especially at the neck, at the top of the shoulders, below the ribcage, along the left rectus abdominis muscle and at BL18 *ganshu*, where I could feel hard and well-defined lumps in the erector spinae muscle. The tissue below the waist was full and lacked tone except for some deep tightness in the groin area. The palpation of specific points produced pain at REN17 *shanzhong*, GB24 *riyue*, LIV13 *zhangmen* and LIV3 *taichong*.

Anger and sex

Summing up the diagnostic findings with Barbara, I emphasised the general feeling of tightness. I asked her if she could see the tightness as a sign of holding something back. 'I don't see myself like that', she commented. 'I'm an outgoing person and quite successful at pursuing my goals. If someone gets in my way, I can be quite aggressive.' Asked if there were exceptions to that general picture, she hesitatingly admitted that she had never been able to express any anger towards her partner, who was 13 years older than her and definitely a kind of a father figure to her.

'My real father died when I was 14 and perhaps I was looking for a substitute', she told me. I cautiously inquired about their sexual relationship and she admitted that sex was very infrequent and not satisfactory. 'It's like a power struggle and I am tired of it.' I sensed some sadness in her voice, but when I shared my impression with her, she became defensive, visibly pulling herself together. At that point I ended the interview by thanking her for her openness.

Summary of clinical manifestations

- Episodic headache on the right side almost every weekend; worse around noon; pulsating pain, concentrated behind the eyes; associated with cold hands and nausea.
- Mouth and tongue ulcers.
- Waking up restless in the middle of the night.
- Palpitations at rest.
- Last three symptoms worse with stress.
- Premenstrual breast pain.
- White, watery leucorrhoea in the second half of her cycle.
- Forceful but restrained.

- Inability to express anger in specific situations.
- Pulse: wiry and a little weak in the proximal position.
- Tongue: redness at the tip.
- Body palpation: coldness around BL17 *geshu* to BL19 *danshu* and in the sacral area; excessive muscular tension above the waist and at the left rectus abdominis muscle; hard lumps on the *erector spinae* muscles; lack of muscle tone and heaviness below the waist, flaccid hips; pain on pressure at REN17 *shanzhong*, GB24 *riyue*, LIV13 *zhangmen*, and LIV3 *taichong*.

Identifying the patterns of disharmony

According to the Eight Principles, Barbara's pattern was an interior one, predominantly of the excess type with some signs of deficiency in the lower burner and a mixture of hot symptoms above and cold symptoms below the diaphragm.

Most symptoms pointed towards a pattern of stagnant and, at times, rebellious *qi*, associated with a Liver and Gallbladder dysfunction. In this context, I saw the cold hands as a sign of stagnant *qi* and Blood rather than a sign of deficiency because they exclusively occurred in conjunction with the excess symptoms of a migraine attack (Hammer L, personal communication, 1992). The coldness around BL17 *geshu* to BL19 *ganshu* is a symptom I frequently find in patients with stagnation of Liver *qi* but it is also found in those with Liver Blood deficiency. The same two patterns can be associated with generalised muscular tensions. In cases of Liver *qi* stagnation, I have found these tensions to be more homogeneous, in severe cases like a rock or a suit of armour, whereas in Blood deficiency cases the muscles appear to be thinner and more stringy. Barbara clearly displayed the first pattern. According to *Nan Jing* abdominal diagnosis, the tension on the left side of the navel also reflects a Liver disharmony (Matsumoto & Birch 1988).

The nausea during a migraine attack is equivalent to Stomach *qi* rebelling upwards due to Liver Invading the Stomach.

The stress symptoms experienced by the patient as a whole were congruent with a pattern of Heart Fire, even though the mouth and tongue ulcers could also have been interpreted as signs of Stomach Fire. There were, however, no other signs relating to that pattern, whereas the red tip of the tongue indicated a Heat pattern of the Heart.

The coldness and heaviness in the pelvic area, together with the white, watery leucorrhoea and the slightly weak pulse in the proximal position, pointed to a pattern of Damp and Cold in the lower burner, with a slight tendency towards a deficiency of Spleen and Kidneys.

The essence of the pattern could be seen as an obstruction of *qi* at the waist level with *yang qi* rebelling upwards excessively and failing to adequately nourish the lower half of the body. This is an essential part of the pathology related to the *dai mai* (Maciocia 1989).

Evidence for the patterns of disharmony

PRIMARY PATTERNS

Liver *qi* stagnation/Liver *yang* rising

Barbara's major pattern was stagnation of Liver *qi* with episodes of Liver *yang* rising along the course of the Gallbladder Channel:

- Episodic headache on the right side (*shao yang* area) behind the eye.
- Worse around noon (*yang* time of day).
- Accompanied by cold hands.
- Nausea (Liver Invading Stomach).
- Premenstrual breast pain.
- Tight body, generalised muscular tension, especially above the waist.
- Hard lumps on the erector spinae muscles.
- Coldness around BL17 *geshu* to BL19 *danshu*.
- Forceful but restrained movements.
- Inability to express anger in specific situations.
- Pulse: wiry.

SECONDARY PATTERNS

Heart Fire

- Mouth and tongue ulcers.
- Waking up in the middle of the night.
- Palpitations at rest.
- Tongue: redness on the tip.

Cold-Damp in the lower burner/ Spleen and Kidney deficiency

The other secondary pattern is Cold and Damp collecting in the lower burner, with a tendency towards Spleen and Kidney deficiency:

- White watery leucorrhoea.
- Coldness in the sacral area.
- Heaviness in the hips and thighs, flaccid hips.
- Tissue below the waist lacks tone.
- Pulse: weak in the proximal position.

Aetiology and pathology

From my point of view, the Liver dysfunction constituted the source of Barbara's problems (Fig. 34.1). In times of relaxation, e.g. at weekends, the

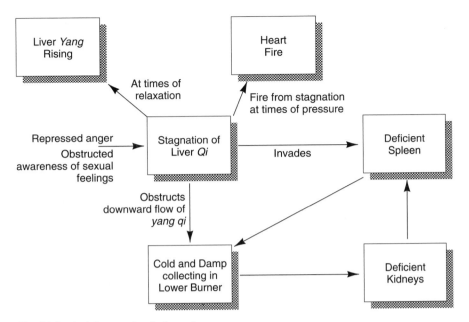

Fig. 34.1 Aetiology and pathology diagram.

bottled-up *yang qi* could no longer be restrained and rose up excessively along the course of the associated Gallbladder channel, causing violent headaches. As long as Barbara pulled herself together in order to achieve a goal, her Liver *qi* remained constrained. The longer this lasted, i.e. in stressful situations, the more the stagnant *qi* transformed into Heat and Fire which was then transmitted to the Heart.

Another aspect of the Liver dysfunction was the obstruction of *qi* at the waist level, i.e. at the level of the *dai mai*. The reduced flow of *yang qi* downwards had the consequence of Cold and Damp collecting in the lower burner. This, together with the negative influence of the Liver dysfunction on transformation and transportation, had started to weaken the Spleen and the Kidneys, perpetuating the disequilibrium in the lower burner.

I was curious as to what had caused the Liver dysfunction in the first place and the nature of the constraining forces within the patient. In an attempt to answer these questions I further analysed Barbara's body structure and her history. As a trained body-oriented psychotherapist, I used these considerations as a bridge between the patient's awareness of herself and my traditional Chinese diagnosis.

I saw a correspondence between the high and sometimes excessive energetic charge of the head and the undercharged pelvic area. I presumed that at a certain point in her life she had sacrificed a lot of her sexual energy for intellectual excellence. The obstruction of the longitudinal energetic currents at the level of the diaphragm and waist then served the purpose of decreasing her awareness of her sexual functions (Lowen 1988).

While palpating Barbara's musculature, I had already drawn her attention to her tensions and blocks. Now I shared with her my impression that they were related to repressed feelings and emotions. In this way I gradually gained her cooperation in elucidating the life events that had distorted her free energetic and emotional flow.

Apparently, as a little girl she had had a covertly sexualised relationship with her father. When she reached puberty, he abruptly distanced himself from her, presumably for fear of acting out his hidden impulses. In an attempt to win back her father's love, Barbara had channelled all her energy into impressing him through intellectual achievements. Before she could find another solution to that conflict, her father had died. She had then found other men to replace him in her attempt to win love by being a 'good girl'.

The other side of the coin was an enormous anger towards her father for not accepting her as a sexual person. This emotion could not be expressed for fear of losing him entirely and had also been transferred to her partners in adult life. So even though she could be very aggressive and pushy in most situations, there was an important part of her life in which she had learned to prevent these impulses from coming to the surface. They were kept inside by a considerable muscular armouring, which is exactly what constituted her pattern of stagnant Liver *qi*.

Her sexuality was covered by the heaviness of her lower body but she had never relinquished it totally. She described how she could like her sexuality at times, 'but then my heart was not open'. This tendency to close her heart in order to protect herself from further hurt was quite evident from the tightness and constriction in her chest.

When I explained that I thought that a long-standing pattern in her life had brought about her present problems, she told me that this made a lot of sense to her.

Treatment issues

Since I saw the stagnation of Liver *qi* as the root of Barbara's problems my central treatment principle was to spread the Liver and to regulate the *qi* of the Liver and Gallbladder. An important part of this strategy would be to open the *dai mai*. In terms of the emotional side of her problems this would mean opening up the avenues to allow her to express anger as well as feelings from the heart.

To address her physical symptoms, namely the manifestation, my secondary goals were to anchor or subdue Liver *yang*, to remove obstructions from the Gallbladder channel, and to disperse Fire from stagnation.

Since her emotional issues were very deep-seated and her migraine condition was quite chronic, Barbara and I agreed to assess the effectiveness of her treatment after a period of 3 months. I told her that she would need to come approximately once weekly, and that each time we would discuss whether the effects of the preceding treatment were still active, or whether a new treatment was required. To engage her actively in the process of finding ways to feel and to express herself differently, I suggested a set of daily exercises.

1 First, she should hit the bed with a tennis racket as a safe, physical way to express anger.
2 Second, she should bend over with her fingers touching the floor in front of her feet. To keep her knees soft, she should slowly and rhythmically bend and extend them slightly, until she felt her legs vibrate. This should create an increased feeling of liveliness in the lower half of her body.
3 Finally she should take some time for deep *hara* breathing to increase the energetic flow into her lower abdomen. For a detailed description of these exercises, see Lowen & Lowen (1977).

Being an active person, Barbara welcomed these suggestions, and, as I discovered later, was quite persistent in carrying them out.

The first treatment

The first treatment took place 3 days after Barbara's first visit. I needled the points listed in the box below and, during the process of insertion and manipulation, I explained some of their actions to her. Her skin was quite sensitive to the insertion of needles but, once inserted, it was easy to obtain a local *deqi* sensation. After a few minutes she reported a streaming sensation in her extremities. She felt relaxed and I let her lie with the needles in place for another 15 minutes. When I removed the needles she told me that she had almost fallen asleep and still felt very tired. 'But it also feels as if something heavy has been taken off my chest', she added.

For me it was important to hear that the treatment had initiated some bodily reactions and even more so that her immediate response had been positive. I explained to her that tiredness after a treatment is a reaction frequently found in people who drive themselves very hard and that it is a sign of letting go.

First treatment procedures

POINTS PRESCRIPTION

- LIV2 *xingjian* subdues Liver *yang* and spreads *qi*, especially effective for cold limbs from stagnation, for migraines, and for Liver Fire affecting the Heart.
- P6 *neiguan* regulates the *qi* of the chest and calms the *shen*, especially effective for tightness in the chest and emotional problems from Liver *qi* stagnation.
- GB41 *zulinqi* spreads Liver and Gallbladder *qi* and opens the *dai mai* (right side only).
- SJ5 *waiguan* is used as the coupled

point to help open the *dai mai* (left side only).

- GB20 *fengchi* and GB8 *shuaigu* subdue Liver *yang* and remove obstructions from the Gallbladder channel (right side only).

Needling technique: I used reducing method on LIV2 *xingjian*, P6 *neiguan*, GB20 *fengchi* and GB8 *shuaigu*, and even method on GB41 *zulinqi* and SJ5 *waiguan*.

Needles: I used 0.25 mm × 40 mm needles which were retained for 20 minutes.

Changes related to sexuality

A week later Barbara reported that the first treatment had really thrown her off balance. She had had problems in accepting her tiredness. She did not have any headaches at the weekend, but had developed a mild attack of aphthous stomatitis. For the second treatment, I therefore used P8 *laogong* instead of P6 *neiguan*, after which the mouth and tongue ulcers healed quickly.

During the next few weeks her headaches became more frequent and she expressed her dissatisfaction with that. On closer inquiry, however, it appeared that the pain was not so strong as it had been previously. She also reported that the situation at home with her partner had become 'very difficult'. She said 'I feel bad, because I think I am responsible'.

After 6 weeks she appeared in my office visibly shattered and told me that after a fight she had thrown her partner out of their apartment. 'Up to that moment I did not know how much anger I had stored up against him', she said. I did not treat her that day, assuming that this strong emotional release was equivalent to free flowing Liver *qi* and that, for the moment, no further release was necessary. Indeed, she did not have any headaches for more than 2 weeks after this event. Also, her vaginal discharge had almost stopped.

Prior to her next menstruation she had another migraine attack, less severe than before, but which was followed by a cramping pain in the groin area lasting until the second day of menstruation. I re-examined her symptoms and found that there was less tension in the diaphragmatic region and no more cold in the sacral area. The points on the lower abdomen, however, were quite painful to the touch. Her pulse was still wiry but no longer weak in the proximal position. Apparently, the main site of the Liver *qi* stagnation had moved down into the pelvis. I assumed that this was related to some change in her sexuality and indeed she told me that she had started to date other men. This was by no means easy for her. 'I feel more pleasure but also a lot of frustration', she said.

I changed the prescription by omitting SJ5 *neiguan* and using GB41 *zulinqi* on both sides instead. I also replaced LIV2 *xingjian* with LIV3 *taichong* and added REN3 *zhongji* as a local point. I treated her during two more menstrual cycles with slow but steady improvement. After this, she decided to go on an extended vacation and discontinued her treatment. Upon her return she decided to move to another city.

More joy in life

I saw Barbara only once more before she moved. She told me that she rarely had headaches, except before her period, but that these were 'manageable without pain killers', and that her premenstrual tension and pains had almost disappeared. There had been no more attacks of mouth and tongue ulcers. She especially emphasised that since I had started to treat her, she had 'found more joy in life' and, at the same time, had become 'more assertive against father figures of any kind'. She was contemplating having psychotherapy in order 'to understand more about myself and how I have developed all these problems'.

I was also very satisfied with the treatment process as a whole because, even though I hadn't cured her migraine problem completely, the treatment had brought about improvements on both a physical and mental-emotional level and had led Barbara to an increased self-awareness and self-expression.

Summary of outcome

- Frequency of migraine attacks reduced by 75%.
- Severity of pain reduced significantly.
- No more attacks of mouth and tongue ulcers (aphthous stomatitis).
- Almost no more leucorrhoea.
- Premenstrual tension reduced significantly.
- More freedom to express emotions appropriately.
- Changed her relationship to her sexuality.

Developing new clarity

I had treated Barbara during a time in my professional career when I was struggling for orientation between the paradigms of Oriental medicine and

Western energetic body-psychotherapy. Even though I was convinced that they were strongly related to one another, I seemed to lack some in-depth understanding that would allow me to use my twofold training during the actual process of assessing and treating my patients. At this point Barbara, and other patients, came to me with problems that somehow revealed themselves from both perspectives. Treating these patients helped me to develop new clarity in my work. Since then I have come to understand more fully the bioenergetic manifestations of patterns of traditional Chinese medicine and vice versa. I am grateful to Barbara, and to other patients, for helping me at this important point in my professional development.

NOTE

1   For information on aphthous stomatitis, see Goroll's *Primary Care Medicine.*

REFERENCES

Goroll A H 1981 Primary care medicine. Lippincott, Philadelphia pp 786–787
Lowen A, Lowen L 1977 The way to vibrant health. Harper & Row, New York
Lowen A 1988 Love, sex, and your heart. Macmillan, New York
Maciocia G 1989 The foundations of Chinese medicine. Churchill Livingstone, Edinburgh
Matsumoto K, Birch S 1988 Hara diagnosis: reflections on the sea. Paradigm Publications, Brookline

■ Jürgen Mücher

Jürgen Mücher became involved with Oriental medicine after he graduated from medical school in 1979. Studying shiatsu with Wataru Ohashi had gradually shifted his focus from scientific to energetic medicine. At the same time, he began to study acupuncture with teachers such as Schnorrenberger, Porkert and Van Nghi.

In 1980, he began training in Western body-oriented energetic psychotherapy at the International Institute for Bioenergetic Analysis in New York, directed by Alexander Lowen. He became a certified therapist in 1986 and a supervisor in 1992.

In 1983, during an extended stay in the United States, he graduated from Ohashi's Shiatsu Education Centre of America, studied at the Tri-State Institute for Traditional Chinese Acupuncture, and continued his acupressure training by studying Jin Shin Do with Iona Teeguarden. He became the first teacher of this bodymind acupressure method in Europe and, later, he was appointed senior staff member at the Jin Shin Do teacher training programme in California.

In 1986, he studied at the Chinese Medical College in Taichung, Republic of China, where he also became interested in Chinese herbal medicine. Since then he has worked as a general practitioner, with a special degree in naturopathy, in Bremen, Germany. In his practice, he mainly uses Chinese medicine and Bioenergetic Analysis.

Among the teachers of Chinese medicine that have been especially influential to him during the last years have been Kiiko Matsumoto, Ted Kaptchuk and Jeremy Ross.

Since 1992 he has been a faculty member of the Deutsche Ärztegesellschaft für Akupunktur, the oldest and most influential among German acupuncture societies.

Managing pharmaceutical drug withdrawal

Dan Kenner SANTA ROSA, CA, USA

The patient's resolve

It always arouses trepidation when a patient comes to me with a need or desire to withdraw from a prescription medication. There are few cases where I feel a prescription drug is really necessary, but asking a patient to withdraw from a medically prescribed drug is fraught with difficulties — emotional, legal and ethical. In this case, the client came to me with a desire to withdraw both from the antidepressant Prozac, which she had been taking at a dose of at least 25 mg a day, and from lithium carbonate, which she had been taking at a dose of 300 mg a day for 4 years. Her condition had been diagnosed as 'manic-depressive bipolar disorder'.

I was personally acquainted with the patient, a 43-year-old mother of two, prior to her appearance at my office, since she had attended one of my nursing classes at the university. Since the patient is a professional nurse, she was well aware of the medical ramifications of her condition. Yet she felt that her condition was deteriorating, and that her treatment had not focused on the core of the problem, from which she had suffered since the age of 16. Despite the insistence of her medical practitioners that there was no other treatment that could be of any potential use, she came to me for treatment with the resolve to withdraw from medication and find another way to deal with the problem.

Her physician was prepared, but reluctant, to cooperate with the drug withdrawal, explaining to me that if unsuccessful, this course of action would adversely affect the patient's self-esteem. With the support of her physician, and the somewhat reluctant support of her husband, we began a course of treatment concomitant with the gradual reduction of the pharmaceutical antidepressants.

The patient had a medium build, mildly corpulent due to weight gain over the past 3 years. She had had a history of asthma since childhood, and still suffered occasional mild attacks. At the age of 7 she had had her tonsils and adenoids removed, at the age of 36 she had had a tubal ligation and, at 39, an excision of basal cell carcinoma with eyelid skin grafts. The first occurrence of her manic-depression was at the age of 16. Episodes of this disorder consisted of a rapid acceleration of thoughts, paranoia, peripheral

hallucinations, anxiety, restlessness and insomnia. Since starting her medication regimen 4 years previously there had been no episodes of manic-
depression but she had felt 'on the edge' of an attack nearly every day.
She still suffered from a low-grade depression, mild confusion and fatigue.
She also complained of frequent headaches behind her right eye, usually
accompanied by nausea.

She suffered from constipation, constant neck and shoulder stiffness,
cold feet, wheezing that would occasionally develop into an asthma attack,
and occasional chest pain with mild tachycardia that was accompanied by
a 'weak' feeling in the chest. Her menstrual cycle was regular. There
was usually mild abdominal cramping at the onset of the menses, flushing,
and often discharge of some dark menstrual blood with a few clots.

Three components to the examination

My examination of her condition consisted of three components: physical
examination, auriculomedical examination of the ear according to the
Nogier method (Nogier 1983), and examination of the blood using dark
field microscopy (Bleker 1993). The physical examination included palpation of the pulse, the abdomen, the affected meridians and areas of physical complaint, and inspection of the tongue. Examination of the ear
involved testing the reaction of the pulse to various stimuli to diagnose the
possible areas of trouble and potential stressful influences. I also use this
method to test the compatibility of the various medications that are under
consideration for use. The dark field examination initially indicates the
nature of the pathological process at the humoral level, and helps future
evaluations of treatment progress. I often examine the blood in cases of
chronic illness. I was not sure of its value in this particular case at first,
but as it turned out, the blood findings were very useful.

The results of the first examination revealed a vacuity in the Pericardium
position of the pulse and a rapid, wiry pulse quality. Abdominal palpation
showed bilateral subcostal pressure pain and the patient reported intermittent discomfort in this area, especially on the right side. There was
extreme tightness along the Gall Bladder channel at the neck and shoulders.
There was also a reddened area at the back of the neck at the level of C3
and C4. The tongue was moderately coated with a white fur. The auricular
examination revealed a field disturbance from a cervical scar (possibily
a tonsillectomy scar), a chronic first rib disturbance (contraction of the
scalenus muscles near the stellate ganglion), laterality instability (which
is fairly common in left-handed individuals), and thyroid dysfunction.
Microscopic blood examination showed clear signs of a tendency toward
fungal infestation.

Summary of clinical manifestations

- Desire to withdraw from prescription medication.
- Suffered from manic depression since the age of 16.
- Believes her condition (diagnosed as 'manic-depressive bipolar disorder') is deteriorating.
- Episodes of this condition used to involve: rapid acceleration of thoughts, paranoia, peripheral hallucination, anxiety, restlessness and insomnia.
- No episodes for 4 years since starting her medical regimen, but feels 'on the edge' of having an episode nearly every day.
- Mildly corpulent due to weight gain during last 3 years.
- History of asthma since childhood, occasional mild attacks developing from wheezing.
- Low grade depression.
- Mild confusion.
- Fatigue.
- Frequent headaches behind right eye, usually accompanied by nausea.
- Constipation.
- Constant neck and shoulder stiffness.
- Cold feet.
- Occasional chest pain with mild tachycardia accompanied by a 'weak' feeling in the chest.
- Regular menstrual cycle, with mild abdominal cramping at the onset of menses, flushing and often discharge of some dark menstrual blood with a few clots.

Physical examination

- Bilateral subcostal pressure pain and discomfort.
- Extreme tightness along the Gall Bladder channel at the back of the neck at the level of C3 and C4.
- Pulse: Vacuity in the Pericardium position of the pulse and a rapid wiry pulse quality.
- Tongue: Moderately coated with white fur.

Auricular examination

- Field disturbance from a cervical scar.
- Tonsillectomy scar.
- Chronic first rib disturbance.
- Laterality instability.
- Thyroid dysfunction.
- Fungal irritation in the large intestine area (appeared by third visit).

Microscopic blood examination

- Clear signs of a tendency towards fungal infestation.

Identifying patterns of disharmony

As an acupuncturist, I do not take what most people would consider an 'oriental medical' approach to diagnosis.[1] I believe that such theoretical considerations are artificial, and that theories are simply 'software' for solving problems. I also believe that the clinical practitioner should collect and combine theoretical models and learn to rapidly generate his or her own theoretical models in order to keep pace with their obsolescence. My Japanese training was very much oriented towards making theoretical considerations subordinate to practical observation. Certainly every experienced practitioner that I met in Japan had his or her own theoretical model and unique methodology. This was a grievous source of frustration for a student such as myself who was seeking the one and only true and correct traditional oriental medicine.

From the viewpoint of auriculomedicine, the right ear is 'dominant' in a right-handed person, and the left ear in a left-handed person. It is not unusual to detect mild laterality disturbances in day-to-day practice. I have found severe laterality disturbances to correspond with severe psycho-pathology or with epilepsy. In this case, at one important stage of recovery immediately after cessation of the pharmaceutical lithium, my patient exhibited a significant laterality disturbance for a few weeks before it spontaneously normalised. Laterality disturbance is considered to be a disturbed function of the corpus callosum, that part of the brain which spans both hemispheres. I do not consider the auricular diagnosis to be conclusive in any way, but it can be correlated with other information. Persistent patterns are important indicators to me, but with these types of 'energetic' diagnoses it is necessary to observe patterns over several sessions. Patterns that are persistent have more diagnostic significance. In this case, from the third visit, the fungal irritation in the large bowel appeared in the auricular diagnosis week after week for over 3 months.

From the viewpoint of microscopic blood evaluation, the clinical picture of a 'fungal terrain' often corresponds with a Phlegm-dampness condition of Oriental herbology. To have subsequent confirmation from the ear examination that there is a fungal condition, and to be able to locate it clearly is very heartening for the sake of diagnosis. Not every case matches up diagnostically as clearly and consistently as this one did. In clinical practice there is usually no shortage of contradictions. Diagnosis, as Kierkegaard would have it, can only be understood in retrospect. He says, in effect, that life can only be *understood* 'backwards' by looking back on events but it has to be *lived* 'forward'.

Motivation

Motivated patients are always a pleasure to work with, because they are willing to take responsibility for the situation. In this case, desperation played a role in her motivation to de-medicate and get well. In addition to that, however, she had worked hard to achieve a fulfilling life despite her difficulties, and was determined to preserve it. She had created a pro-fessional career for herself and a contented family life. Her rapport with her children was easy and natural and when she spoke of her husband, it was with affection. I believe she also wanted to make some improvement rapidly to appease both her husband and her physician, and to prove to them that she really could live without drugs.

My methods of treatment for this case had several facets. Treatment of points on the ear was carried out during most of the patient's visits using a mild (microampere range) electrical stimulation. This type of treatment is extremely useful for many forms of depression, immune system dysfunction and pain. Body acupuncture was also useful in this case, especially for the headaches and acute anxiety. I usually recommend dietary reform, or at least an identification process whereby the patient is asked to discover which foods or other substances have a deleterious effect on the condition being treated. In most cases, once this process has begun, I then use herbal formulae, essential oils, mineral salts and isopathic remedies (Prescription Book of Sanum Preparations 1985).

For the first treatment SP4 *gongsun* and P6 *neiguan* were used in combination. After this, 'draining' (sedation) of the shoulder points was carried out and a few drops of blood were squeezed from DU15 *yamen*. The patient's condition was acute and because of this dietary reform experimentation was postponed in favour of symptomatic relief. The patient was given aloe tablets to assist bowel elimination and capsules of California poppy to promote deeper sleep.

First treatment procedures

BODY ACUPUNCTURE

SP4 *gongsun* and P6 *neiguan,* a pattern for treating one of the extraordinary vessels (the Penetrating vessel). I often use this pattern for a patient who is exhausted, often with a vacuous Pericardium pulse position, or with Liver dysfunction, according to Dr Yoshio Manaka's method of application of extraordinary vessel treatment.

GB21 *jianjing* is a particularly important shoulder point. Releasing tension here releases the first rib (which is so important in auriculomedicine), improves circulation to the head, and creates a profound relaxed state. In this patient, there was tightness along much of the Gall Bladder channel, especially in the neck and shoulders. Other points drained included BL15 *xinshu*, BL19 *danshu*, BL22 *sanjiaoshu* and BL29 *zhonglushu*.

DU15 *yamen* (a few drops of blood were squeezed from this point). The patient exhibited a reddened area on the back of the neck at about the third and fourth cervical vetebrae. I was taught in Japan that this is a sign of Blood stagnation in the neck and head and an excessive concentration of *ki (qi)* in the upper body. Draining a few drops of blood has a calming effect, and is often used along with cupping for lowering high blood pressure.

AURICULAR ACUPUNCTURE

Auricular points that were frequently indicated included neck and head points in different phases, and liver, duodenum, pancreas and thalamus points.

Needling methods

I use almost exclusively Japanese #2 and #4 needles with a guide tube. I almost never obtain *de qi* sensation with the needling. With this patient, I actively attempted to release, with manipulation of #4 needles, tension in the trapezius muscles at GB12 *wangu* and GB21 *jianjing*. When the channel 'released', there was often a sensation. When I used LU5 *chize* to treat dyspnoea, there was a spontaneous release of tension locally and throughout the chest, but the art is to know when to sedate by the way the point feels under light palpation. Many Japanese acupuncturists believe that you should never drain (sedate) the channels, but I often feel that it is necessary.

ESSENTIAL OILS

1   Aloe tablets: to assist bowel elimination.
2   California poppy capsules: to promote deeper sleep.

I find that essential oils act very quickly. For this reason I use them for crisis situations: anxiety attacks, acute

infections, etc. I do not recommend using massage-grade oils internally. I use only pharmaceutical-grade oils for oral or rectal administration. The auriculomedical protocol is useful in determining which oil or oils are most likely to be helpful when there are several to choose from.

DIETARY REFORM

The focus of the treatment was on symptomatic relief. Dietary reform experimentation was postponed.

Subsequent visits

On the next visit, the patient was very tired because she had been up most of the previous night with her son, who had suffered an asthma attack. She had also suffered some bronchial constriction and had used a medicated inhaler twice during the night. She was given a very light acupuncture treatment using several points: GB41 *linqi*, SJ5 *waiguan*, BL19 *danshu*, BL22 *sanjiaoshu*, BL43 *gaohuangshu*, GB21 *jianjing*, GB12 *wangu* and DU17 *naohu*. She was also given capsules containing essential oils of niaouli and eucalyptus in a base of flax seed oil for her respiratory distress.

By the third visit, she was down to 10 mg of Prozac a day and 100 mg of lithium carbonate a day. Her pulse was very wiry, rapid and replete. Ear examination this time revealed a fungal focus in the large intestine area. This point would appear in subsequent auricular examinations consistently for several months. The patient was given capsules containing a combination of oil of rosemary and oil of peppermint for headaches and to soothe the nervous system. She was also given capsules of essential oil of bitter orange and granules of Bupleurum and Citrus, Pinellia Formula (Japanese: *yokkansan ka chinpihange*; Mandarin: *yi gan san jia chen pi ban xia*) for hyper-excitability of the nervous system and panic attacks (Hong-yen Hsu 1980).[2] In addition, she was given lithium orotate to take as a supplement during withdrawal from the pharmaceutical lithium. Lithium orotate is absorbed much more efficiently by the body than lithium carbonate or acetate and therefore doesn't accumulate in the blood and damage the kidneys. It is not necessary with lithium orotate, then, to monitor the blood levels of lithium as it is with the carbonate or acetate salts. The patient was advised that lithium orotate was a 'nutritional lithium' from which she could withdraw voluntarily at any time without repercussion.

Dietary reform

Once the chronic fungal infection had been identified, the issue of dietary reform became one of great urgency. I recommended an elimination diet for 5 days excluding all fats, oils, animal protein, sugar, coffee and alcohol. In addition, I advised eliminating all fruit and fruit juice. We had previously discussed the need to identify any irritating dietary factors, and this diet was used to sensitise the patient to irritants, enabling her to identify them more easily. She was very motivated to adopt any approach that could help. Body acupuncture and auricular treatments were given weekly, and she received essential oils for crisis management and Pefrakehl rectal suppositories (Prescription Book of Sanum Preparations 1985), an isopathic remedy for fungal infections.[3]

Five days into this diet a skin rash appeared on the arms in areas corresponding to the Lung and Large Intestine channels. On the first day that she stopped the elimination diet, the patient suffered wheezing which was relieved by capsules of essential oils of pine and hyssop in combination.

Complete withdrawal from medication

Five weeks after the start of treatment, she was completely off the Prozac and by 3 months she had completely stopped the pharmaceutical lithium and was using lithium orotate only as an occasional supplement together with capsules of oil of bitter orange when she felt 'shaky'. Approximately coinciding with her complete withdrawal from lithium, auricular treatment shifted from dominance in her left ear to dominance in her right. Normally, the left ear is the dominant ear in a left-handed person and this shift to the right indicated a significant laterality disturbance. It persisted for about 4 weeks, and then the dominance reverted to the left ear. During this time there were several important occurrences.

The patient discovered a significant allergy to wheat and dairy products. I had, of course, recommended stopping oils and animal proteins as part of the elimination diet, but the patient discovered her sensitivity to wheat by herself. When she ingested wheat, dairy or sugar etc. she would immediately experience anxiety, rapid heartbeat and an uncomfortable feeling of detachment ('spaced out'). This was a very fortunate discovery. After a couple of weeks of avoiding wheat and dairy products, she experienced a new sense of wellbeing 'somatically', as she described it, but anxiety and 'emotional pressure' remained a daily problem. She experienced immediate relief from headaches, which were diminishing in severity and frequency, by using rosemary-peppermint capsules and relief from anxiety using bitter orange capsules and Bupleurum and Citrus, Pinellia Formula (Hong-yen Hsu 1980). Her sleep was deeper and more satisfying when she was 'eating well'. At this time she also experienced another flare-up of asthma. From our previous discussions she was reasonably convinced that the asthma attack was not a setback. Her pulse was slippery and Lung position vacuous. The asthma was relieved by treating LU5 *chize*, ST37 *shangjuxu*, DU20 *baihui* and DU23 *shangxing*, and deep points medial to GB21 *jianjing*. Capsules made from essential oil of lavender provided subsequent relief at home.

Steady improvement

Five months after treatment began we increased the interval between visits to 2 weeks, and a month after that to 3 weeks. I consider the patient to be stable and under control, because she has completely withdrawn from the pharmaceutical medications, has had only one headache in the last 3 months and has not had any asthma attacks during the autumn which, in the past, has been a difficult time for her. She has significantly lower levels of anxiety, and is able to recognise much earlier when a problem is building up and thus take countermeasures with dietary change, or herbal supplementation.

Seven months after her first visit, the patient still has a slight inclination towards fungal infection which is apparent from her blood picture. The ear still sometimes tests positive for fungal irritation in the Large Intestine, but the problem now seems sporadic instead of constant. I encouraged the patient to use capsules of grapefruit seed extract on a daily basis for several weeks at a time to help eliminate the fungal problem. At the present time the patient feels confident about her life and believes in her own ability to steadily improve her condition through her own efforts. She is still observing strict dietary practices whenever possible and takes Bupleurum and Citrus, Pinellia Formula on a regular basis and/or lithium orotate as needed. She comes for acupuncture treatment for stress management usually once but sometimes twice monthly.

Summary of outcome

- Patient now considered stable and under control.
- She has withdrawn completely from all pharmaceutical medications.
- She is 'eating well'.
- Sleep is deeper and more satisfying.
- Only one headache in the last 3 months.
- No asthma attacks during the autumn, a time when she has been susceptible in the past.
- Significantly lower levels of anxiety,

and is able to recognise much earlier when a problem is building up.
- Slight inclination towards fungal infection is apparent in the blood picture.
- Ear still sometimes tests positive for

fungal irritation in the Large Intestine.
- Confident about her life now.
- Believes in her own ability to steadily improve her condition through her own efforts.

Patient empowerment

This was not an easy case, and the patient's distress at each visit challenged me to provide the best relief and safest direction for her to follow. I should point out that I had previously seen cases like this one where lithium was being used to control a bipolar disorder when the actual cause of the problem was a chronic fungal infection with food allergies. This is not to say, of course, that this is the sole cause of manic depression, but it illustrates, I believe, an important principle: that drugs are useful only for temporary states of extreme distress or for dangerous situations. It is a fantasy to believe that psychopharmaceutical intervention is corrective when there are other, less dangerous, methods which deal somatically with nervous system complaints.

My philosophy of acupuncture treatment, as well as herbal and dietary treatment, is to train the patient to be in charge. The ultimate outcome with this patient is that she knows when she needs me. If she needs acupuncture, herbs, advice or encouragement, she now feels empowered to make these decisions by herself.

NOTES

1 In my own notes and reports on patient visits, I don't really use a 'diagnosis' or attempt to reduce a patient's condition to a single description of a basic pattern of disharmony. Of course, when I teach or write I, by necessity, try to codify patterns and teach students how to recognise patterns. I don't believe that it is futile to teach or learn formalised pattern recognition, but it is part of the paradox of what one Japanese *kampo* master termed the 'theoretical-clinical dichotomy'. In theoretical texts, we are in an idealised conceptual world which is very different to the one we inhabit in the clinic. An important feature of this book is that it clearly demonstrates this point. However, I cannot avoid the fact that I use different methods of investigation, creating a theoretical 'Macedonian salad'. I do actually occasionally treat cases that follow a standard pattern of one *ism* or another, but they are usually uninteresting. I have chosen this case study to demonstrate more clearly the range of treatments I like to call upon in a difficult case.

2 From an oriental herbal medicine model, I felt that this patient was suffering from an excess of dampness and exhibited symptoms of Wind-heat and

disturbance of the *shen*. In *kampo*, the Japanese method of herbal prescription, I felt her pattern fit was with the *sho* or 'conformation' of Bupleurum and Citrus, Pinellia Formula. The formula is used to Harmonise the Liver and to Stop Wind, along with other functions, and for the treatment of anxiety, insomnia, restlessness, headaches and dizziness, among other symptoms. I recommended that the patient used this formula when she began to feel anxiety and restlessness because, in my experience, it is faster-acting than either the oil of bitter orange or the lithium orotate.

3 My sense of her pattern of disharmony, as it developed over the months, was that her manic depression was actually the result of toxicity to the nervous system and thyroid gland due to the chronic fungal infection. Calming the nervous system and Harmonising the Liver and Wind symptoms alone would not correct the problem. It would also be necessary to cleanse the Dampness, or accumulated mucus and fluid, which provided the environment for fungal growth to proliferate. This was accomplished through dietary change, a herbal formula (which also contained herbs for clearing out Dampness), and the isopathic medications, particularly Pefrakehl and Fortakehl (Prescription Book of Sanum Preparations 1985). Isopathic medications are fundamentally 'symbiotic' microbes, the purpose of which is to break down pathogenic microbes in a pathological terrain.

REFERENCES

Bleker M 1993 Examination in dark-field microscopy according to Professor Guenther Enderlein. Semmelweis-Verlag, Hoya

Hong-yen Hsu 1980 Commonly used Chinese herbal formulae. OHAI Press, Los Angeles

Nogier P 1983 From auriculotherapy to auriculomedicine. Maisonneuve, Paris

Prescription book of Sanum preparations 1985 Sanum-Kehlbeck GmbH & Co. KG, Postfach 322, D-2812 Hoya

FURTHER READING

Kenner D, Requena Y 1994 Botanical medicine: a European professional perspective. Paradigm, Brookline

Nieper H 1981 Dr Nieper's revolution. MIT Verlag, Oldenburg

Wiseman N, Ellis A, Zmiewski P 1985 Fundamentals of Chinese medicine. Paradigm, Brookline

■ Dan Kenner

Dan Kenner trained at the Meiji College of Oriental Medicine in Osaka followed by an internship at Osaka Medical University Pain Clinic and an internship with Dr Tamotsu Mii, founder of the Pulse Diagnosis Research Association. He subsequently worked with Dr Shigeru Arichi, head of Oriental Medicine at Kinki University Medical Teaching Hospital, south of Osaka, in Japan. He is licensed to practise acupuncture in both Japan and California. He has studied European botanical medicine in France and is author with Yves Requena of *Botanical Medicine: a European Professional Perspective*. He runs training seminars for health care practitioners in both European and Oriental botanical medicine, and imports pharmaceutical-grade botanical products. He teaches classes in alternative health care through the nursing and psychology departments at Sonoma State University, California. He is on the Board of Directors of the Meiji College of Oriental Medicine in San Francisco, and is a founding member of the National Society for Acupuncture Research.

Solidity and fragility

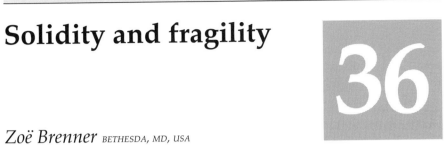

Zoë Brenner BETHESDA, MD, USA

Anne is a heavy woman in her late forties who dresses well, with carefully applied make-up and neat hair, but who seems uncomfortable in her body. At first I felt a solidity about her and then realised that I was catching glimpses of fragility. She seemed very open, present and reasonably at ease.

A major depression

I was quite surprised when Anne told me that she had been in a private psychiatric hospital for 4 months that year for a 'major depression'. She was also a recovering alcoholic. She spoke of lacking emotional feeling and not caring about anything, which surprised me as it did not show. She obviously had a good mask and had learned not to give many clues as to what was going on internally. However, she was fairly free with verbal information and wanted me to know that, as a result of the hospitalisation, she was beginning to know what made her vulnerable. She had just stopped taking lithium and Prozac and was tapering off Xanax which she had been prescribed in the hospital.

Asthma and allergies

Anne's other major complaint was asthma, which had developed at the age of 30, 'but I ignored it and thought it was in my mind'. Eight years ago, she was in intensive care for 3 weeks with an asthma attack and there were many physical side-effects from the medication. Prednisone, which she took in high doses, gave her most problems. At first she had found it to be life saving but then it had made her feel quite worn out. She had also received allergy shots that had been initially effective but had not really helped in the long term. She noted that stress and allergies, which manifested with hay-fever symptoms and colds, could initiate the asthma.

The allergy season for her, 'started in February but was worst from August to October . . . I have had a lot of losses in my life'. That was an amazing connection for her to make. When I asked her to explain she replied simply that there seemed to be a connection between the asthma and stress from losing her son and grandchildren, who had just moved across the country, and from losing a grandchild when her daughter miscarried.

Abuse and hiding

We then talked about the stresses to which she was so vulnerable. She said that she worked for a crazy organisation and that her direct boss was very abusive, but she added that she had been there for 15 years. 'I was a high school drop-out and worked my way up to executive positions. I never thought that I was as good as anyone else'. She now held a college degree. I was not surprised. Anne was obviously used to abuse and hiding, but when did it start?

She described her mother as a volatile perfectionist, who blamed her children abusively and would even tie them to a pole in a parking lot when she went to the store. She described her mother as 'sadistic'. And where was her father? 'He was a wimp who was nice to the outside world. I wanted to yell at people who thought he was good. He preached a rigid religion'. Her brother was born when she was 12 and she then went 'wild'. She figured out when to get pregnant and did, and then got married and thus escaped.

Not worthy enough to complain

Anne described a lot of other symptoms that were important to the whole picture and these are listed in the box below. What I found interesting was the way in which she expressed her symptoms as if she did not feel worthy enough to complain.

What I was beginning to sense was that Anne was one of those patients with whom it is a great privilege to work. Here was a very bright woman who was really sensitive and intuitive about her own being but unsure of herself. The therapies and drugs she had already tried had not worked well for her. As she said herself, she tended to 'drop out of a lot of therapies'. She was indeed one of those individuals who tends to fall through the cracks when set theories and treatments are applied. To be able to help her I had to be fully present with her and follow her very sensitive lead. The exciting pay off for me was that I learned a lot about acupuncture.

Physical examination and referral

In the physical examination, I discovered that her pulse was floating in the third position on the left. I have found this to indicate the floating nature of the Lung *qi* which is not descending to the Kidneys and which should be felt at that depth.

Not surprisingly, Anne apologised to me for reacting to the pain when I checked the *mu* points and the abdominal diagnosis[1] and did the Akabane test.[2]

When I felt Anne's back, I found the muscles to be very tight, especially at the neck, and her head was not able to fully rotate. These chronic difficulties with her back and neck led me to recommend a referral to an osteopath in the near future. Prior to referral, I wanted some time to observe her response to the acupuncture treatment. She told me that she had tried chiropractic treatment and found it to be harsh and unhelpful. However, she said she would be willing to try osteopathy. I told her the osteopath to whom she would be referred did a very sensitive type of work.

Diet, medication and herbs

Anne said that she had gained a lot of weight since stopping drinking because she now substituted sugar for alcohol. When I questioned her about her diet, it seemed that she was living on carbohydrates, so I recommended that she ate more vegetables and protein to stabilise her blood sugar level and to reduce her hunger. She was receptive to this suggestion. Regarding medication, she would continue to reduce her Xanax dosage and continue with her asthma medications as directed.

Anne said that she knew I worked with herbal medicine as well as acupuncture, but would rather not take herbs because she was already taking medication. I think she also wanted to see how the acupuncture treatment would work. I was a little disappointed because I knew herbal treatments that might help, but I valued her judgement.

Summary of clinical manifestations

- 'Major depression', flatness of spirit, no joy.
- History of emotional abuse and neglect.
- Asthma, with phlegm when very bad.
- Allergies, especially in the autumn.
- History of frequent upper respiratory infections.
- Fluctuating moods.
- Severe lack of self esteem.
- Masked emotional presentation.
- Has difficulty crying or mourning, but has had 'a lot of losses'.
- Irritable.
- Anxiety, like 'jumping out of the skin', and rising agitation from the lower abdomen ('running piglets').[3]
- Very sensitive to people, impressions and treatment.
- Weight gain, desire for sweets.
- Recovering alcoholic.
- Low back pain.

- 'Aches in the arms like headaches', mostly on the Large Intestine meridian.
- Neck pain, with two disintegrated cervical discs.
- Insomnia, waking at 2 to 4 a.m. and often not returning to sleep.
- Irritable bowel, anxiety causes more explosive diarrhoea.
- Fibrocystic breast disease.
- Some hot flushes.
- PMS, with mood swings, nervousness and breast pain.
- Clotting and cramping with menstrual flow.

- **Abdominal diagnosis:** GB, LIV, LU, LI , KID, BL are sensitive points.
- *Mu* **point** of Lung is sensitive.
- **Akabane test:** Kidney (left) deficient and Spleen (right) deficient.
- **Facial colour:** green and shiny white.
- **Voice:** shouting frequently but also weeping.
- **Odour:** mildly rotten.
- Pulse: left middle position wiry, right middle position slippery, empty first position, especially on the right, and left third position floating.
- Tongue: red body with some blue; little coating but moist.

Identifying the patterns of disharmony

My usual practice is to play with different models of patterns until something fits. In this case, I saw signs of Liver *qi* stagnation, congealed Blood, Lung *yin* deficiency, countercurrent of Lung *qi* and disturbed *shen*, plus more. Somehow, however, this pattern seemed too fragmented for Anne and I would be chasing symptoms all over the place. In addition, there appeared to be a lot of contradictions. When this happens, my first response is to opt for the simpler concepts and assess the patient's reaction to treatment.

The most prominent pattern that I saw was a basic disruption of the upward and downward movements. This could be seen from the Five Phase pattern as a disturbance of the balance between the upward thrust of Wood and the downward concentration, controlled by the Lung. This model, in its simple form, actually allowed me to explain much of what I saw in my patient. However, when I looked at the details of the patterns in each of the phases, there were further contradictions and difficulties.

I was confident enough to use the simple model as a starting point even though I was unable to explain how everything fitted together. I often think of my diagnosis as a working hypothesis and I discover how things fall together (or not) as I treat and assess the patient's response.

I now had to decide which was the primary element — Wood or Metal? I certainly felt more clearly drawn to the weakness of the Metal and the patient's difficulty in descending the *qi*. However, her vulnerability and lack of self worth were more like Wood characteristics, due either to deficiency of Gall Bladder *qi* or deficiency of Liver Blood. With her asthma, I saw an interplay between the Metal (Lung) not descending the *qi*, the Kidney not grasping the *qi* and bringing it downward, and the Liver, in countercurrent, forcing the *qi* upward. All three play their part in the essential upward and downward movement of *qi*.

Evidence for the patterns of disharmony

Metal imbalance: countercurrent of Lung *qi* and deficient Lung *yin*

- Asthma.
- Allergies, especially in the autumn.
- Unable to weep or mourn.
- Severe lack of self esteem; puts up a mask.
- Insomnia, wakes between 2 a.m. and 4 a.m. (during the transition between Liver and Lung time).
- Hot flushes.
- Extreme sensitivity.
- **Facial colour:** shiny white.
- **Voice:** weeping.
- **Odour:** mildly rotten.
- **Abdominal diagnosis:** LU and LI sensitive.
- *Mu* point of Lung sensitive.
- Pulse: floating left third position (a 'Lung type' pulse), empty Lung position.

Wood imbalance: stagnant Liver *qi*, congealed Blood, Liver *qi* countercurrent

- Fluctuating moods.
- Irritability.
- PMS with breast pain and nervousness.
- Clotting and cramping with menstrual flow.
- Very tight muscles in the neck and low back.

- Rising agitation from the base of the abdomen ('running piglets').[3]
- Asthma (from countercurrent of *qi*).
- Irritable bowel syndrome.
- **Facial colour:** green.
- **Voice:** shouting frequently.
- **Abdominal diagnosis:** GB and LIV sensitive.
- Pulse: wiry in the Liver position.

Fire imbalance: *shen* disturbance, deficient Heart Blood

- 'Major depression' — a flatness of spirit and no joy (*bu le*).
- Extreme sensitivity.
- Masking of emotions.

Water imbalance: Kidney *yin* deficiency, Kidneys not grasping the *qi* and upsurging Kidney *qi*

- Hot flushes.
- Anxiety, with rising agitation from the low abdomen ('running piglets').
- Asthma.
- **Abdominal diagnosis:** KID and BL sensitive.

Earth imbalance: deficient Spleen *qi* with Dampness

- Desire for sweets.
- Weight gain.
- Phlegm.

Aetiology and pathology

What seemed to be the deepest issue for Anne was her lack of trust and belief in herself which stemmed from abuse and neglect as a child. She protected herself by putting up a mask whilst remaining fragile, weak and not feeding her internal self, particularly the sensitive *zang* (Lung and Heart). I believe the result was the countercurrent of Lung *qi* and deficiency of the quiet, deep *yin* aspect of the Lung.

Her healthy assertiveness and frustration were often quashed, thereby constraining the Liver *qi* and eventually affecting the flow of Blood. The unevenness of the flow of the Liver *qi* caused an uprooting of the *qi* affecting the Kidney, and an invasion of the Spleen, and also affected the clarity and spark of the Heart *shen*. In addition, her Heart must have been injured from an early age because of the depth of her feelings of inadequacy and self-doubt, almost to the point of being out of touch with reality.

There were obviously other factors as well. The use of alcohol had affected the *yin* and the Liver. There were also structural problems that had originated perhaps from the constrained *qi* or other factors.

In Five Phase terms there was a basic disruption of the entire *sheng* cycle. Most phases, because of their own disruption, were not fully generating the activity of the next phase. Figure 36.1 shows this simple basic concept and a complexity of connections.

Treatment issues

Since I had decided to work initially with the simplest part of the pattern, my procedure was to address the Lung difficulties first and foremost, starting with the right-left Akabane imbalance. I planned to treat the Lung to see what effect this would have in balancing the other aspects. I believe that in such complex and sensitive cases, if too many patterns are treated to begin with, one loses track of what is effective and what is not. In Anne's case, I would assess her response to each treatment and would move on to other treatments in addition to or instead of the original Lung treatment as necessary.

I discussed the treatment plan with Anne, emphasising that we would need to find out, over time, what was most effective in treating her overall condition. I was concerned to highlight this since she had found a number of previous therapies to be unsuccessful in the long term and because the problems she was experiencing were fairly serious. Acupuncture has many variables and many ways of treating conditions, so if my best judgement took us in one direction and that was not wholly successful, there were other options. I would do my best to find the most effective treatment for as many aspects of her discomfort as possible. I also explained that I aimed to treat the patterns of imbalance that were underlying the symptoms. She seemed pleased with this and I think hopeful because of the nature of our interaction.

I told her that I would start with once or twice weekly treatments, de-

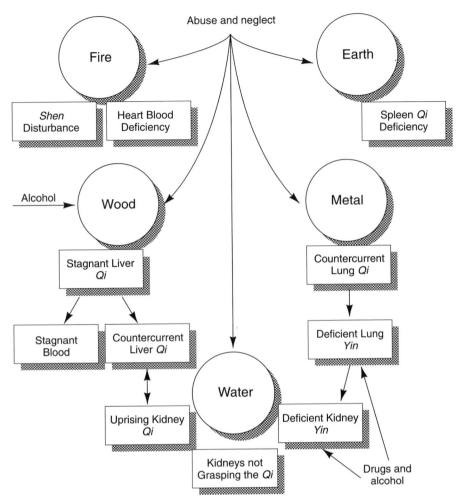

Fig. 36.1 Aetiology and pathology diagram.

pending on her response, and would then progress to treatment every other week and move on from there. I explained that my experience of depression and asthma was that these conditions rarely cleared within a few treatments and that many people attended for treatment on an on-going basis. I explained that she was free to discontinue treatment whenever she wanted to, and that some people with chronic conditions saw treatment as part of their health maintenance. She was ready to start. Money was not an issue at this point; she said her wellbeing was very important.

As I mentioned before, I recommended some dietary changes and planned to refer her, in the future, to an osteopath for structural work. I expected also that there would be some changes in her future relationships. It seemed that she felt most conflict with her boss and I wondered how this would change as her self esteem improved. There might also be changes in her family relationships.

Returning for the first treatment

There was a 2-week gap between the first consultation and the first treatment. In the week before the treatment Anne had a 'major asthma attack', triggered by stress at work and pollen. She was tapering off taking prednisone and had also tried my dietary suggestions, reporting that her cravings were diminishing (even with the prednisone).

I explained each step of the procedure as we went along. Some of it was explained in the consent form that I had given her to read and sign at the first visit. Interestingly, this time there was a thick, slightly yellow coating on her tongue. At our first meeting, Anne's tongue had been without a coat, so the evidence of phlegm was now more apparent.

I repeated the Akabane test. When I started treatment to balance the Akabane she responded strongly to the needles and apologised for her reaction as if she had done something wrong. I assured her that her response was okay, that it was a good sign of her sensitivity to herself and that many people responded in that way.

After needling LI11 *quchi,* I went on to treat LU2 *yunmen,* followed by LU3 *tianfu,* and Anne reported easier breathing. A few minutes after LU3 *tianfu* she said she felt really peaceful; and after the next point, LU9 *taiyuan,* she said that my ceiling tiles were in sharper focus! She was very clear about her responses. When I got lost, I only had to listen to my patient and she would tell me what was happening.

I felt a big change in her pulses, especially in the Lung position, but also her Liver and Gall Bladder pulses were much less wiry. The floating quality of the 'Lung pulse' in the left third position was gone and the Kidney pulse felt more appropriately lower. Her green facial colour had completely cleared.

I was very pleased and so was she. Even though she had responded well, I knew it would not all be so easy and I felt myself waiting for the difficulties. So far, however, all my questions had received good answers.

First treatment procedures

POINTS PRESCRIPTION

Listed in order of use:
- KID4 *dazhong* (left).
- SP4 *gongsun* (right).

Both points were used to balance the Akabane. For each meridian, the *luo* point is tonified on the deficient side in order to create balance. The meridian is then re-tested. If the deficiency remains, the source (*yuan*) point is then treated on the deficient side. If it persists in its imbalance, the next step is to disperse the *luo* point on the other side for a few minutes and then re-tonify the deficient side.

In stubborn cases I even use the *shu* points on the back to balance the right and left of the meridian.

- LI11 *quchi* is the tonification point of the Large Intestine and disperses Damp-Heat; also, being on the Metal, it helps to clear the Lung.
- LU2 *yunmen*, 'Cloud Gate', clears the clouds, i.e. the dampness of the Earth that was blocking the descending movement of the Lung (Rochat de la Vallée 1991).
- LU3 *tianfu*, 'Heavenly Palace', is the first point on the Lung meridian to descend and is thus very powerful in initiating downward movement. It is also known to help balance the up and outward movement of the Wood, with this downward movement from the top of the Lung meridian.
- LU9 *taiyuan*, 'Great Abyss', is a source point and so balances the whole function of the Lung and also very powerfully moves the *qi* down and inward, as into an abyss.

These last three points helped free up the blockage and re-establish a good and balanced downward movement of the *qi* to correct the countercurrent of the Lung *qi*.

Needles and needling technique

I used 12 mm, Japanese size 1, metal-handled needles for all the points except LI11 *quchi* and LU3 *tianfu*, for which I used 25 mm needles of the same type. For the Akabane treatment I used a tonification technique of insertion, half turn clockwise and rapid withdrawal. For LI11 *quchi* I used a technique which I call 'rapid dispersion' and in which I insert the needle in dispersing mode and then give a strong half turn counter-clockwise to release the blockage with some force, after which I remove the needle. For the other points, I used a gentle tonification, inserting in the direction of the meridian flow, feeling the *qi* and gently turning clockwise and then removing quickly. I have found that it can make a noticeable difference in the efficacy of the treatment if I visualise and feel the physical movement of the *qi* that I want to achieve.

A calling out of Wood

Anne returned, saying that she had been able to expectorate well immediately after her first treatment. She had been even-tempered, surprisingly her boss had noticed, and her anxiety level had been better. So I continued to work with her Lung-Metal Phase for several treatments. Then Wood started calling out more strongly, manifesting in irritability and muscle mobility complaints.

So it was now time to treat the Wood Phase. At first I treated the source points of the Liver and Gall Bladder, using my 'rapid dispersion' method (see box above), because I thought that, primarily, the Liver *qi* was stagnant. I then tonified points on the Heart and Small Intestine to give the Wood *qi* somewhere healthy to go. I included the Lung source point. This helped, but soon after the treatment Anne returned to the same state of irritability. However, there was a change in her. She had been for a job interview for the first time in 10 years saying, 'I didn't have the nerve before'.

I continued to work in the same way but still something was wrong. So I tried a different needle technique on the Liver and Gall Bladder, leaving the needles in sedation mode for 30 minutes. This technique has a more calming effect and is less actively dispersing. However, a few days after the treatment, the 'jumpiness', muscle tightness and irritability returned. I also used an even needling technique to no particular avail. I used P6 *neiguan* to free the constrained *qi* and I needled DU20 *baihui* to see if that would calm the Liver *qi* in its countercurrent. In fact, as a result, Anne seemed to have more anxiety reactions, together with the rising jitters from her pelvis ('running piglets'), which I then tried to treat as a blockage of Kidney *qi*.

The problem remained that I needed to free the Liver *qi* without sedating it so strongly that, through suppression, it intensified the Liver symptoms of irritability and anger. There were times when the Liver *qi* stagnation, combined with difficult external circumstances, resulted in *shen* disturbance where Anne reported severe lack of feeling and when she would just shut down into a depressive state. Anne would recover from this state, to her surprise, very quickly with treatment of her Heart and has not considered re-taking antidepressants.

Return to the Metal phase

Meanwhile I stopped using Lung points after having used them in every treatment up to this point. At the next treatment, Anne reported some breathing problems, and had an asthma attack immediately after the treatment. I felt that I was really losing control. So I returned to treat the Lung. There was not much improvement until I treated LU9 *taiyuan*, when she said, 'The ceiling tiles are clearer again!'. At the next treatment, I used some other Lung points and left her resting for 30 minutes to see how she felt. She reported that her breathing was still shaky, so I treated LU9 *taiyuan* again and she was immediately much better and remained so for the next 2 weeks. I discovered that, for the time being, she was much better if I treated LU9 *taiyuan* every time. The constant reusing of a point is not my usual method, but it worked for Anne for some considerable time. This also confirmed that, whilst other aspects needed to be addressed, reinforcement of the healthy downward direction of the Lung was crucial.

When I was having negative or not very good results, Anne would say, apologetically, that she felt bad. I assured her, however, that I really needed the information, because I could not treat her without it. It was incredible to her that I wanted negative feedback and yet did not feel personally criticised or insulted. I told her that it was part of the treatment process and that if I did react by feeling insulted, we would never find out what was effective and what was not. This was a very important part of her healing process, on many levels. She really needed to be heard and respected and to realise that it was okay to say what was wrong for her.

Being right there with her

In fact, this has been the key to her treatment. I had to be right there with her at every point to make sure that the rising and falling of the *qi* was balanced. The slightest little bit too much in one direction or another would throw her off balance. Her sensitivity and responsiveness required me to be very clear and precise about my intention regarding the action of the needle. When I was keenly present, the same points and needle actions would work much better.

Recently, I have been working with the Water phase to balance the rising and falling of *qi* within the balance of the *yin* and *yang* of the Kidney. It has been very useful to use upper Kidney points, together with lower ones, to assist the Lung in descending the *qi*, to stabilise the Water and to free up the return of the rising aspect of the Kidney. This then supports the good movement of the Liver.

Anne's assessment

I talked with Anne about this case history project and asked for her assessment. She said that she was 'more full of life' and had 'stopped beating myself up'. She also said that, for her, acupuncture was an incredible form of healing and she could not understand why more people didn't use it. When I asked her what aspect of her treatment was not working, she said that it was difficult to explain that, for example, her anxiety had improved whilst her insomnia worsened.

Overall, she is much improved. Her asthma attacks are infrequent, less severe and more easily treated and her recovery is quicker. She is also less reactive to circumstances which include stress, people and 'allergens'. A big part of her recovery is that she feels more entitled to her perceptions and accepts that they can be respected, and responded to, in a way that is not abusive and actually can be helpful.

Summary of outcome

- 'I feel more full of life.'
- Asthma attacks are less frequent, less severe and more easily controlled.
- 'I've stopped beating up on myself so much.'
- Still has some bouts of insomnia and anxiety but less out of control.
- Depression is infrequent and feels no need for medication.
- Feels better at work and knows she can look for another job if necessary.
- Her reactiveness is less dramatic externally and she seems to trust her inner perceptions more.

Being connected to the moment

I knew when I first met Anne that I was going to learn a lot by treating her. Some of the learning included the techniques of treatment. A larger part involved my being very present with her in order to know what to do. It was not the technique that made the difference, it was more a case of being really connected to what was happening at the moment and watching and eliciting reports of subtle changes. The same points or needling techniques were more successful when I was really with her. When I was tired, not clear in myself or just paying attention to the symptoms, she would clearly worsen in some way. This case reinforced my knowledge of how important it is to be as present as possible in order to assist in a person's healing.

NOTES

1   These are tender points on the abdomen, using the basic map found in the Nan Jing in Difficulty 16 (Unschuld 1986). The diagnostic technique became popular in Japan from the 17th century onwards. The areas that are tested for sensitivity are not the same as *mu* points. There are descriptions of various types of abdominal diagnosis in Shudo Denmai (1990), Fukushima (1991) and Matsumoto & Birch (1988). The actual map of the abdomen that I use is the one taught by J R Worsley, personal communication, 1976.

2   The Akabane technique starts with a test that is basically a passing of an incense stick close (about 3 mm) to the nail points of the right and left fingers and toes. The stick is passed back and forth, counting the number of passes, until a threshold of heat is reached and the patient tells you it is too hot. Comparing the response on the left to the right, the side with the greater number of passes is deficient. In this case that was true for the Kidney and the Spleen. I should add that the results of the Akabane test are often not relevant to the diagnosis as a whole except in certain cases. I use it more to help clear the meridians before treating them. The test was developed by Akabane Kobei (1895–1983) (Worsley 1990).

3   'Running piglets' or *ben tun* is a sensation of rising agitation from the lower abdomen to just under the heart with possible palpitations, difficultly breathing, dizziness, countercurrent of *qi* and eventual weakening of the bones (Huang Fu-Mi 1980 and 1994).

REFERENCES

Fukushima K 1991 Meridian therapy: a hands on text on traditional Japanese *hari*-based pulse diagnosis, Part 1. Toyo Hari Medical Association, Tokyo

Huang Fu-Mi 1980 *Zhen jiu jia yi jing jiao shi.* (The acupuncture and moxibustion classic, collated and annotated.) Edited by Shangdong College of Traditional Chinese Medicine. People's Hygiene Press, Shangdong

Huang Fu-Mi 1994 The systematic classic of acupuncture and moxibustion. Yang S Z, Chace C (trans). Blue Poppy Press, Boulder

Matsumoto K, Birch S 1988 Hara diagnosis: reflections on the sea. Paradigm, Brookline

Rochat de la Vallée E 1991 Les points du taiyin de main, poumon, Vol 1. Institut Ricci, Paris

Shudo Denmai 1990 Introduction to meridian therapy. Trans. Brown S. Eastland Press, Seattle

Unschuld P U (trans) 1986 Medicine in China: Nan jing the classic of difficult issues. University of California Press, Berkeley

Worsley J R 1990 Traditional acupuncture, Vol 2: traditional diagnosis. The College of Traditional Acupuncture, Leamington Spa

■ Zoë Brenner

I had a BA in anthropology with a minor in psychology and 2 years of training in body-centered psychotherapy when I decided to study acupuncture in 1976 with J R Worsley. After several years of practice and trying to solve clinical problems, I heard Peter Eckman and Stuart Kutchins speak about Eight Principle acupuncture and realised how much of it made sense from clinical experience. So I started studying every book in English I could find, most of which were in the style of Traditional Chinese Medicine.

About the same time, in 1981, I met Father Claude Larre who had been studying the Chinese language and classical literature for more that 30 years. I began my study of Chinese medical literature with him and Elisabeth Rochat de la Vallée. This orientation towards the classical medicine and philosophy has made a huge impact on the way that I understand, think and practise Chinese medicine. I continue that study and currently I have been working on texts regarding point usage. I lecture alone and with Elisabeth Rochat on the classical and modern uses of points.

In 1983, I began to study Chinese herbal medicine with Ted Kaptchuk. That class began a dialogue between us that has been an exciting and enriching experience in our exploration of our understanding of Oriental medicine and that dialogue continues as we now teach Chinese herbal medicine together.

I continue to expose myself to other aspects of Oriental medicine by taking classes in different styles of Japanese and Chinese treatments and observing many different practitioners. I believe the practice of this type of medicine has to be a continually developing experience. I like to challenge my understanding and practice to keep it vital and fresh.

Anxiety, agitation and angry determination

Richard Blackwell YORK, UK

This terrible anxiety

Mary was 64 years old, a retired teacher and mother of three. As I entered the waiting room, she was telling the receptionist about the difficulties of her journey to the clinic, how she had got lost and had been terribly worried that she might be late or might not be able to find her way. Once in the consulting room she was clearly very tense and agitated, and so I just let her talk for a while about how anxious she was, especially about any journey. I could sense that she was finding it difficult to feel at all at ease, and her tension made her whole body look clenched. She had a dull, sallow face which seemed strained and pinched, but at the same time she definitely had some sparkle in her eyes. Her body shape was quite trim, and physically she seemed younger than her years, although her face looked older. Despite her anxiety, I felt she also possessed a kind of angry determination which had helped her to battle with her fear of coming to the clinic, where another person might easily have given up.

Mary told me that her problem was 'this terrible anxiety' and asked 'do you think there is anything you can do to help?'. I replied that anxiety often responds well to acupuncture and explained the need for more details to get 'a picture of how your whole system is working'. Mary was badly in need of reassurance that something could be done, and she asked me five or six times during this first consultation whether or not I could help her. I found this quite difficult. Individual responses to acupuncture treatment vary a great deal and, although I give new patients an estimate of the number of treatments needed, I emphasise that the prognosis is clearer after 5 or 6 treatments. In this case I found myself responding to Mary's desperate need for reassurance by saying that acupuncture could definitely help, that I was sure it would make a big difference, but that she would need to attend for 4–5 weeks, initially twice weekly, before she would feel the benefit. I explained my concern that she might become discouraged too quickly, and that I was particularly confident of her case because I had had good results with the treatment of anxiety, and I sensed that she actually had quite a lot of strength of spirit. Nonetheless, I was aware of a slight feeling of trepidation. Having promised so much, I would hate to disappoint.

Mary's story unfolds

Gradually, with much digression and careful reassurance, Mary's story unfolded: she had had a breakdown 8 years ago when she had experienced 'nights of utter terror' and had stayed in bed for weeks. Her husband was alive then and gave her a great deal of support; they were very close and they used to do everything together. She gradually recovered, at least partially.

Her husband died of cancer 2 years ago and 6 months later she had another breakdown: she was afraid to be on her own (her adult son lives with her), afraid to go out, and panic-stricken at night. She had thought that she was gradually improving, but over the last few months all these symptoms had become severe.

I asked her about physical symptoms and she responded by saying that she was particularly terrified of being ill, and especially of having cancer. She went on to tell me that she suffered from 'burn-ups' where she felt as if she was on fire. These lasted for about 15 minutes and were at their worst when she was in bed, after waking up in the morning. (She was taking an antidepressant at night which helped her to sleep.) The burn-ups affected her entire body from the waist upwards.

At times, she also suffered from nausea, which meant that she was unable to eat, and she often had belching and flatulence. Further questioning elicited the other clinical manifestations which are listed in the box.

I also asked Mary what her temperament had been like in the past, before she had became so anxious. She explained that she had been quite confident — indeed as a teacher it had been necessary for her to be so. Many aspects of Mary's lifestyle were quite encouraging. She ate a good diet, with plenty of fresh vegetables and reasonably small amounts of fats and sugar. She didn't smoke and hardly ever drank alcohol. I asked her if she used to be good at relaxing and she replied that she'd had an interest in yoga but had always driven herself hard. I was delighted to learn that she had been a keen practitioner of yoga for many years and had even been a yoga teacher. Although she had not felt able to practise her yoga for several years, I felt that this would prove an extremely valuable asset once she did feel well enough to practise again.

Tongue and pulse

I asked Mary to stand near to the window to show me her tongue, explaining the importance of good light. Her tongue was generally pale, purple, and dry. The edges were especially pale. In contrast to the rest of the tongue, the centre of the root was red, peeled and dry. This peeled area was surrounded by a wider area of rootless coating. The coating over the tongue was generally thin and yellow.

I then asked Mary to sit comfortably and rest first one hand and then the other on my small corner table, so that I could take her pulse. The pulse rate was 76 beats per minute, which I would consider to be within the normal range. The overall quality was thready and wiry. However, both third (*chi*) positions were empty. I like to conduct a detailed analysis of the different pulse positions, but in this case little more was found, showing that the overall qualities were most significant.

Summary of clinical manifestations

- Anxiety and agitation.
- Panic-stricken at night.
- Afraid to be on her own and afraid to go out.
- Terrified of being ill.
- 'Burn-ups', at their worst in the morning.
- Physically tense.
- Dull, sallow face.
- Nausea, poor appetite, belching.
- Loud tinnitus affecting the right ear had recently worsened.
- Loose bowels with flatulence; worse for eating fruit, also from hot, spicy and pickled foods.
- Sleep is OK for the first few hours if an antidepressant is taken; thereafter restless and fitful sleep, and the burn-ups begin.
- Feels totally exhausted.
- Thirsty; partly due to the antidepressant, but has recently worsened.
- Weak low back which easily aches.
- High blood pressure.
- Angry determination, drives herself hard.
- Tongue: pale, purple, and dry. Edges especially pale. Centre of tongue root is red, peeled and dry. Peeled area surrounded by a wider area of rootless coating. Tongue coating thin and yellow.
- Pulse: Rate 76/min. First and second positions (*cun* and *guan*) on both sides thready and wiry. Both third (*chi*) positions empty.

Medical history and medication

Mary had lost one kidney in childhood, due to tuberculosis. In the past she had had low blood sugar problems, with fainting after eating if she went too long between meals. In terms of medication, she was on Dothiepin, an antidepressant. This recently had been changed to a beta blocker but the new drug left her without energy and so Dothiepin was prescribed once more. She was also taking Endopamine, a diuretic.

Three months ago she developed midcycle bleeding. Her GP had been concerned and, in response, had taken Mary off hormone replacement therapy (HRT) which she had been on for some time for recurrent cystitis and vaginal dryness. There had been no recurrence of the midcycle bleeding since stopping the HRT. Although, in this case, the midcycle bleeding was probably caused by the HRT, it can also be an early warning of endometrial carcinoma. I therefore made a mental note to ask her occasionally about any further bleeding she experienced.

I had ambivalent feelings about the HRT and its cessation. I knew that in some ways it would be easier to treat Mary without HRT, which would otherwise remove some of the symptoms of heat and dryness, making it difficult to see the true picture. On the other hand, it was immediately apparent that the deterioration she had experienced over the last few months coincided with discontinuing the HRT. Given that hormonal treatments are known to affect mood in some cases, a causal relationship seemed likely. I put this to Mary and she was surprised to hear that stopping the HRT could have worsened her anxiety and 'burn-ups'. She was, however, also relieved that there may have been a reason for her deterioration. Of course, my hope was that acupuncture would improve the symptoms which HRT had been controlling. In an ideal world, however, I would have liked to have treated Mary for a month or so first, to calm her Spirit (*shen*) and strengthen her system, before she withdrew from the HRT.

Once Mary's symptoms had clearly and consistently improved, my first priority regarding medication would be to suggest that she gradually reduced the dosage of Dothiepin, in consultation with her GP. I was less concerned about the diuretic. Although this might weaken the Kidneys slightly in the long term, in the short term it controlled her blood pressure well and was not my primary concern.

Identifying the patterns of disharmony

In this case the patterns were clearly internal and did not involve invasion by pathogenic factors. I therefore differentiated according to the patterns of the *zangfu*. Details of the diagnosis are given in the box below. The primary diagnosis was Kidney and Heart *yin xu* (Beijing College of TCM 1980, Ross 1985, Maciocia 1989). The only confusing aspect was the way in which the 'burn-ups' were at their worst in the morning, upon awakening. The most likely explanation for this was that the Dothiepin was suppressing the Empty Heat symptoms of night-sweats and insomnia and these symptoms re-emerged as the drug wore off. Mary may also have become tense upon awakening because of the thought of having to face another day.

The secondary patterns were less clear cut. The tinnitus, which I attributed to Liver *yang* rising, could be seen as a Kidney *yin xu* symptom. However, the tinnitus was quite severe, and unilateral. Also, there was the yellow tongue coating, a wiry and thready pulse and evidence of Liver *qi* stagnation and Liver Blood/*yin xu*. The latter two symptoms are common preconditions for Liver *yang* rising (Maciocia 1989). The digestive system symptoms pre-dated the rest of the picture and I suspected that she had had *qi* deficiency of Stomach and Spleen with Liver invading for many years. The Stomach and Spleen *qi xu* was probably the origin of the Liver Blood *xu*. There were however no symptoms of the *qi* deficiency, because it had been obscured by the much more dramatic and more recent *yin xu* picture. The Blood deficiency, however, clearly showed in the unexpected finding of a pale tongue. I expected that, in time, the more typical *yin xu* appearance of the base of the tongue would spread to the whole tongue (Maciocia 1987, Song 1986).

All of these secondary patterns were somewhat uncertain, partly because I was looking back at older patterns which were somewhat buried beneath all the Empty Heat. I was happy to wait and allow these patterns to become clearer as time passed and the treatment took effect.

Although it is not my specialty, I do find that differentiation according to the Five Elements can also be of value, particularly in cases with a strong involvement of the emotional level. In Mary's case, Water was the element most evidently distressed, manifesting in all the fearfulness and the need for reassurance. I also felt that there were pointers to a long-standing Wood imbalance, given my sense of her determination and her description of the need to drive herself hard. A consideration of the aetiology suggests that, constitutionally, Water was the primary element and was failing to nourish Wood. A more recent, secondary, development was Water failing to control Fire, with the overactive Fire then further damaging Water.

Evidence for the patterns of disharmony

Kidney and Heart *yin xu* with Empty Fire blazing

- Anxiety and agitation.
- Panic-stricken at night.
- Afraid to be on her own and afraid to go out.
- Terrified of being ill.
- 'Burn-ups', at their worst in the morning.
- Restless at night; fitful sleep.
- Thirsty.
- Weak low back which easily starts to ache.
- Tongue: Centre of root red, peeled and dry. Peeled area surrounded by a wider area of rootless coating.
- Pulse: Both third (*chi*) positions empty.

Liver *Yang* rising

- Loud tinnitus affecting the right ear, which had recently worsened.
- 'Burn-ups', worst in the morning.
- Angry determination, drives herself hard.
- Tongue: coating thin and yellow.
- Pulse: First and second positions (*cun* and *guan*) on both sides thready and wiry.

Liver *qi* stagnation and Liver Invading Stomach and Spleen (with Stomach and Spleen *qi xu*)

- Physically tense.
- Nausea, poor appetite, belching.
- Loose bowels with flatulence; worse for eating fruit, also for hot, spicy and pickled foods.
- Tongue: purple and pale.
- Pulse: wiry in the first and second positions (*cun* and *guan*) on both sides.

Liver Blood *xu*
- Dull, sallow face.
- Tongue: pale and dry; edges especially pale.
- Pulse: First and second positions (*cun* and *guan*) on both sides thready and wiry.

Aetiology and pathology

The primary aetiological factors here were, of course, emotional. As I got to know Mary better, her story gradually emerged of how, for 2 years, she had cared for her husband as he slowly died a painful death. One can easily see how her anxieties about illness and cancer had arisen, and obviously the emotional strain and physical demands during this time had put heavy demands on her *yin*.

It is more difficult to be sure of the causes of the earlier breakdown, but we do know that she had childhood tuberculosis (TB) and had lost a kidney. TB nearly always produces a *yin xu* picture, so it is reasonable to assume that Mary had suffered a tendency to *yin* deficiency ever since childhood. The restlessness characteristic of *yin xu* would have led her to overwork and would have made it easy for her to push herself, denying her true needs. These behaviours then further depleted her Blood and *yin*. The failure of the Blood to soften the Liver made her increasingly prone to Liver *qi* stagnation. She then reached her menopause and the Kidney *yin*, already weakened, became deficient enough to produce marked symptoms and to undermine the stability of her *shen*. The interaction between the patterns is shown in the diagram in Figure 37.1.

Treatment issues

My treatment principle was to nourish the Kidney and Heart *yin*, clear Empty Fire, calm the *shen* and subdue Liver *yang*. I decided to leave the other Liver and Spleen/Stomach patterns for later.

I proposed an initial treatment plan of at least 15 acupuncture sessions, twice weekly for 2–3 weeks and once weekly thereafter, with a review of progress after eight treatments. This was acceptable to Mary as long as I thought I could help her. I made clear my concern that she might become discouraged too soon, since her progress was likely to be up and down.

I asked Mary to ensure that she had a really good nourishing diet while I

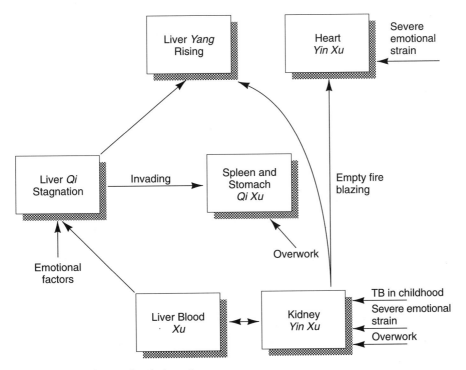

Fig. 37.1 Aetiology and pathology diagram.

treated her, and I encouraged her to begin her yoga again. She didn't feel ready to do her *hatha* yoga, but we agreed to a daily, 20-minute programme of deep relaxation. I encouraged her to start practising the *hatha* yoga again as soon as she felt able. In this way, increasingly, she would be able to help herself.

The first treatment

Mary was of course very anxious about being needled. I find it helps patients if they feel they have some control over the process, so as well as describing exactly what to expect, I told Mary that, if she asked at any time, I would stop the treatment at once. Also, it is my usual practice to use Japanese needles with an insertion tube, which I find minimises the pain of insertion. Mary allowed the needling to proceed normally, although she was still distinctly sensitive to the needle insertion. However, she was now even more anxious than before and I was concerned that her tense state would inhibit the movement of her *qi* and hence reduce the effectiveness of the treatment. Therefore, once the needles were in, I gave Mary a *shen tao*[1] neck release. It involves extremely gentle touch on pairs of acupuncture points, often those of the extraordinary meridians.

The neck release is used to finish off a full *shen tao* treatment, but it is also deeply relaxing in its own right. The points are contacted in pairs in the following order: SI10 *haoshu*, SJ15 *tianliao*, GB21 *jianjing*, GB20 *fengchi*, DU16 *fengfu* with DU20 *baihai*, then DU20 *baihui* then *Yintang*, and then finishing with *Yintang* alone. *Yintang* is often treated 'off the body', and this was appropriate here since it had already been needled! Each pair of points is held with a light touch for a minute or two until the practitioner feels a balancing out of the *qi* in the points.

Within 10 minutes Mary was in a deeply relaxed state. I left her for a while with the needles in place, and when she was ready to leave the clinic she already felt a lot better. The neck release was so helpful for her that it became a regular part of her treatments. Interestingly, apart from the energetic effects of the treatment, Mary commented that, since her husband had died, nobody touched her any more, and how nice it was to be touched again.

First treatment procedures

POINTS PRESCRIPTION

- KID6 *zhaohai* nourishes Kidney *yin*, clears Empty Heat and calms the *shen*.
- HE8 *shaofu* clears Heat from the Heart and calms the *shen*.
- P6 *neiguan* calms the *shen*.
- *Yintang* calms the *shen*.
- LIV3 *taichong* subdues Liver *yang* and moves Liver *qi*.

Rationale: The focus here is on strongly clearing Empty Heat and calming the *shen*, in order to quickly ease the severe anxiety state. Hence the unusual needling of HE8 *shaofu*, which is more commonly used for Full Heat patterns but can also be used for Empty Heat (Maciocia 1989). It is also indicated for sorrow and fear (Ellis et al 1988, Deadman & Al-Khafaji 1995).

Needles: I used Japanese needles 40 mm × 0.26 mm, except for HE8 *shaofu* and *Yintang* where I used 30 mm × 0.22 mm.

Needle technique: *De qi* was gently obtained, then needles were left in place for 20 minutes.

Auxiliary treatment: *Shen tao* neck release.

Responding but variably

Mary returned 2 days later. She had not experienced any burn-ups that morning and after the treatment she'd felt so good that she'd gone to the pub with her son and had a ginger ale! She was delighted, but I was wary since part of the effect may have derived from the intense nature of the first consultation. I warned her that she might have some bad patches yet to come.

A major problem was Mary's continuing anxiety about treatment, and particularly her sensitivity to needle insertion. I reduced the needle size to 30 mm × 0.22 mm and used techniques such as massaging the points before insertion and stretching the skin over the point with one hand while tapping the needle in with the other. The *shen tao* helped Mary to relax again as soon as the needles were in.

After four treatments I changed HE8 *shaofu* to HE6 *yinxi* and added ST36 *zusanli* and GB20 *fengchi*. After ten treatments she was having several good days each week without anxiety, the bad days were not as bad as before, and there were fewer burn-ups of less severity. She had begun to get mouth ulcers, which I perceived as an encouraging movement of the Heat from the emotional to the physical level. The digestive symptoms were continuing to worry her, and I began to use points like ST25 *tianshu*, LIV13 *zhangmen* and SP6 *sanyinjiao*. I also used *Sishencong* and KID9 *zhubin* in some treatments (Ellis et al 1988, Maciocia 1989). Since she was responding well but overall still variably, we continued with twice weekly treatment for 20 sessions. Between the twelfth and fourteenth treatments she experienced a deterioration, with the burn-ups and digestive symptoms worsening once more. Once again her GP prescribed HRT, this time as transdermal patches. I would have liked Mary to have persevered with the acupuncture alone, but she had always been quite keen on the HRT and had never wanted to stop it. Predictably, the burn-ups did subside. Her anxiety continued to improve, and was clearly much better than before, when she had been treated with HRT but without acupuncture.

A turning point in her recovery

After 20 treatments Mary was well enough to go on holiday in Denmark with her daughter's family, and to feel 'very confident' whilst driving. This was a turning point in her recovery and we agreed to treat once weekly from then onwards. After 25 treatments she felt well enough to reduce the Dothiepin from 150 mg to 125 mg, and after 30 treatments to 100 mg. After 30 treatments she had driven several hundred miles on her own to visit her other daughter's family, and she described herself as very much improved. She was keen to visit people and to attend yoga and keep-fit classes. Even though her abdominal symptoms recurred at times, she no longer felt panicky and agitated about them. She felt ready to stop treatment, and we agreed that in future she would only come in for a treatment when she felt the need.

When she first consulted me, Mary was one of the most agitated and anxious patients I had ever seen. Over a 6-month period she recovered much of her confidence and enthusiasm and began to feel like her old self again. The most recent aspect of the pathology (Empty Fire severely disturbing the *shen*), had cleared, and some of the underlying *yin* deficiency had also improved. Other aspects of the pathology could have benefited from further attention, but the patient was satisfied with the outcome at this point.

Summary of outcome

- Major improvements in levels of anxiety, agitation and number of burn-ups.
- No longer afraid of being alone or going out.
- Less worried by physical symptoms.
- Back pain improved.

- No change in tinnitus.
- Less tense.
- Digestive symptoms still recurring, but less often.
- Better facial colour.
- Tongue: less pale and dry, less purple, centre of root less red.

Wholeness re-emerging

This case made an impression on me for several reasons. When seeing patients I always find it helpful to remember that there is a part of each of us which always remains untarnished and undamaged, however harmed we may be in other ways in body and in spirit. Sometimes it is difficult to remember this but in Mary's case, as soon as I met her, I found I could glimpse her untarnished spirit shining out through all her distress, and it was particularly rewarding to see the clouds of distress gradually dispersing and Mary's strength and wholeness emerging again.

Secondly, this was a case where it was particularly apparent that, whilst the diagnosis, point selection and acupuncture treatment were very important, especially to achieve long-term benefit, the 'non-specific' aspects of the treatment were also important. In particular, the creation of a calm and meditative atmosphere during the *shen tao* treatment had an immediately settling effect, and seemed to enable Mary to re-establish contact with the peaceful and expansive aspects of her spirit. These quiet and centred moments were important to me too, and always left me recharged and refreshed for the next patient.

NOTE

1 *Shen tao* is a treatment method derived from the Japanese system of *jin shin do* and developed in the UK by Jo Harvey, Chris Lowe and colleagues (Teeguarden 1978, Shen Tao Foundation 1986).

REFERENCES

Beijing College of Traditional Chinese Medicine, Shanghai College of Traditional Chinese Medicine, Nanjing College of Traditional Chinese Medicine, The

Acupuncture Institute of the Academy of Traditional Chinese Medicine 1980 Essentials of Chinese acupuncture. Foreign Languages Press, Beijing

Deadman P, Al-Khafaji M 1995 The treatment of psycho-emotional disorders by acupuncture: with particular reference to the Du Mai. Journal of Chinese Medicine 47: 30–34

Ellis A, Wiseman N, Boss K 1988 Fundamentals of Chinese acupuncture. Paradigm Publications, Brookline

Maciocia G 1987 Tongue diagnosis in Chinese medicine. Eastland Press, Seattle

Maciocia G 1989 The foundations of Chinese medicine. Churchill Livingstone, Edinburgh

Ross J 1985 Zang Fu — the organ systems of Traditional Chinese Medicine. Churchill Livingstone, Edinburgh

Shen Tao Foundation 1986 Three-Season seminars' course notes

Song T B 1986 Atlas of tongues and lingual coatings in Chinese medicine. People's Medical Publishing House, Beijing & Editions Sinomedic, Strasbourg

Teeguarden I M 1978 Acupressure way of health — Jin Shin Do. Japan Publications

■ Richard Blackwell

Richard Blackwell began his career conventionally at the University of Nottingham Medical School in the UK, with a view to possibly specialising in psychiatry. Although his 3 pre-clinical years were an academic success, in his spare time he was reading major critiques of orthodox medicine and psychiatry by the likes of Illich and Laing. The award of a first-class honours degree in medical science provided the opportunity for an honourable exit before the gruelling and constraining process of clinical training began.

As a medical student Richard had visited the acupuncture practice of his cousin Ralph Perks. Ralph had been one of the small band of students who had studied acupuncture in the UK in the sixties, and he had numbered J R Worsley and Sidney Rose-Neil among his fellow students. Richard was particularly impressed to meet a patient with badly arthritic hands who told him that, since being treated by acupuncture, she could knit again.

With a long-standing interest in Buddhist, Hindu and Taoist philosophy and the beginnings of an orthodox medical background, a move into Chinese medicine seemed to be written in the stars. Richard studied for 3 years at the British Acupuncture College in London, obtaining the LicAc in 1982. Feeling that he had been introduced to part but by no means all of this massive subject, he went on to study for a year with Vivienne Brown, Peter Deadman, Giovanni Maciocia and Julian Scott. These four were teaching the material they had brought back from China, which had only recently opened up to foreign visitors. Richard was astounded and delighted by the wealth of information they provided and the way it made sense as a coherent whole. He felt that he now had a solid basis on which to build his practice, which he did over the following 9 years whilst also further expanding his knowledge. Among others, he studied acupuncture with Dr Chen Qing Hua and Dr Su Xin Ming, and Chinese herbal medicine with Ted Kaptchuk. In 1988 he spent 5 weeks of clinical study at the affiliated hospital of the College of Traditional Chinese Medicine in Nanjing, China.

Also in 1988, Richard was invited to teach with Vivienne Brown, Peter Deadman, Julian Scott and Mazin Al-Khafaji in London, and at the Northern College of Acupuncture in York. As most teachers find, his own understanding and knowledge began to take another major leap forward through teaching. Indeed, he enjoyed teaching so much that he had little hesitation when offered the chance to move to York, where he continues to practise acupuncture and Chinese herbal medicine and works as Deputy Principal of the Northern College of Acupuncture. In this role he played an important part, with Hugh MacPherson, in obtaining university validation for the award of an MSc in acupuncture, the first university validated degree in acupuncture in the UK.

A clear case of possession

Angela Hicks READING, UK

George was 26 years old when he came for treatment. His father came from Trinidad and his mother from England. He was casually dressed. Superficially he seemed at ease but underneath he was more nervous. He would say a few words and then would look at me from the corner of his eyes or look intently as if to size up how I was reacting to what he said. I noticed that his eyes looked very glazed and dull.

We initially chatted. It became apparent that he was pleased to be able to hold down his job as a porter in a hospital but that he didn't enjoy his work. For the previous 4 months he had been in a relationship with a nurse at the hospital and this was important to him. He said, 'She goes about her own life regardless, whilst I wear my heart on my sleeve. I easily imagine offence when it's not there.'.

Reason for coming for treatment

He had come for treatment because:

Of late I've been getting panicky and my moods have been changeable, then I get depressed. I have aches and pains in the back of my chest and I also have headaches. I'm developing a very pessimistic attitude to the future. I feel I'm bound to fail. That passes, but it comes back. I've always had some mild apprehension but over the last 10–12 weeks it's been escalating. Panic wells up out of nowhere. Over the last 2 years a lot has happened — a few disappointing love affairs, my father developed stomach cancer and had to retire. I can't watch the news. If something horrendous is on, I feel angry and useless and go into a mild depression.

Panics

When I panic my breathing becomes irregular and I have to concentrate on breathing regularly. The muscles of my face and neck become tense. Overall I have a feeling of weakness like someone has pulled the plug out. It lasts for anything from 5 minutes up to 60 minutes. Sometimes I manage to catch on to it and stop it before it develops. If I'm doing something at the time I try to carry on doing it, to break my attention from the panic. Recently I've been drinking more as it clouds the mind. I'm feeling close to the edge.

Headaches

My headaches are an intense pain more on the left side of the head and round the ear. With the headaches light and noise become quite irritating. The pain is often pounding. I never feel sick with them. I'm not sure if there's any special time when they start, maybe when I am more depressed or panicky.

He also told me that his headaches could come on anything from one to three or four times a week but they had been more or less continuous for 5 days now, from Sunday night until Thursday. He had been suffering from headaches for the last 2 years.

Aches in chest

They're like a lump in the middle of my chest but towards the back. It feels like something is stuck in there. It comes and goes according to how I'm feeling. I've never had palpitations with the sensation or the panic.

Additional information

Whilst taking his case history I noticed that his emotions seemed most out of balance around issues of fear. When I gave him reassurance he became uncomfortable and was unable to accept it. It was as if his fear was preventing him from taking in any relevant information. I also noticed that his predominant face colour was blue-black, especially around the eyes. His voice tone was 'groaning' and his odour was 'putrid'.

He told me his sleep had not been good recently and that he woke up around 3 a.m. and then wouldn't get back to sleep until 5, 6 or 7 in the morning. 'I feel a bit dazed when I wake up. Sometimes I lie there and think and it gets oppressive, so I make a cup of tea or listen to a record.' He also said that he had vivid dreams which were quite 'varied and random'. He would usually take a glass of water to bed as sometimes he felt thirsty when he woke. If he was uptight in the morning he would sometimes break into a sweat. He told me he would also sweat during a panic attack. He also occasionally perspired during the night.

He said his bowels and water works were 'fine'. His appetite was also usually fine but he often skipped lunch and he was quite 'addicted' to fried breakfasts. An evening meal would usually consist of meat, vegetables and rice. Although he sometimes felt hot, especially in his head, he hated the cold weather and didn't like the damp much either. His blood pressure was 160/90. Towards the end of the case history he told me more about why he had been getting these symptoms.

Drugs

He looked nervous as he told me, 'Until 1 month ago I was taking a lot of drugs, and have done so since the age of 14'. I asked him which drugs and he said, 'Dope, amphetamines, LSD, psylocibin, opium and various combinations. I've taken acid 50–60 times and have been comatosed on hash'. He told me that he had originally taken them out of 'curiosity'. He had stopped suddenly as he was feeling unwell and knew the drugs were partly to blame and also because his girlfriend didn't like him taking them.

His internal state

He then went on to say, 'I feel as if I have a nastiness inside me that's been there for a long time. I get outbursts of rage as though I am possessed, then I get sad and experience a resigned despair'. A little later he told me, 'I get voices inside my head harassing me, telling me things about myself that I can't dispute. It feels like there's something inside that I'm doing battle with'. At this point I began to realise that as well as being generally depleted, he possibly was also what could be termed 'possessed'.

Family life

He still lived at home.

> *My father doesn't make me feel very comfortable. There used to be tremendous arguments. He used to scare the living daylights out of me. He beat me for about 20 minutes when I was small for knocking over some paint. I feel sorry for him since he's been ill. I should feel affection for him but I've never regarded him as a friend.*

When he talked about his mother, on the other hand, he told me, 'Mum's the closest person I've met to being a saint'. He described her as a contented person and said that he felt very protective towards her.

Pulse and tongue

George's pulses were all floating and rapid. The middle positions on both sides were full. All of the other pulses were empty. In the middle position, the left-hand side was wiry. George's tongue was red, more so at the tip and sides and it was very dry.

Summary of clinical manifestations

- Panics with irregular breathing, face and neck muscles becoming tense.
- Feel weak like 'someone's pulled the plug out'.
- Moods changeable, then gets depressed.
- Ache in the back of chest which feels like a lump and comes and goes.
- Headaches: intense pain on the left-hand side and around the ear, worse when depressed or panicky.
- High blood pressure, 160/90.
- Very pessimistic attitude to the future; feels bound to fail.
- Mild apprehension which is escalating.
- Can feel angry and useless and go into mild depression.
- Wears his heart on his sleeve, imagines an offence when it's not real.
- Wakes in the middle of the night around 3 a.m.

- Eyes look dull and glazed over.
- Sweating from panic.
- Some night sweats.
- Occasionally thirsty at night.
- Seems out of balance around issues to do with fear.
- Blue-black facial colour.
- Putrid odour.
- Groaning voice tone.
- Feels he has 'a nastiness' inside him.
- Outbursts of rage as though he is possessed.
- Gets voices 'telling me things about myself that I can't dispute. It feels like there's something inside that I'm doing battle with'.
- Pulses: floating and rapid, middle positions full, other pulses empty: middle position on left-hand side wiry.
- Tongue: body red, more so at the tip and the sides; tongue very dry.

Identifying the patterns of disharmony

The main patterns that were showing in the diagnosis were an underlying constitutional imbalance in the Water element (the Kidney and Bladder) and Kidney *yin* deficiency with some Heart *yin* deficiency leading to Liver *yang* rising. The Kidney and Heart *yin* deficiency had caused *shen* disturbance. He was also 'possessed' and he had some Liver *qi* stagnation. For more details see the box below.

Evidence for patterns of disharmony

'Possession'

- Feels he has 'a nastiness inside'.
- Outbursts of rage 'like being possessed'.
- Gets voices 'telling me things about myself that I can't dispute. It feels like there's something inside that I'm doing battle with'.
- Eyes glazed.

Constitutional imbalance in Water Element (Kidney and Bladder)

- Blue-black facial colour.
- Groaning voice tone.
- Seems most out of balance around issues of fear and also has panic attacks.
- Putrid odour.

Kidney *yin xu*

- Panics (and Heart *yin xu*).

- Feels weak like someone's pulled the plug out.
- Some night sweats.
- Occasionally thirsty at night
- Pulses: floating and rapid.
- Tongue: body red, tip and the sides more red; dry.

Liver *yang* rising

- Headaches: intense pain on the left-hand side and around the ear.
- High blood pressure.
- Outbursts of rage (could also be possession).
- Occasionally feels hot in his head.
- Pulse: wiry, middle left-hand position.
- Tongue: red sides to tongue.

***Shen* disturbance**

- Panics (Heart and Kidney *yin xu*)

- Wears his heart on his sleeve, vulnerable, imagines offence when it is not real.
- Wakes in the middle of the night around 3 a.m.
- Vivid dreams.
- Sweating from panic.
- Eyes glazed and dull.

Liver *qi* stagnation

- Moods changeable, then gets depressed.
- Ache in the back of chest which feels like a lump and comes and goes.
- Very pessimistic attitude to the future; feels bound to fail.
- Mild apprehension which is escalating.
- Headaches worse when depressed.
- Pulse: in the middle position of the left-hand side wiry and full.

Sources of this diagnostic approach

This style is an integration of styles derived from two sources: Traditional Chinese Medicine (TCM) as it is currently taught in China and Five Element acupuncture as taught by J R Worsley (personal communication, 1975).

Five Element acupuncture

The Five Element style of acupuncture places emphasis on finding the patient's underlying constitutional weakness. It is assumed that each patient has a slight imbalance in their *qi* which will result in subtle changes in the facial colour, the voice tone, the odour and the appropriateness of the emotion. A constitutional diagnosis can be made whether a patient has symptoms or not. Focusing the treatment in the direction of this original cause can often help to create deep and profound changes in the patient at all levels: physical, mental and spiritual.

Traditional Chinese Medicine

The TCM diagnosis takes into consideration the patient's signs and symptoms and the patterns that these form. Unlike the constitutional imbalance which does not change, these patterns may come and go. TCM is immensely helpful in dealing with specific diseases, full and empty conditions, substance disharmonies and in refining the appropriate treatment within the constitutionally weak Element. It also helps the practitioner to determine the patient's needs in terms of lifestyle changes and to clarify prognosis.

Possession in Chinese medicine

The concept of a person becoming 'possessed' is a very old one in Chinese medicine. Unschuld (1985) states:

> *The belief that demons could cause illness is widely documented in literature of the later Chou period as well as during the subsequent Ch'in and Han dynasties. Han Fei (died 233 BC) expressed the prevailing attitude of the age when he concluded: 'When a person falls ill it means he has been injured by a demon'.[1]*

Acupuncture can be used to clear possession. The concept is still important today.

Aetiology and pathology

Aetiology

The two main causes of George's symptoms were his emotional problems in childhood and his previous drug intake (Fig. 38.1). At this stage I was unsure of his prognosis as it was difficult to say how much irreversible physical damage the drugs had created. I told him that he needed to stay off drugs if he was to regain his health and he reassured me that he was determined to do so.

The difficulties that he had had with his father when he was a child were probably key factors in his inclination to take drugs and, in order for him to become wholly better, the resulting fear needed to be healed. I felt that this could be achieved by treating him at the level of his constitutional imbalance.

Pathology

George's constitutional imbalance lay in the Water Element and thus he was unable to experience fear appropriately and to develop normal behaviour when he felt threatened.[2] This had put further strain on his Kidney and Bladder.

The syndromes from which George had suffered can also be connected to the constitutional imbalance. In George's case the weakness in his Kidney and Bladder had caused a deficiency of the Kidney *yin* which had been exacerbated by the use of drugs. This had, in turn, caused the Liver *yang* to rise up creating headaches, high blood-pressure and outbursts of

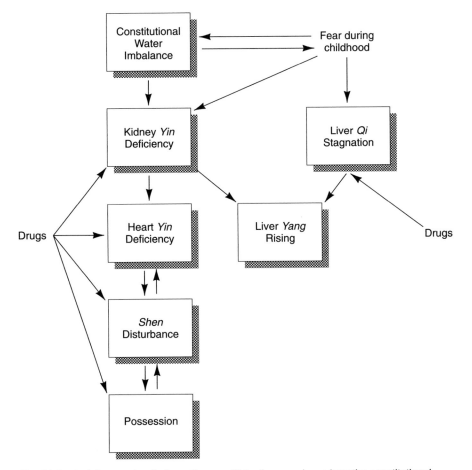

Fig. 38.1   Aetiology and pathology diagram. This diagram shows how the constitutional cause in the Water Element was exacerbated by fear during George's childhood. This fear is then likely to have also contributed to the Kidney *Yin Xu* and Liver *Yang* Rising. The drugs then created further Kidney *Yin Xu* and Liver *Yang* Rising and also the disturbance of the *Shen*. Because *Shen* is disturbed it is easier for him to become 'possessed'.

anger. The disturbance of the Kidney *yin* had also caused the Heart to become *yin xu* and had therefore caused the *shen* to become disturbed. The drugs had also caused the Liver *qi* to stagnate.

In this case the syndromes are the *biao*, coming from the *ben* of the Water imbalance. A further *biao* at this point in time was the 'possession'. When a patient's *shen* or spirit is not properly 'rooted' in the Heart, the patient is more vulnerable to an 'attack' by an outside 'demon'. Unschuld clarifies this:

> *When the spirit and influences are not protected, evil is able to enter the body. Thus it is written for example in the 'Directions for restoring losses by means of acupuncture', that when someone suffers from depletion he loses his spirit, for it has not been preserved; this enables evil demons to attack the body from the outside.*[3]

Where does the possessing spirit comes from? 'Possession' has been a cause of disease in most cultures (except in the West this century) and has been the subject of much speculation, even in ancient times.[4] It could be said to be merely an External Pathogenic 'Evil', or an emotional 'Evil'. The Chinese also believe that the *po* (the corporal soul) is the part of a person that disintegrates at death, as opposed to the *hun* (the spiritual soul) which survives death. The *po* can haunt or possess another person if the spirit isn't settled after death. The word *po* has '*gui*' (demon) as a main part of its character.

Treatment principles

The main treatment principles in order of importance at this point in time were:

1 Clear possession.
2 Tonify Water Element (Kidney and Bladder) and Kidney *yin*.
3 Calm the *shen*.
4 Subdue Liver *yang*.
5 Clear Liver *qi* stagnation.

The possession needed to be cleared first as it was a secondary cause of disease, i.e. it created symptoms in its own right and would possibly have caused obstruction to any further treatment until it had been dealt with. I expected that this could take more than one treatment to clear completely as a patient who has been possessed sometimes has more than one 'demon' needing to be cleared. This treatment, in its appropriate context, can stimulate very dramatic changes.

The treatment principle of tonifying the Water Element was very important as it affected the constitution and would therefore strengthen the patient overall by treating his underlying weakness. In George's case there was prolonged deficiency caused by weakness from childhood as well as from drugs, so I would expect the Kidneys to be strengthened only by the use of long-term treatment.

Calming the *shen* and subduing the Liver *yang* would be important if they were not dealt with by treating the Kidney and Bladder. I decided to move the Liver *qi* if it didn't naturally move on its own accord as treatment progressed.

Presenting the treatment plan

I told George that he needed to attend treatment on a weekly basis initially and less frequently once treatment progressed. I also explained that after treatment some patients felt no change at all, some patients felt a slight exacerbation of symptoms which usually diminished within 24 hours and some patients immediately felt much better. I wanted George to know that he might react immediately to treatment (especially as I was about to give him a strong treatment) and I didn't want him to think that this was unusual. I also let him know that he could ring me if he had any cause for concern. I told George very little else prior to starting treatment because first, I didn't want to put ideas either of 'possession' into his head beforehand, or of what might happen to him as a result of treatment, and, second, he was in a poor state of mental and physical health and the best course of action seemed to be immediate treatment.

Seven dragons for the seven demons

I treated him on the same day that I took his case history. By this time I was confident from what he said and how he looked that he needed treatment to release the 'seven dragons for the seven demons'. I was also sure that he trusted me sufficiently and that he had some faith in the treatment he was going to receive. He had opened up to me and told me a lot about himself and in order for him to do this we needed to have good rapport. I explained that I was about to put in some needles and would be leaving them in for a while. Before the treatment he seemed quite tense and his pulses were more floating and rapid than before.

When the needles were in, he visibly relaxed and his breathing slowed. During the treatment his pulses slowed down, became much less floating, and felt stronger. When the treatment had finished and the needles were out I left him lying down until he was ready to get up. When he did get up he commented that he felt extremely peaceful.

First treatment procedures

POINTS PRESCRIPTION

The point combination used was the 'seven dragons for seven demons':

- REN15 *jiuwei*.
- ST25 *tianshu*.
- ST32 *futu*.
- ST41 *jiexi*.

This point combination is said to release the 'seven dragons that will destroy the seven demons'. It is used if a patient has signs and symptoms of what could be called 'being possessed by a demon'.

These points can be used to awaken what are called the 'internal dragons'. There is also a treatment to awaken the 'external dragons' (points: DU20 *baihui*; BL11 *dazhu*, BL23 *shenshu* and BL61 *shenmai*). In reality it is often difficult to decide whether a 'demon' is internal or external and therefore the internal dragons are awakened first if a possession treatment is thought to be needed.

Point location

The location of the internal dragon points is on the front of the body, the *yin* side, whilst the location of the external dragon points is on the back, the *yang* side.

In Chinese medicine it is said that the pure goes upwards and the impure downwards. Note that these point combinations take the energy in a downwards 'V' to the feet to take the impure (demons) in a downwards direction and possibly expel them from the feet.

Point order of use

The points are used in the order listed above, starting with REN 15 *jiuwei*, i.e. from the top down to the bottom.

Needle length, gauge and action

I used 25 mm, 34 and 36 gauge needles on points REN15 *jiuwei* and ST41 *jiexi* and 40 mm needles on the deeper points, ST25 *tianshu* and ST32 *futu*. Although I had to clear an external invasion I used an 'even' needle technique, as the patient's underlying energy was weak. I left the needles in place for about 30 minutes by which time the patient's pulses had settled and his eyes had become less glazed.

Internal and external dragons

After the first treatment George reported that he had initially felt much better and more relaxed but that he had got very drunk 2 days later and now felt much the same as he had done previously. I repeated the 'dragons' treatment, this time suggesting that he didn't drink for the next 24 hours and in future to only drink a little if at all. He agreed to this. I realised that I should have warned him to cut down on his drinking when I had talked to him about drugs. After repeating the treatment he reported that the voices were still there but, 'I didn't pay as much attention to them as before'. I then used the 'external dragons' at the third treatment followed by the 'internal dragons' at the fourth treatment. After the fourth treatment George reported that he wasn't being troubled by the voices much at all. We were both pleased with this progress. He was still having some panics and the headaches continued though less frequently. Overall he said he felt much better.

Treating the constitutional imbalance

The next few treatments were aimed primarily at treating his Kidneys and Bladder and specifically at nourishing the Kidney *yin*. At this stage I wanted to find out how much only treating of the Water Element, as the constitutional imbalance, would affect the Liver *yang* and the Heart *shen*. Over the next few treatments George's panic attacks continued to decrease, his blood pressure went down to 130/80 and his chest pains became what he called 'minor'. He was still inclined to be nervy and anxious and was still getting headaches. After treatment his pulses would all become less floating and rapid and his Liver pulse would also become less full. However, by the time he returned a week later his pulses were often rapid again and the Liver had returned to a full pulse.

I then moved Liver *qi* and calmed the *shen* (using points such as LIV3 *taichong*, P6 *neiguan*, H7 *shenmen* and REN14 *juque*) as well as continuing to treat the Kidney and the *yin*. I would use points such as KID6 *shaohai*, KID3 *taixi* and BL23 *shenshu* as well as points such as KID24 *lingxu*, the 'spirit burial ground' to strengthen his *shen* and his Kidneys. I also used the 'dragons' treatment twice more when the voices returned after a temporary set-back during treatment.

The whole treatment as an exorcism

He came for weekly treatments for 4 months, then for treatment every 2 or 3 weeks as he improved and, for the final 6 months, he attended monthly. Altogether he received treatment for one and a half years. He never took drugs again and his life changed considerably. He then moved away from the area and I haven't heard from him since. By the time he moved he described himself as 'pretty steady and calm'. He no longer had headaches, chest pains or panic attacks. At one point during the course of treatment he even said about his father, 'He's not a monster, I feel quite good about him now'. He had started a training course in carpentry which he was enjoying and was buying a flat with his girlfriend. Over the course of the treatment he had experienced times of great stress in his relationship with his girl-friend, often thinking that they were going to split up. However, they had come through this and seemed to be more settled together. He described himself as feeling dependent on others for happiness at times and could still be critical of himself, though never again in an extreme way as at the start of his treatment when he had been harassed relentlessly by voices.

At one time towards the end of his treatment he commented that, 'To me this whole treatment has felt like an exorcism'. I was very surprised by this remark as I had never told him about his treatment for 'possession'. This comment came directly from his experience of the treatment.

Summary of outcome

- Life is now 'pretty steady and calm'.
- Blood pressure is now 130/80.
- No further headaches, chest pains or panic attacks.
- No further harassment by voices.
- Worried that he is dependent on others and still somewhat critical of himself.
- Feels differently about his father, 'He's not a monster'.
- Training in carpentry and buying a flat with his girlfriend.

NOTES

1 See Unschuld (1985), chapter 2, page 37.

2 Everyone feels emotions when it is appropriate, but the emotion connected to the constitutional imbalance may also be felt inappropriately, e.g. people who are born with a Fire imbalance are often less able to feel warmth, love and joy. They may feel habitually sad, or excessively, but superficially, joyful. People who are born with an imbalance in the Metal element will often feel that something is missing inside for no reason; this can be something indefinable and may be experienced as an emptiness or grief. Any subsequent losses will reinforce this feeling.

3 See Unschuld (1985), Appendix, page 329.

4 See 'On injuries caused by evil' in Unschuld (1985), Appendix, page 325.

REFERENCES

Unschuld PU 1985 Medicine in China, a history of ideas. University of California Press, Berkeley

■ Angela Hicks

I am Joint Principal of the College of Integrated Chinese Medicine in Reading, England. At the College we teach an integration of two styles of acupuncture. One is known as Five Elements acupuncture, the other is based on TCM which is currently taught in China.

I qualified at the College of Chinese Medicine in Leamington Spa in 1975. I then worked in a group practice in Oxford with seven other acupuncturists. We shared learnings and insights into our patients and explored our own personal growth which we valued highly as part of our ability to treat patients.

I then taught and supervised clinical training at the college in Leamington Spa. I observed J R Worsley and I especially respected his ability to detect the underlying 'constitutional imbalance' of a patient. This gave me the ability to help patients to change at deep levels although there were still patients I did not feel confident in treating.

I then went on a course in Traditional Chinese Medicine (TCM) run by the Journal of Chinese Medicine which increased my confidence to treat a wider range of patients. I spent the next year using TCM and Five Element acupuncture together as well as teaching TCM to a small group of 12 students. In 1988, I went to China for clinical training. I was very appreciative of Dr Gu Yue Hua, an associate professor at Nanjing College of Traditional Chinese Medicine, whose skills demonstrated to me the effectiveness of TCM.

Up to this point in time, western practitioners had mainly practised using TCM or the Five Elements. Enjoying the best of both styles seemed a better option. In 1989, with my husband John, we created a postgraduate course, teaching TCM and an Integrated Clinical Course, thus bringing together the two styles for those who had trained only in Five Element acupuncture. In 1993, we opened the College of Integrated Chinese Medicine (CICM) where students learn both styles seamlessly.

Most recently, I have learned *qi gong* and specifically, *tai xi wu qi gong* and *bu qi*. These are ways of developing one's *qi* for more effective needling and healing. My teacher is Dr Shen Hongxun, who now teaches at CICM. I also learned Ki Aikido to the grade of 2nd Dan and the 'ki' exercises have made an impact on how I use my body and mind when practising, especially in my use of needle technique and pulse taking.

Finally, one of the people to influence me most was a healer called Rose Gladden who taught me about possession and healing. I spent a year working with her when she taught me more about the light and the spirit in relation to healing than anyone else I have ever known.

Fleas, ponies, doctors, angels

39

Harriet Beinfield SAN FRANSCISCO, USA

A great healer does not work alone;
A great angel is always by her side.[1]

Diana

Diana's shoulders hunched protectively, cradling her chest. Although her eyes met mine, it seemed they were peering through an invisible wall of armour. Pale ivory cheeks were softened by a thin rose blush. Encircling her eyes was the colour of ashen snow. Undressed, Diana's 47-year-old body was well-proportioned with appropriate amounts of flesh hugging her bones, yet it hung without tenacity, somewhat spongy to the touch.

In April, 5 months before her acupuncture visit in October, Diana had been bitten by a flea. Diana's internist surmised that this was the cause of her irritatingly itchy allergic red rash which covered her arms, legs, and back. At that time, he prescribed a 10-day course of steroids which made the rash all but disappear. When Diana had finished the medication, however, the rash resumed, twice as virulent as before. Although Diana had continued to use antihistamines and medicated lotions, the rash had persisted and now covered her arms, legs, back, and chest.

Exasperated, Diana complained:

> *The antihistamines leave me feeling drained and hung over. I have become so used to itching that I behave like a chimpanzee and, without thinking, reach up under my sweater to scratch, even when I'm in a business meeting. I'm at my wits end — my doctor said the rash is chronic and simply renewed my prescription for antihistamines.*

In addition to the rash, Diana also complained of right hip pain (aggravated by weekly horseback riding), left elbow tendonitis (exacerbated by long hours on the computer), and weakness with limited range of motion in her right wrist (which she had fractured the year before). Each of these, together with mood swings, were stirred up by PMS. When asked if there was anything else I should know, Diana said her father drank too much and her mother had been depressed and emotionally neglected. Diana was also a single parent of a 10-year-old daughter, and had been in psychotherapy for the previous 5 years.

Summary of clinical manifestations

- Itchy red rash on arms, legs, and back, worse premenstrually.
- Pain and stiffness in right hip and left elbow.
- Recurring hives.
- Premenstrual mood swings.
- Irregular, painful periods with premenstrual mood swings since birth of daughter 10 years previously.
- Scanty menstrual flow since menarche.
- Hot flushes in last year.
- Head and pubic hair turning grey.
- Skin losing tone, smoothness, elasticity.
- Muscles flaccid, tender.
- Tension, muscle cramps, pain in neck and shoulders.
- Easy chilling and mottling of limbs.
- Chronic scoliosis.
- Poor skin healing.
- Dry skin and hair.
- Sore, hardened breasts.
- Palpitations and restlessness with upset or fatigue.
- Occasional vertigo.
- Sensitive to wind, heat, noise.
- Oral herpes triggered by exposure to sunshine.
- Frequent nausea and intestinal wind.
- Difficulty waking, morning fatigue.
- Easily irritated, sensitive to insult, pain.
- Sensitive, easily moved emotionally.
- Easily startled and frightened.
- Disconcerted by major or sudden change.
- Morbid thoughts about dying at an early age.
- Depression accompanied by melancholy, rage, despair.
- Often worried and anxious.
- Awkward when expressing feelings.
- Feelings of social inadequacy, paucity of friends.
- Pulses: weak, thin and tight. Middle position left especially tight. Distal position right also weak and small.
- Tongue: body pale, scalloped edges, white fur.

Treatment

Diana described her experience of the first acupuncture treatment as follows:

> I lay down on a purple-covered table, my head resting on a small red pillow, with Eastern melodies softly filling the room. The needles went in with a faint prick, each one followed by a different sensation. One felt like a dull ache, rippling out from deep under my skin, like a pebble thrown into a pond, with a power that made me catch my breath. Another felt as if the part of my body surrounding the needle had been dipped in cold water, leaving a tingling sensation close to the surface. Lying there I felt myself turning inward, losing interest in my surroundings and instead becoming highly conscious of my thoughts, feelings, and body.

For me, Diana's treatment was interrupted by Jill, a patient in an adjoining room, who cried out suddenly for help. Having suffered as a child, Jill was unexpectedly remembering being held upside down, her head dunked repeatedly in the bathtub. She was scared to revisit this experience alone so, placing my hand on Jill's abdomen, I listened. Returning to Diana I apologised for leaving suddenly, and explained that sometimes acupuncture dislodged buried memories and feelings, and that such an event had just occurred in the room next door.

On the next visit, Diana said, 'I was so grateful to learn that it's natural for acupuncture to precipitate a tumult of emotions. Nobody ever mentioned that to me and it has helped me account for my own response to treatment'. Diana reported that she liked the herbal extract I had prescribed to help her skin and that drinking two squirts from the dropper, diluted in hot water, 5 times a day had definitely stopped her itching. Usually before her periods the rash got worse, but this time, it had improved. Diana also related that immediately after her initial treatment she had felt depressed, spacey, and off-centre, although a week later, on her second visit, she was feeling more like herself.

Diana's journal entry after the first treatment reads:

It is as if I have gone inside myself, closed the door, and can't come out. I simply cannot focus on the world outside. I keep reliving old memories, becoming entirely caught up in their emotions. This has not been without cost. This afternoon at the stables, my horse reared up as I was bridling him and crushed me against the fence. Instead of calming him and freeing myself, I found myself screaming, 'Help me, won't somebody help me?' which is exactly what my mother cried out when the nurses turned her over, shortly before she died, because the movement was hurting her so much. In my mother's cry I heard all the resentment and betrayed hope of a lifetime. And in my cry, to my huge embarrassment, I heard the same. I was a pile of raw emotion, awed that after 5 years of therapy, there were still so many demons on the loose. Until now, however, I have rarely talked about my mother's death which was more than 20 years ago, when I was 23.

After the second treatment, Diana reported impressive relief from her rash, saying:

If I take the herbs, the itching seems to stop, although I still feel it lurking beneath the surface. My hip is extraordinary — I rode without pain or the usual hour of limping after dismounting. My chest, too, feels better although my shoulder hurts, with pain travelling to my head.

Diana wrote about another aspect of her experience in her journal, saying:

What is really remarkable to me is how much my life has changed since I've begun acupuncture. Frankly, I don't understand my sometimes overwhelming psychological reactions to this treatment. In 5 years of therapy I've never been so turned inside-out. The last session left me with a wonderful sense of wholeness within myself and a rather mystical separateness from the world around me — as if I'm a genie and can appear and vanish at will. At the same time, I feel friendly and tolerant toward co-workers and am full of good intentions about eating right, working sensible hours, and offering my gifts to the world. For years I had trouble washing the dishes right after supper. I was too tired and I could not see the point. Now I realise that I was probably too depressed. I think I have been depressed for longer than I like to admit, probably since my mother's death, and there is nothing like depression to sap energy. Now, I'm playing the Marriage of Figaro, singing as I wash away . . . Ever since I can remember I have been shy, like my mother, and dreaded going to parties. I used to pluck up all my courage just to walk through the door. Then, tonight I was invited to a gathering and not only did I enjoy it, I looked forward to it all day. I feel as if a new person has come and lodged inside me, someone not shy at all.

In the middle of December, 6 weeks after beginning treatment, Diana was told by her gynaecologist that he had found abnormal cells on her pap smear. Her mother had died of cervical cancer, so this threw Diana into a panic. In her diary, Diana wrote:

I haven't been to work for 3 days. One thing seems clear — I don't want to die. When I went for my acupuncture treatment today, Harriet told me in no uncertain terms that I am not my mother; that I can take a different path. I liked the idea, although the anguish I felt as I lay there full of needles was almost too much to bear. Both my mother and father died terrified of death, isolated in their fear while everyone around them pretended they were going to get well. Today I stared at the devil and the devil blinked. I believe I can live longer than my mother.

Later it was established that the abnormal cells were neither problematic nor pathological.

Two months after receiving weekly acupuncture and drinking herbal extracts daily, Diana said her rash was gone, her wrist was better, and her hip and elbow were no longer in pain. She also said, as the effect of acupuncture wore off, that:

I find myself at war between my three separate parts — my sense of wholeness disintegrated. On Monday my mind took over and I stayed up all night writing, skipping dinner and breakfast. On Tuesday my body demanded attention, craving dinner at a good Thai restaurant and 15 hours of sleep. On Wednesday the day went by and I did not write at all — instead I wrestled with my spiritual demons, perched by my ear whispering to me that I had no talent. I was acutely aware that my mother, who dropped out of nursing school, never found her vocation before she died. Was I afraid to succeed where she had failed? Despite this turmoil, I am grateful for the new vigour and awareness that comes with it.

After 30 acupuncture visits and a year of drinking herbs, Diana reflected:

My physical ailments are no more, but even more importantly, I am no longer the person I was a year ago. Now I have the energy to get through each day, weathering ups and downs more cheerfully, and surprisingly, I am much more outgoing. It seems clear to me that more than infected fleas were the culprits. I believe many problems were the result of a long overdue conversation between my body, mind, and soul — the result of which was a mutiny. They had to get my attention somehow (and having succeeded, they have been warring like jealous siblings ever since). Or was it my mother, soul to soul, so to speak, who put them up to it?

First treatment procedures

POINTS PRESCRIPTION

LU7 *lieque* or 'broken sequence' is also known as *tongxuan* or 'child mystery'. It is a *luo* point that activates the Conception Vessel (*ren mai*). Sedation of this point loosens the Lung *qi*, allowing the chest to open and the pectoral or *zong qi* to disperse and descend. Combined with P6 *neiguan*, the diaphragm relaxes, permitting natural peristalsis and respiration to resume. The name 'child mystery' may suggest that this point helps one gain access to early, forgotten, or hidden information.

P6 *neiguan* or 'inner pass' is a *luo* point that activates the Penetrating Vessel (*yin wei mai*). Sedation aids the relaxation of the chest, diaphragm, oesophagus and stomach. This point calms the Mind, and promotes harmony between the Heart and Spleen by regulating the *qi* of the Upper and Middle Burners. It restores the buffer between the *shen* and the body and between the *shen* and the external world. The combination of P6 *neiguan* with LU7

lieque also harmonises the relationship between the *shen* and the *po*, the psychic aspects of Fire and Metal.

LI11 *quchi* or 'pool at the bend', also known as *shangsanli* or 'upper three mile', is an Earth point and a helpful local point for the elbow. When combined with ST36 *zusanli*, it helps tonify *qi* and Blood by promoting the digestive and eliminative functions of the Stomach and Intestines. Tonifying the Earth points on these two channels enhances the relationship between Earth (Spleen) and Metal (Lung). In addition, LI11 *quchi* is one of the Thirteen Ghost Points and is named *guichen* or 'ghost minister'. The ghost points have the purported ability to expel either obstinate negative influences that have penetrated the individual from the outside world, or persistent negative thoughts that have formed inwardly as a consequence of psychological trauma, e.g. clinging to the memory of a deceased loved one as if she were still alive. This point was used on the left.

ST36 *zusanli* or 'leg three mile', also known as *xiaqihai* or 'lower sea of qi', is an Earth point and is the major point on the Stomach channel for strengthening and harmonising the Spleen and Stomach. Combined with P6 *neiguan* (which is sequentially connected with the leg *jue yin* Liver channel) it helps to encourage normal peristalsis and appetite, and allays nausea caused by visceral tension and emotional friction between the Heart, Stomach and Liver. Tonifying ST36 *zusanli* also promotes the generation of postnatal Essence which helps to restore the Essence of the Kidney. S36 *zusanli* is another of the Thirteen Ghost Points known as *guixie* or 'ghost evil'.

KID7 *fuliu* or 'recover flow', also known as *fujiu* or 'deep lying mortar', is a Metal point. Tonifying this mobilises the relationship between the Lung and Kidney (Metal supplements Water) which strengthens the Kidney, anchors the Kidney and Lung *qi*, fortifies the *zhi* (will or primal instinct), and helps the Lung to release its fixations and disperse stagnant *qi*. The alternative name 'deep lying mortar' suggests that this point can influence the deep Essence or Marrow (*sui*), the foundation substance that sustains the body's structural components including the brain, bones, and joints.

GB30 *huantiao* or 'jumping circle', also known as *shuzhong* or 'pivot centre', is a major point for clearing obstructed *qi* of the Gallbladder and Bladder channels, especially in the area of the hips, pelvis, legs, and lumbar region. Static Liver *qi* is often shunted into the Gallbladder channel as a result of long-term frustration, emotional restraint, or over-control. This point relaxes muscles, tendons, and ligaments, soothes nerves, and defuses pent-up rage. The names 'jumping circle' and 'pivot centre' suggest that this area of the body is central to the organisation of flexibility, agility, and the coordinated movement so essential for adapting to the inner and outer vicissitudes of daily life including coping with obstacles and transitions. This point was used only on the right.

Needles: were 32 gauge, 25 mm and remained in place for 30 minutes with the lights dimmed, music playing, and a heat lamp over the legs for warmth.

CHINESE HERBS

Diana's herb prescription consisted of two separate formulae from 'Chinese Modular Solutions'.[2] The first formula addressed the rash and consisted of the modules 'Purge External Wind (*qu wai feng*)', 'Strengthen Lung (*qiang fei*)', 'Harmonise Heart and Lung (*tiao he xin fei*)', and 'Comfort *Shen* (*an shu shen*)'. It was to be used before breakfast and as needed during the day. The second formula was to be used before bed and contained 'Harmonise Liver and Spleen (*tiao he gan pi*)', 'Tonify Blood (*bu xue*)', 'Strengthen Liver (*qiang gan*)', and 'Comfort *Shen* (*an shu shen*)'.

The herbal formulae support the acupuncture treatment by helping to sustain its effects and accelerate the process of change and resolution. In this case the morning formula addressed the acute condition and the evening formula the chronic constitutional pattern. Whilst the morning formula concentrated on correcting the disturbances of the Heart and Lung networks whose *qi* was waxing in the early part of the day, the evening formula concentrated on rectifying the deeper distortions of the Liver network whose *qi* was ascendant at night. Together the formulae addressed deficiencies and excesses, stagnation and instability, psyche and soma.

Patterns, aetiology, and pathology

Diana can be identified as a Wood type, a person moved by the yearning to break through whatever limits or confines her.[3] Resolve is characteristic of Wood types. Diana continued to horseride, undaunted by the fact that doing so aggravated her hip and made her vulnerable to injuries such as the crushed ribs and broken wrist. She was a single mother with a professional career and a fervent desire to make her life count in an individually creative way.

The organ network of Wood, the Liver, is responsible for mobilising activity by creating pressure. Pressure is mounted by regulating the volume and force of Blood and *qi*. People instinctively seek out circumstances that permit or encourage them to do what comes naturally and easily. Wood types exhibit certain proclivities. Often those good at building pressure and galvanising power are not equally adept at relaxing and resting. Under prolonged or extreme stress they become tense and fatigued, which leads to the craving for more stimulation to maintain their customary level of performance and arousal. This process eventually leads to their becoming erratic, irritable, volatile and weary.

Organ network disharmonies

Liver dominance

- Irritable.
- Sensitive to pain, wind, heat, noise, sun.
- Muscle cramps.
- Easily startled.
- Depression with rage.
- Hot flushes.
- Painful, stiff hips.
- Elbow tendonitis.
- Painful, irregular periods.
- Premenstrual mood swings.
- Symptoms worse premenstrually.
- Dry skin and hair.
- Chilly mottled limbs.
- Pulse: tight in the Liver position.

Heart *shen* disturbance

- Anxiety.
- Sensitive to insult.
- Easily moved emotionally.
- Palpitations.
- Easily frightened.
- Hot flushes.

Spleen deficiency

- Weak, tender muscles.
- Sensitive to pain.
- Worry, upset by change.
- Socially deprived.
- Nausea, gas.
- Tongue: scalloped.
- Pulse: thin, weak.

Lung fixation

- Sensitive to insults.
- Morbid thoughts.
- Depression with melancholy.
- Stiffness of body.
- Poor healing of, and dry, skin.
- Itching, hives, rash.
- Inhibited expression of feelings.
- Sadness, grief.
- Pulse: Tight, weak in the Lung position.

ACUPUNCTURE IN PRACTICE

Kidney weakness

- Stiff, painful hips.
- Increasingly irregular menstrual cycle.
- Chronic scanty menstruation.
- Early greying of head and pubic hair.
- Loosening of skin and muscles.
- PMS since childbirth.
- Hot flushes.
- Chronic scoliosis.
- Difficulty arising in morning.
- Fear and expectation of early death.
- Despair and hopelessness (can't imagine a future).
- Social isolation.
- Pulse: thin, weak.

The power of Wood is in ascendence in spring, a time when existing disharmonies of the Liver network become accentuated. Incited by an infected flea bite during this season, Diana's Liver engendered Heat and Wind which assaulted the Lung network, producing an irritable, red, itchy rash. Initially Diana's determination to become free of this problem led to an escalating level of frustration. Eventually, because she would not accede to a poor prognosis, she ventured into the unfamiliar territory of Chinese traditional medicine. Already we have a vivid picture of the power of Wood to disrupt the status quo and propel an individual forward into a new realm of experience. It is as if her vital force would not settle for a simple and direct outcome — what appears to be a superficial Wind Heat rash has become a somatic metaphor for a deeper, older, buried struggle between movement and stasis, growth and resistance.

Diana had a history of chronic dryness, probably due to deficiency of Blood. Her skin and hair were dry, her menses scanty, her skin healed slowly, she had palpitations, restlessness, emotional reactivity and sensitivity, and occasional vertigo. Her tongue was pale with scalloped edges and white fur and her pulse tight, especially in the positions of the Liver and Lung. Dryness due to Blood deficiency adversely affected the Liver, creating a propensity for the generation of internal Heat and Wind. She also began experiencing signs of menopausal deficiencies such as greying hair, hot flushes, mood swings, anxiety, depression, and increased premenstrual distress.

Patterns of disharmony

Deficient Blood

- Dry skin and hair.
- Scanty periods.
- Poor skin healing.
- Muscle cramps.
- Palpitations.
- Irritability.
- Stiff, pained hips.
- Emotionally sensitive.
- Easily startled, frightened.
- Tongue: pale.
- Pulse: thin, tight.

Deficient *qi*

- Morning fatigue.
- Loss of skin and muscle tone.
- Poor skin healing.
- Sensitive to insult and pain.
- Tongue: scalloped.
- Pulse: weak.

Deficient essence

- PMS since childbirth.
- Irregular periods.
- Early grey hair.
- Poor skin and muscle tone.
- Chronic scoliosis.
- Hot flushes.
- Despair and hopelessness.

- Expectation of early death.
- Pulse: thin and weak.

Stagnant *qi*

- Nausea, gas.
- Neck and shoulder tension.
- Premenstrual mood swings.
- Painful, irregular periods.
- Awkward expression of feelings.
- Pulse: tight.

Wind-heat in the skin

- Itching red rash.
- Recurring hives.
- Sensitivity to heat and sunshine.
- Sensitivity to wind.

Like other Wood types, Diana tends to rob herself of Blood and Moisture, and squander *qi* as a result of her drive to maintain a high degree of internal pressure and level of striving. As a Wood type, Diana also swings between states of *collapse* and *exaggeration*. *Collapse* means that Diana behaves like a Water type, retreating to her inner world, feeling shy, retiring, self-enclosed, grumpy, grim, and preferring solitude to socialising. *Exaggeration* means that she behaves like Fire, rushing about in a hyperactive, manic state, unable to find time to sleep or eat with regularity, preferring stimulation and activity to quietude.

Organ conflicts and tensions

Lung-Liver disharmony

- Depression with feelings of rage, sadness.
- Dermatitis with predominance of itching, dryness.
- Unpredictable moods.
- Physical, emotional stiffness and inflexibility.
- Hypersensitive, highly reactive to outside influences.
- Muscle cramps.

Kidney-Heart disharmony

- Fear, anxiety about future.
- Lack of self-confidence and optimism, despair.
- Hot flushes.

Heart-Lung disharmony

- Easily hurt, insulted.
- Suppressed grief, pain.
- Melancholy.
- Vulnerable to outside influences.

Diana's primary conflict was between the Liver and Lung, initiated by suppressed grief and rage over her mother's death (Fig. 39.1). Treatment addressed this central dynamic as well as the deficiency and stagnation of

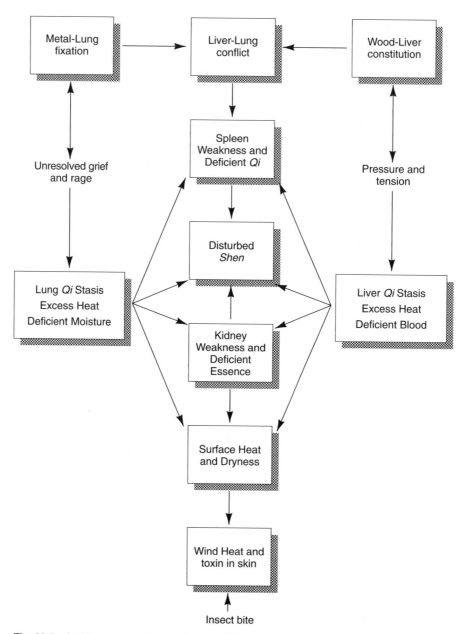

Fig. 39.1 Aetiology and pathology diagram. Diana, being a Wood type, is predisposed towards pathogenic Heat and Dryness which, together with suppressed and unresolved grief and rage, overinhibit Liver-Wood and create stagnation of Lung-Metal. Injuries by insect toxins induce an external Wind-Heat illness that, in turn, brings out the chronic underlying disturbances. Long-term Lung-Liver constraint and conflict lead to depression and isolation, with consequent weakening and instability of the Heart, Spleen and Kidney (*shen, qi, jing*). Chronic *Yin* deficiencies (Blood, Moisture, Essence) set the stage for aberrations of *Yang* activity (Heat, Wind, panic, rage).

qi and Blood. The secondary tensions between Lung-Heart and Kidney-Heart contributed to Diana's depression, evidenced by her hypervigilance, anxiety about the future, hopelessness, melancholy, and fear of death. Disorganising the pattern of conflict between the Lung and Liver loosened the other knots that had developed between the other organ networks, especially the Kidney and Heart.[4]

Interpretation and discussion

In Chinese medicine, pathology and ontology are inextricably linked — how we get sick is tied to *who we are*. If we assume that a pattern of illness arises from the distortion of a person's *true nature*, then illness becomes a heuristic window through which the imperative of the vital force may be observed. Within a constitutional approach, the process of resolving symptoms becomes one of reinvigorating a person's promise or destiny (*ming*).

The routes by which people find their way toward healing are both intriguing and mysterious. Diana's story is exemplary of the seemingly — always in retrospect — fortuitous sequence of events that initiated not only recovery, but also a process of reclamation.

Very soon after beginning acupuncture treatment, Diana is faced with powerful memories of her mother's death, the recognition of her unabated grief, and the spectre of her own fear of dying like her mother. She is surprised, having presumed that this had all been reconciled through psychotherapy. Perhaps the trauma had been resolved at a mental or cognitive level, but not in the spiritual and bodily realms.

Loss and its consequent feelings of sorrow and emptiness injure the Lung. If such experiences are not integrated at all levels of the self, a lesion or scar is created that becomes an area of stasis, a part of bodily life that is cut off from sensory and emotional experience. This is what occurred in Diana at the age of 23. When pain is felt as unbearable, the body adapts by contracting in the area of pain in order to squeeze off the feelings and sensations. As a result, a kind of fixation develops that not only obstructs the circulation of *qi* and Blood, but inhibits the developmental process of growth and maturity. Diana informs us that, immersed in the upheaval of her thoughts and feelings about her mother and her death, she is feeling like her younger self.

This can be viewed as a successful effort by the Liver — her organising force — to undermine the Lung's fixation. She began to free herself from her identification with, and loss of, her mother. What carried her through the ensuing period of turmoil was a clearer sense of herself, her capacity, and her own destiny. Once the lesion was opened, the vital force asserted itself, expressed as the beginning of being 'at war between my three separate parts — my mind, body, and spirit'. Out of this struggle emerged self-assurance and renewal. A disorganisation, reorganisation, and re-integration of the tripartite self — the *shen*, *qi*, and *jing* — is underway, which in spite of its discomfort, is felt as fundamentally affirming and unifying.

Upon regaining self-confidence, Diana became more gregarious, and immersed herself in her *deeper, inner nature* which she described as her *spiritual side*, imagining a future in which she would be alive and well past the age at which her mother succumbed to a life of 'resentment and betrayed hope'. It dawned upon her that she was strong where her mother was weak; she was determined where her mother was resigned; she had a life full of possibilities, while her mother relinquished her yearnings to fate. Upon uncovering her hidden self, her mission was clarified and she decided that she no longer required treatment. She had become realigned with her *true nature* and empowered to pursue its fulfilment on her own.

In this scenario, the dynamic dual nature of illness can be seen. On the one hand it is a perverse force that can drive Diana into submission and despair, and, on the other hand, it is a subversive force that coerces Diana into radically rearranging herself.

The surge of the forces of Liver-Wood ultimately undermined the chronic Lung-Metal fixation. Out of this struggle emerged a new sense of expanded boundaries and a sort of reembodiment — a decision to 'breathe into the outlines of my body' and to 'stay rooted' within it. This represents a return of liveliness and elasticity in Lung-Metal which stretches the skin — the tangible limits of the self — to make room for increased energy and excitement. The original insult to Diana's Lung (Metal) which obstructed her emotional and spiritual growth, is recast by a more mature awareness.

Progress and outcome

- 'Massive amounts of energy'.
- More cheerful and outgoing.
- 'Feeling better than I have in 20 years'.
- Skin clear, no wrist or hip pain.
- 'Sense of being more in control of my life'.
- Began journalism and creative writing class.

The purpose of medicine

To treat illness is to liberate primordial energies. Chinese traditional medicine not only undermines the organism's ill habits, countering the momentum of illness, it also advances the intrinsic design — the *li*[5] — freeing the *true self*, replete with its drive toward self-realisation (Fig. 39.2). Health is wholeheartedly pursued only when it is recognised as the way to satisfy one's deepest needs and yearnings. It is first imagined, and then assembled out of the fabric of our lived experience. While our failures and traumas may indicate how we lack competence and resilience, our achievements, however small, and our moments of transcendence, however brief, point the way back to the primal force which unconditionally affirms us, steering us further and deeper into life.

Medicine is science, art, and above all else, a language which generates a hypothesis that a given problem is caused by X, so intervention Y will antidote it. The only way to test our hypothesis is by clinical trial. However, when we do so, there are countless non-specific influences that elude control. In the end we do not know whether it is the needle in its position with such and such manipulation which is the positive trigger, the herbal formula with its composition, form, and frequency, or our intention to be helpful and wish for a right outcome that has provoked a course of change. There is an ineffable magic in medicine. Perhaps we merely offer an opportunity for the transformative process, already underway, to unfold.

The healing relationship dwells in sacred space. Like romantic love, it grows out of trust, derives power from the process of being heard, known, and touched, and demands a willingness to risk exposure. It is a co-operative venture in the misty realm of the unpredictable that involves the coming together of subjectivities, ours as healers with those of our patients, and the commingling of our destiny.

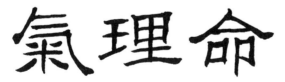

Fig. 39.2 Chinese letters for *qi*, *li* and *ming*.

NOTES:

1 Adapted from the Talmud.

2 'Chinese Modular Solutions' is an integrated herbal system formulated by the author and Efrem Korngold. Each formula is organised around a specific diagnostic-therapeutic focus. The category-specific formulae (modules), such as 'Tonify Blood', can then be mixed and matched to compose a prescription that more closely fits the problem or person.

3 Each person can be identified as embodying the power of one of the Five-Phases (*wu xing:* Wood, Fire, Earth, Metal, Water). These types represent five metaphors for the emotional, physical and spiritual dynamics that organise us. Each type has idiosyncratic traits, motivations and dilemmas — five styles of being in the world. Predisposition towards illness and predilection for the cultivation of virtue can be anticipated for each of the five. By helping people to recognise their type, habits of suffering can be interrupted and self-awareness can be enabled, preparing the ground for self-acceptance and mastery. For a complete discussion, see Five-Phase Archetypes in Beinfield & Korngold (1991).

4 The Heart harbours the *shen* (psyche, heaven) and the Kidney preserves the *jing* (soma, earth). *Shen-jing* is the embodiment of *yin-yang*. It is the marriage of our endowment at birth, our original nature, our potential *(jing)*, with how we express that nature, or actualise it *(shen)*.

5 *Li* can be understood in this context as the individual pattern that original *(yuan) qi* fashions in each person, also known as one's nature.

REFERENCES

Beinfield H, Korngold E 1991 Between heaven and earth: a guide to Chinese medicine. Ballantine

■ Harriet Beinfield

Harriet Beinfield, LAc, wrote *Between Heaven and Earth: A Guide to Chinese Medicine*, *Chinese Modular Solutions Handbook for Health Professionals*, and the pamphlet *Chinese Medicine: How It Works* with her husband, Efrem Korngold, LAc, OMD. Having initially trained in England, she has been in practice since 1973 at Chinese Medicine Works in San Francisco. Beinfield and Korngold have blended their interest in psychology with their understanding of the many explanatory models within the Chinese medical paradigm to form their own perspective. This is articulated by the Five-Phase Archetypes discussed in *Between Heaven and Earth*. With Efrem Korngold, she is coformulator of an integrated herbal system called *Chinese Modular Solutions*. Beinfield has lectured, given seminars, written articles, and appeared on American radio and television in order to share Chinese medicine with both health care providers and the American public. Beinfield represented Chinese medicine at the July 1994 National Institutes of Health Conference on Examining Research Assumptions in Alternative Medicine.

Headaches, angels and guiding spirits

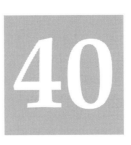

Jacqueline Young LONDON, UK

Teresa had a waif-like, almost ethereal quality to her. When she entered the room she appeared 'mousy', with drab clothes and a slightly cowed posture. Her build was slight and she was pale and softly spoken. Yet, when she finally made eye contact, I was struck by her brilliant blue-green eyes.

Incapacitating headaches

A 24-year-old trainee florist of Irish descent, Teresa came to see me complaining of persistent headaches of several months duration. The pain was boring, intense and intermittent and initially located frontally but, more recently, had also spread to the temporal and parietal regions. The headaches would come on 'for no apparent reason', though they were often worse at night and when she was on her own. They often lasted for many hours and were starting to affect her concentration at work. She had already taken time off work on several occasions when the pain had become really incapacitating and her employers were beginning to lose their patience. She feared losing her job as a trainee florist and, with it, her future work prospects because she had no other skills.

Teresa had made several visits to her GP who had examined her thoroughly and had put her condition down to 'stress'. He had given her some tablets, which she had forgotten the name of, but she had stopped using them after a short time because they brought little relief and upset her stomach. She had tried over-the-counter remedies too, including Anadin and Neurofen, but again these had brought little relief and she generally felt worse after taking them. She had tried acupuncture once before but had also found that unhelpful.

Teresa said she could not associate anything in particular with the initial onset of the headaches, or any current pattern to them, but she had tried altering her diet after a friend suggested that food allergies might be involved. After experimenting a little she had found that an excess of dairy products or chocolate did seem to contribute to the headaches but these were not the only factors.

An old head on young shoulders

Teresa's mother was Irish and both she and her younger sister had been born in Ireland. However, the family had moved to London when Teresa was a young child because her British-born father had wanted to return to the capital to find work. Teresa's mother had had psychiatric problems for as long as Teresa could remember, with alternating depression and mania. For the most part, this had been contained at home but more recently her mother had been admitted to hospital on several occasions. She was currently in a psychiatric unit where she had been for several months. Teresa and her 16-year-old sister lived at home with their father, but he was unemployed and was often drunk, so they saw little of him except in the evenings. They would try to get to bed before he came home in order to avoid seeing him.

For as long as Teresa could remember she had looked after her younger sister and had taken care of the household. She had also, to some extent, been responsible for her parents, especially her mother whom she would help to dress and take to hospital appointments, etc. In many ways, Teresa seemed to have an old head on young shoulders and appeared careworn with little joy in her life. She admitted being a 'worrier' and expressed anxiety about each member of her family.

She did enjoy working with flowers, and obviously found the creative stimulus at work a welcome break from home life, but she did not get on well with her employer, who was often domineering and impatient with her.

Her closest contact was her sister, of whom she was very protective. She was close to her maternal grandmother, whom she only saw once yearly during summer visits to Ireland. Her boyfriend was also in Ireland and their contact was only occasional. She had a few friends in London but little social life because of limited finance and the need to take care of the home and her sister.

After a long wait she had been referred to a counsellor through her GP and had found the sessions helpful in working through family problems. She felt that the counsellor had given her more confidence in herself and had helped her to become more assertive, but she was disappointed that the sessions had been terminated because the doctor's surgery only allowed six sessions at a time.

Timidity and depletion

Although an occasional spark of humour would come through in Teresa's conversations, for much of the time she was timid and quiet, and there were many signs of physical weakness. Her digestion was poor, with little appetite and feelings of nausea, and her abdomen felt soft and weak to the touch, with some bloating. She often 'forgot' to eat or ate very little and her body had very little energy or vitality. Her periods were scanty with a short cycle and she felt weak and debilitated pre-menstrually when her moods would swing from feeling depressed and hopeless to feeling tense and irritable.

Teresa often had difficulty falling asleep and her sleep was frequently disturbed by dreams. Most of the time she felt tired. Her pulse was wiry in the Liver position but weak and deep overall. Her tongue was pale and flabby with a thin, clear, greasy coating in the centre and a red tip.

Body scanning

While studying acupuncture in Japan I learned how to 'scan' the body. This involves running the palm of the hand just over the surface of the body to detect energetic imbalances and blockages in specific meridians, as well as to 'see' these blockages by looking at the energetic emissions, or lack of them, in the electromagnetic field around the body (Young 1988).

Looking at Teresa as we spoke, it became obvious to me that there was a tremendous block of energy concentrated at the front of her forehead, the area known as the brow *chakra* or 'third eye'. There was also corresponding weakness in her abdomen, in the area of the solar plexus *chakra*. When feeling over these areas with the hands, there was a constricted and hot feeling over the brow and an empty and cool feeling over the abdomen.

Sensing a hidden potential

Teresa summed herself up by saying:

> *I'm not sure how I feel about life. I feel I haven't found my way. There are things I want to do but they don't seem to work out somehow and most of the time I just feel tired, worn-out and worn down with the pain of the headaches.*

I was intrigued by Teresa. Her appearance was drab and timid and yet her eyes revealed a brilliance within. There was a real sense of hidden potential about her that was masked by her present suffering and vulnerability. I felt sure that her headaches were the tip of the iceberg and that, in treating them, we would together pave the way for deeper transformation.

Summary of clinical manifestations

- Waif-like and pale with cowed posture.
- Brilliant blue-green eyes, difficulty making eye contact.
- Headaches: intense and boring, initially located frontally, but more recently are in the temporal and parietal regions, intermittent pain, worse at night, impaired concentration.
- Some improvement to headaches by avoiding dairy products and chocolate.
- Poor appetite and feelings of nausea, poor digestion.
- Bloated abdomen, soft and weak to the touch.
- Scanty menses with a short cycle.

- Premenstrual debility and mood swings between mild depression and feelings of hopelessness, alternating with tension and irritability.
- Insomnia with disturbing dreams.
- Fatigue and weakness.
- Anxiety and worry.
- Timidity, softly spoken.
- Constricted and hot feeling over the brow.
- Empty and cool feeling over the abdomen.
- Pulse: weak and deep but wiry in the Liver position.
- Tongue: pale and flabby with sticky, greasy coating in the centre, also red tip.

Patterns of disharmony

In traditional Chinese medical terms, the patterns of disharmony in Teresa's case appeared to be fairly straightforward. It was clear that her headache was endogenous, rather than exogenous, because of its protracted nature with intermittent, intense pain. Several of her more recent symptoms provided evidence of hyperactivity of the Liver *yang*, namely the boring, one-sided parietal or temporal pain of the headaches together with feelings of nausea, disturbed sleep, irritability, PMT, sticky tongue coating and wiry pulse in the Liver position. There was also clear evidence of underlying deficiency of both Kidney and Spleen *qi*, which was reflected in her lethargy and fatigue, pallor, loss of appetite and poor digestion, menstrual insufficiency, insomnia, pale and flabby tongue and generally weak pulse.

However, it was also apparent to me that her 'symptoms' went deeper than a basic traditional Chinese medical analysis allowed and that other concepts of disharmony had to be considered, namely problems of a psychic origin. According to the Japanese scientist, researcher and psychic, Dr Hiroshi Motoyama, with whom I have studied and worked for many years, each of the meridians are connected with specific *chakras* or 'energy centres' of the body (Motoyama 1981, Young 1989)[1]. Each *chakra* stores the seeds for particular physical imbalances, emotional patterns and also for certain psychic 'traits' that relate to the development of consciousness. According to this theory, Teresa's symptoms related to dysfunction in the *ajna chakra*, located in the middle of the forehead, and also the *manipura* and *svadhisthana chakras*, located in the abdomen. On a meridian and physical level, the former links with a Liver and Gall Bladder meridian imbalance, and with headaches, menstrual problems and irritability, whilst the latter relate to Stomach, Spleen and Kidney meridian imbalances, and to digestive problems, menstrual insufficiency, worry and anxiety.

At the same time, strong activity in the areas of these *chakras* is generally indicative of psychic function in the individual. Based on many years of both acupuncture and parapsychological research, Motoyama argues that, as the person evolves spiritually, the activity of different *chakras* becomes heightened, leading not only to physical, emotional and meridian changes, but also to the appearance of certain so-called 'psychic' abilities. Specific paranormal activities are associated with each *chakra* (Motoyama 1988, Young 1989). In Teresa's case the imbalance in the *svadhisthana* and *manipura chakras* would be associated with experiences of uncontrolled ESP (extrasensory perception) and telepathy or intuition while the *ajna chakra* activity, which was most pronounced in her case, would be associated with visions and powerful dreams. From the picture she presented I was fairly sure that she had inborn psychic ability that had been firmly repressed and that the repression and blockage were contributing to her present symptoms.

Evidence for the patterns of disharmony

Liver *yang* rising

- One-sided, parietal or temporal headaches.
- Intermittent, boring pain, worse at night.
- Constriction and feeling of heat over the brow.
- Nausea.
- Disturbed sleep.
- PMT, mood swings from feeling depressed and hopeless to being tense and irritable.
- Tongue: red tip.
- Pulse: wiry in the Liver position.

Kidney *qi* deficiency

- Lethargy and fatigue.
- Menstrual insufficiency.
- Pallor.
- Cowed posture.
- Timidity and soft voice.
- Anxiety.
- Empty and cool feeling over the abdomen.
- Tongue: pale.
- Pulse: weak and deep.

Spleen *qi* deficiency

- Loss of appetite.
- Poor digestion.
- Bloated abdomen, soft and weak to the touch.
- Menstrual insufficiency.
- Insomnia.
- Frontal headache, poor concentration.
- Headaches improve with exclusion of dairy products.
- Tongue: pale and flabby.
- Pulse: weak.

Angels and visiting spirits

While Teresa relaxed on the couch during her first treatment, she told me a little more about her dreams. She said that she often felt a 'presence' in them, but then would feel afraid and wake up. I asked her if she ever experienced visions while in a waking state. At first she was evasive and just mumbled 'sometimes', but when I reassured her that many people have this type of experience and asked if her visions went back to childhood, she visibly relaxed and began to pour out her experiences.

As a little girl playing in the garden she had first become aware of seeing 'moving strands of light' and 'fairy-like figures'. They had been her play companions and she had not been afraid of them. Gradually, she had also become aware that if she closed her eyes she could see pictures, as if projected on to a screen in her mind's eye. Sometimes the pictures were of far-off places and made no particular sense to her, but at other times they involved people she knew and, on a few occasions, the pictures she 'saw' actually happened in reality some time later.

At night time she would gaze at the ceiling in the half-light and, on two occasions, saw angelic beings. One night, however, when she was a teenager, she had woken to the presence of the ghostly figure of a man standing at the foot of her bed. She was so terrified by this experience that she had been unable to sleep without a light in the room from then onwards and had decided, out of fear, to suppress or stop any visions appearing before her. In effect, she had unconsciously tried to 'shut down' her psychic ability. At times she was successful in doing this, but at other times she could not prevent the visions. She became increasingly anxious about these phenomena, especially in view of her mother's psychiatric history. She feared that she was going 'mad' and told me that, until this conversation, she had never dared mention these experiences to anyone, for fear that they would think her mad.

I reassured Teresa that these experiences were not abnormal and asked her to tell me what she 'saw' when she closed her eyes and focused her concentration on the centre of her forehead and then on her abdomen (the areas of the *ajna* and *svadhisthana chakras* respectively). She told me that she saw a moving, smoky, purple light in the area of her forehead and a glowing, fire-coloured ball of light in the area of her abdomen. Although she herself had no knowledge of the *chakras* at this time, these descriptions are typical signs of activated *ajna* and *svadhisthana chakras* (Motoyama 1981, 1988) (Table 40.1).

An understanding of these experiences, and a knowledge of how to control and develop them therefore needed to be an integral part of

Table 40.1 The Chakras

Physical imbalances	Psychic traits
Ajna chakra Disturbance of the Liver meridian Headaches Irritability	Visions of angels and fairies Visions projected on to the mind's eye Precognition Perception of a smoky, purple light in the area of the *chakra* on the brow
Manipura chakra Spleen meridian imbalance Poor digestion Worry and mood swings	Clairvoyance (psychic vision) Awareness of spiritual beings Strong intuition
Svadhisthana chakra Kidney meridian imbalance Menstrual insufficiency Anxiety	Uncontrolled extrasensory perception Perception of glowing, fire-coloured light in the area of the *chakra*

Teresa's treatment, in addition to meridian balancing and a strengthening of her physical body.

Aetiology

Teresa is typical of an individual who is born with certain psychic abilities but who attempts to repress them because she does not understand them. She has not been taught how to control and develop them, with disastrous results.

In her case, the fearful experience of the 'man' at the foot of the bed was pivotal. She had already been anxious about some of her dreams but the 'reality' of the presence in her room so frightened her that, from then on, she actively tried to suppress the appearance of any visions. This affected the functioning of the brow *chakra*, leading gradually to a build up of energy in the region of the brow and culminating in the increasingly severe headaches. In addition, the shock and fear of the experience, and her subsequent and increasing anxiety, affected the functioning of the *svadhisthana* and *manipura chakras*.

Disruption of the *chakra* function in turn affected meridian function and the Liver, Spleen and Kidney meridians became progressively imbalanced. The problem was further exacerbated by other external factors. The stress and strain of her family situation produced additional fear and anxiety, weakening the Kidney meridian and leading to her current symptoms of tiredness and anxiety. Similarly, all her emotional worry and poor eating habits further weakened the *qi* of the Spleen and contributed to the frontal headaches. In addition, her increasing frustration and irritation damaged the Liver (Fig. 40.1).

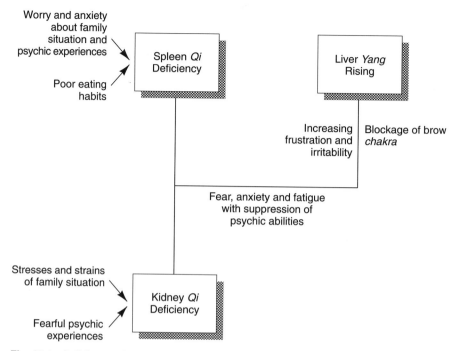

Fig. 40.1 Aetiology and pathology diagram.

As the Liver and Gall Bladder disturbance began to occur, the frontal headache began to spread to the temporal and parietal regions. At the same time, the symptoms of irritability, depression, poor digestion, PMT and sleep disturbance developed.

Treatment issues

I was interested to learn that Teresa's previous treatment with acupuncture had been unsuccessful. I felt this was most likely due to three factors:

1 Insufficient treatment was given (she had only attended two or three times).
2 The selection of points was inadequate. I was unable to contact the acupuncturist who had treated her because he had gone abroad. However, from the points she described from memory, it would appear that she had been treated correctly for Liver/Gall Bladder imbalance. However, the underlying imbalances of Spleen and Kidney *qi* deficiency may not have been fully addressed.
3 No attention was given to the psychic aspects of her case.

I decided to select points to tonify the *qi* of the Kidneys and the Spleen and to sedate the *yang* of the Liver, as well as to help develop *chakra* function. I wanted to teach Teresa meditation techniques to ease energetic blockage of the brow *chakra* and promote circulation through all the *chakras*. I also selected reading material that she could use to gain a greater understanding of the *chakras* and her psychic abilities. Finally, I wanted to help her re-establish support systems with other health professionals, such as the counsellor, to enable her to continue to work through family issues.

The first treatment using the extraordinary vessels

In our first session together I instructed Teresa in simple relaxation and breathing techniques as she lay on the couch. This practice is widely adopted at the start of Japanese acupuncture treatment in order to enhance and maximise the acupuncture effects (Matsumoto & Birch 1985). She was not afraid of the needles and said she was 'looking forward to the treatment'. I explained that I would use several points on both the front and back of the body to balance the Liver and digestive system and that my intention was to relieve the headaches, balance digestion, restore menstrual function and improve vitality.

My root treatment was based on a Japanese acupuncture technique that utilises pairs of opening and coupled points in order to treat through the extraordinary meridians. The opening and coupled points of the *dai mai*, or girdle vessel, were selected as particularly appropriate for Teresa's configuration of symptoms. In Japanese acupuncture, this combination is often used for headaches caused by a combination of Liver *yang* rising and an underlying deficiency of the Kidneys. This idea is supported by Maciocia's interesting proposal of extraordinary vessel 'types' (Maciocia 1989). One of his girdle vessel types is 'Young women with headaches, menorrhagia . . . and a full pulse, especially in the Liver position'.

Treatment involved first applying gentle fingertip pressure to the opening point GB41 *zulinqi* bilaterally to determine which had the strongest 'pulse', i.e. the most *qi*. This point was then needled very superficially, barely penetrating the skin. The needle was inserted slightly obliquely in the direction of the flow of the meridian and to a depth of no more than 1 mm, into what is known as the *wei qi* area of the skin.[2]

Care was taken to insert the needle on the exhalation of the patient and then, as both the patient and the practitioner inhaled, to draw *qi* into the point in order to obtain a tonification effect. There was no attempt to tonify or disperse through needle stimulation techniques. Instead, the emphasis in this technique is on the sensitivity of the practitioner's fingertips and on mental intention to sense and draw the *qi* to the point. Once the *qi* is felt in the fingertips the needle is withdrawn as the patient inhales. This approach is based on the principles of Japanese meridian therapy (Denmai & Brown 1990).

The same technique was then applied to the coupled point SJ5 *waiguan* on the opposite side of the body, then to the untreated side of GB41 *zulinqi* and finally to the untreated SJ5 *waiguan*. The needle was retained until the arrival of *qi* could be sensed in the fingertips.

On completion, the four points were again palpated and the wrist pulses checked. The process can be repeated, as necessary, until the pulses feel balanced. Utilising these points in matched pairs and treating obliquely in diagonals across the body is said to help balance the upper and lower portions and the left and right sides of the body. This is particularly useful in the case of headache and syndromes caused by rising Liver *yang* and deficient Kidney *qi* as these are characterised by an excess of energy and heat in the upper part of the body and deficiency and coolness in the lower body.

In Japanese subtle acupuncture techniques, the opening and coupled points are thought to be particularly good for treating problems of a psychic origin because the extraordinary meridians also link powerfully with the *chakras* and with different levels of consciousness.

Summary of treatment procedures

FIRST TREATMENT

- GB41 *zulinqi*, opening point of the *dai mai*.
- SJ5 *waiguan*, coupled point of the *dai mai*.

SUBSEQUENT TREATMENTS

I continued to use the above opening and coupled point combination on several occasions. I also selected a few additional points each time, according to the predominance of Teresa's different symptoms and to her tongue and pulse picture:

- LIV2 *xingjian* and GB34 *yanglingquan* to pacify the *yang* of the Liver.
- KID3 *taixi* and BL23 *shenshu* to strengthen the *qi* of the Kidney.
- SP6 *sanyinjiao* to strengthen the *qi* of the Spleen.
- *Taiyang* (extra), GB20 *fengchi*, DU20 *baihui* and LI4 *hegu* to relieve headache symptoms.
- REN6 *qihai* and ST36 *zusanli* to improve general vitality.

Needling technique: The needles in the additional points were retained for 15–20 minutes and tonification (Kidneys and Spleen) and sedation (Liver) effects were achieved through breathing rather than through needle techniques. The needles were held, but not moved.

Needles: I used Taga, 30 mm, silver Japanese needles[1] of the finest gauge (size 0), inserted with a stainless steel guide tube warmed in the hand. I chose silver needles for their tonification properties.

Cutaneous needles: Treatments were completed by placing small, Japanese cutaneous needles on a few selected points to maintain treatment over a longer period of time (Young 1989). On a few occasions I used Japanese magnets (600 gauss with north and south poles on the same side), retained with sticking plaster on BL23 *shenshu*, to further boost the Kidney function.

A tremendous weight is lifted from her shoulders

I saw Teresa ten times on a weekly basis and, as part of each session, she was given meditation instructions to practise during the following week, together with reading material from Motoyama's books (Motoyama 1981, 1988)[3] to enable her to better understand her experiences. She was first taught the technique of *'sushumna purification'* which involves purification of the central channel in the spine and connects to each of the *chakras,* and then a *daoist* technique, called 'circulation of light', which helps to regulate the activity between the *chakras.* Later, she was given specific meditation techniques for balancing the *ajna* and *svadhisthana chakras* (Motoyama 1988).

From the first treatment session Teresa reported that she felt as if a tremendous weight had been lifted from her shoulders. For the first time, she had been able to talk about her psychic experiences and understand them better. She was enjoying reading the literature and learning more about the nature of psychic and spiritual development, and was practising the exercises keenly. She was less worried about 'going mad' and was feeling more self-confident and able to cope. She felt less tired and her headaches were beginning to ease.

By the third session, Teresa had been able to re-establish contact with her counsellor and, in talking with her, had been fascinated to learn that she too experienced telepathy and spiritual dreams which gave her insight. This further strengthened Teresa's confidence and, by the following week, she had joined a training course on spiritual healing.

The counsellor also helped Teresa to re-establish her role in the family and to reassess her own needs. As her energy began to increase, Teresa was more able to contemplate moving away from home. After a short time in a squat, Teresa and her sister were able to rent a flat together, which brought new-found independence and gave them a starting ground on which to develop a better relationship with their parents.

Transforming fear

An important development came during the sixth session. While Teresa's needles were in place, and she was relaxed, I gently took her back to the experience in her bedroom of the ghostly figure at the bottom of the bed. Reassuring her to stay calm and relaxed, I encouraged her to actually look at the man rather than to panic. After a while she was able to do this and suddenly she opened her eyes in surprise, telling me that she recognised the man as her grandfather who had died when she was a young girl.

She developed this theme at her healing class a few days later when the instructor talked about 'spirit guides' and how they came to help and to guide, and were often deceased family members, linked through a bond of love. This enabled Teresa to transform her fear of her experience all those years ago and instead to feel that she was surrounded by love and was being helped. This gave her confidence to develop her healing abilities still further.

Teresa continued to work as a trainee florist during the day time and undertook healing training in the evenings. Her headaches gradually became less and less frequent and severe, and she began to rebuild her health and vitality, taking more care with diet and nutrition and spending more time being happy. Her digestion improved and her menses normalised. After a while she moved back to Ireland and we lost contact.

Summary of outcome

- Headaches improved.
- Pallor gone.
- Energy increased as Kidneys tonified.
- Will and sense of purpose and decisiveness increased as the Spleen strengthened.
- Menses and digestion improved.
- Calmer sleep with fewer dreams; remaining dreams were instructive or pleasurable.
- Able to recognise the 'ghost man' as her grandfather and as a guiding spirit; became encouraged by his support and love.
- Improved relationship with her sister and father; counsellor helped separation from her parents; now able to visit mother and give loving support, but does not feel responsible for her or to blame.
- Moved to her own flat with her sister; developing a new relationship with her father.
- Joined a healing group and learning to become a healer whilst continuing as a trainee florist; hopes to run her own florist shop one day and continue healing work in her spare time; interested in investigating the healing power of plants.
- Returned to live in Ireland where she feels most comfortable.
- More confident, self-reliant and joyful.
- Retrieved her sense of self and purpose in life.
- Pulses: improved, Liver pulse no longer wiry, and overall pulses stronger and more energetic.

A blossoming

Teresa transformed during her treatment from a timid, cowed and unhappy girl, borne down with the weight of her responsibilities and anxious about herself and others, to a more confident, self-reliant and joyful young woman. In her own words, 'I know I'm not there yet but I feel I'm on the way to where I want to be. I've got a sense of myself back and my purpose in life, and I'm enjoying myself too!'.

I enjoyed all my contacts with Teresa and the pleasure of watching her blossom towards her true potential. Our experience together confirmed for me the importance of holistic treatment, taking into consideration all aspects of the person and his/her life. In Teresa's case, acupuncture treatment was certainly important in re-establishing meridian balance and relieving many of her physical symptoms but I believe the headaches would have remained if she had not had the opportunity to explore and understand their psychic origin and work on her spiritual self at the same time. The counselling support she received was also crucial to increasing her confi-dence and ability to make changes in her life. The acupuncture supported this work by providing her with more energy to explore issues and make changes.

I don't know what's happening to Teresa these days but I hope she's continuing to progress and that those blue-green eyes are shining!

NOTES

1 Motoyama and Young publications are out of print but available from: Health Systems, PO Box 2211, Barnet, Herts EN5 4QW, UK.

2 See the reference to Japanese acupuncturist, Shohaku Honma's technique in Matsumoto & Birch 1985, pages 162–3.

3 I do not use disposable needles, unless the client specifically requests them, because of the poor quality of materials used in their manufacture. Having trained in Japan, I have been taught that the quality of the needle is as important as the acupuncture that is performed with it. So, instead, I buy high quality needles from Japan which are sometimes handmade and, since I incorporate their cost into the treatment fee, I am free to dispose of them. Alternatively, I retain personalised, individual sets of needles that are stored in sterilisable, labelled tubes. The needles are then rigorously sterilised between treatments and are only ever reused for the same client. With this system, sterilisation and hygiene standards are strictly observed but so too is the Japanese idea that the needles build up their own relationship with the client, over time, in rather the same way that the practitioner does.

REFERENCES

Denmai S, Brown S (trans) 1990 Introduction to meridian therapy. Eastland Press, Seattle

Maciocia G 1989 The eight extraordinary vessels. Journal of Chinese Medicine 30: 3–8

Matsumoto K, Birch S 1985 Five elements and ten stems. Paradigm, Boston

Motoyama H 1981 Theories of the *chakras*. Theosophical Publishing House, Illinois

Motoyama H 1988 Guidelines for awakening the *chakras*. International Association for Religion and Parapsychology Journal 18

Young J 1988 Subtle acupuncture, part 2: diagnosis. International Register of Oriental Medicine Review 3: 13–17

Young J 1989 Subtle acupuncture, part 3: treatment. International Register of Oriental Medicine Review 4: 12–16

FURTHER READING

Motoyama H 1990 Towards a superconsciousness, meditation theory and practice. Berkeley

Young J 1988 Subtle acupuncture, part 1: preparation and needle technique. International Register of Oriental Medicine Review 3: 13–16

Young J 1989 Subtle acupuncture, part 4: understanding the subtle body. International Register of Oriental Medicine Review 5: 10–15

■ Jacqueline Young

Jackie originally completed undergraduate and masters degrees in psychology and qualified as a clinical psychologist in the UK National Health Service. From 1981–1985 she lived in Japan, where she studied and worked extensively with Dr Hiroshi Motoyama, a leading international scientist, acupuncture specialist and parapsychologist. During this period she graduated from the International Institute for Oriental Medicine, Tokyo, trained with several master Japanese acupuncturists and completed the second International Advanced Course in Acupuncture at the Academy of Traditional Chinese Medicine in Beijing, China.

After returning to England in 1985, she cofounded the Whole Woman Clinic, an integrated health care clinic for women in London, and became a guest lecturer, and later Faculty Coordinator, at the International College of Oriental Medicine in East Grinstead. She has taught Japanese acupuncture and practitioner development courses at several UK and European acupuncture colleges, and is currently a visiting lecturer at the Centre for Complementary Health Studies at Exeter University.

She is a past member of the Executive Committee of the British Acupuncture Association and Register, and was a founder member of the European Journal of Oriental Medicine. She has taken a keen interest in both the development of the profession and the promotion of Japanese acupuncture techniques. She is the author of several books and numerous articles on Oriental medicine and currently teaches, writes and runs a consultancy practice in London.

Index